CT FOR THE NON-RADIOLOGIST

The Essential CT Study Guide

THIRD EDITION

ROCKY SAENZ, D.O. FAOCR

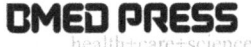

BMED PRESS
health+care+science

For more information about this book:

BMED Press LLC
700 Everhart
Suite H1
Corpus Christi, Texas 78411
Phone: (817) 400 -1639
www.bmedpress.com
customer-service@bmedpress.com

Copyright © 2024 by Rocky Saenz, D.O., FAOCR
All Rights Reserved

ISBN - 978-1-7349618-4-3 (paperback)
ISBN - 978-1-7349618-5-0 (digital)

All rights reserved.

No part of this book may be reproduced without written permission of the publisher

AUTHOR AND EDITOR

Rocky Saenz, D.O., F.A.O.C.R.
Chairman, Department of Radiology, Corewell Health East, Farmington Hills Hospital
Assistant Program Director of Diagnostic Radiology Residency
Clinical Assistant Professor, Michigan State University College of Osteopathic Medicine
Director of MRI & MSK Imaging, Corewell Health East, Farmington Hills Hospital
28050 Grand River Ave.
Farmington Hills, MI 48336

ASSISTANT EDITOR

Jordan Skrivanek, D.O., M.S.
Adjunct Clinical Faculty, Michigan State University College of Osteopathic Medicine
Radiology Resident, Corewell Health East, Farmington Hills Hospital
28050 Grand River Ave.
Farmington Hills, MI 48336

CONTRIBUTING AUTHORS

Reehan M. Ali, D.O.
Clinical Assistant Professor, Michigan State University College of Osteopathic Medicine
Director of CT & Thoracic Imaging, Corewell Health East, Farmington Hills Hospital
28050 Grand River Ave.
Farmington Hills, MI 48336

Elias Antypas, M.D., PhD
Clinical Assistant Professor, Michigan State University College of Osteopathic Medicine
Chief of Interventional Radiology, Corewell Health East, Farmington Hills Hospital
28050 Grand River Ave.
Farmington Hills, MI 48336

Rajeev Aravapalli, D.O.
Diagnostic Radiologist, X-Ray Associates of Port Huron
Port Huron, MI

Tammam Beydoun, D.O.
Director Pediatric Interventional Radiology
Children's Hospital Orange County
1201 W. La Veta Ave.
Orange, CA 92868

Lauren Corley, D.O.
Women's Imaging Fellow, University of Alabama-Birmingham
1802 6th Ave S.
Birmingham, AL 35233

Zachary Franks, D.O.
Clinical Body MRI Fellow, Stanford Health Care
500 Pasteur Drive
Stanford, CA 94305

Juliann Giese, D.O.
Diagnostic Radiologist, SDI Radiology
Tampa, FL

Colby J. Jones, D.O.
Chief Radiology Resident, Corewell Health East, Farmington Hills Hospital
28050 Grand River Ave.
Farmington Hills, MI 48336

Maqsood A. Khan, D.O.
Radiology Resident, Corewell Health East, Farmington Hills Hospital
28050 Grand River Ave.
Farmington Hills, MI 48336

Michael J. Legacy, D.O., M.B.A.
Diagnostic Radiologist, X-Ray Associates of Port Huron
Port Huron, MI

Naveen Malay, M.B.B.S.
Clinical Assistant Professor, Michigan State University College of Osteopathic Medicine
Diagnostic Radiologist, Corewell Health East, Farmington Hills Hospital
Director Neuroradiology, Corewell Health East, Farmington Hills Hospital
28050 Grand River Ave.
Farmington Hills, MI 48336

Zophia I. Martinez, D.O.
Diagnostic Radiologist, Radiology Imaging Associates
Daytona Beach, FL

Andrew Mizzi, D.O.
Clinical Assistant Professor, Michigan State University College of Osteopathic Medicine
Diagnostic Radiologist, Corewell Health East, Farmington Hills Hospital
28050 Grand River Ave.
Farmington Hills, MI 48336

Timothy McKnight, D.O.
Program Director of Radiology Residency, Corewell Health East, Farmington Hills Hospital
Clinical Assistant Professor, Michigan State University College of Osteopathic Medicine
Director of Nuclear Medicine & Radiation Safety, Corewell Health East, Farmington Hills Hospital
28050 Grand River Ave.
Farmington Hills, MI 48336

Gregory D. Puthoff, D.O.
Assistant Professor, Department of Radiology, Medical University of South Carolina
96 Jonathan Lucas St., MSC 323
Charleston, SC 29425

Ahmed Tahawi, D.O.
Clinical Assistant Professor, Michigan State University College of Osteopathic Medicine
Radiology Resident, Corewell Health East, Farmington Hills Hospital
28050 Grand River Ave.
Farmington Hills, MI 48336

Jordan Verlare, D.O.
Adjunct Clinical Faculty, Michigan State University College of Osteopathic Medicine
Radiology Resident, Corewell Health East, Farmington Hills Hospital
28050 Grand River Ave.
Farmington Hills, MI 48336

Matthew Waldrop, M.D.
Radiology Resident, Corewell Health East, Farmington Hills Hospital
28050 Grand River Ave.
Farmington Hills, MI 48336

Madison Kocher Wulfeck, M.D., M.B.A.
Cardiothoracic Radiologist

CONTENTS

Author And Editor iii
Forward xv
Introduction xviii
Chapter 1: Head Ct 1
    Head 2
    Case 1 4
    Abscess 5
    Case 2 6
    Giloblastoma Multiforme 7
    Case 3 8
    Cerebrovascular Accident 9
    Case 4 10
    Hydrocephalus 11
    Case 5 12
    Hypoxic Ischemic Injury 13
    Case 6 14
    Epidural Hematoma 15
    Case 7 16
    Subdural Hematoma 17
    Case 8 18
    Intraventricular Hemorrhage 19
    Case 9 20
    Subarachnoid Hemorrhage 21
    Case 10 22
    Hypertensive Bleed 23
    Case 11 24
    Cerebral Contusion 25
    Case 12 26

Diffuse Axonal Injury 27
Case 13 28
Orbital Fracture. 29
Case 14 30
Globe Rupture. 31
Case 15 32
Preseptal Cellulitis 33
Case 16 34
Temporal Bone Fracture 35
Case 17 36
Tripod Fracture 37
Chapter 2: Neck Ct. 39
Neck Ct. 40
Case 18 42
Peritonsillar Abscess 43
Case 19 44
Sinusitis. 45
Case 20 46
Metastatic Squamous Cell Carcinoma 47
Case 21 48
Sialolithiasis. 49
Case 22 50
Epiglotitis 51
Case 23 52
Carotid Artery Stenosis 53
Case 24 54
Soft Tissue Hematoma. 55
Case 25 56
Vestibular Abscess 57
Chapter 3: Spine Ct 59
Spine. 60
Case 26 62
Multiple Myeloma. 63
Case 27 64
Cervical Disc Herniation 65
Case 28 66
Disc Bulge. 67
Case 29 68

Discitis Osteomyelitis	69
Case 30	70
Occipital Condyle Fracture	71
Case 31	72
Atlanto-Occipital Dissociation, Aod	73
Case 32	74
C1 Fracture (Jefferson)	75
Case 33	76
Dens Fracture	77
Case 34	78
Clay Shoveler Fracture	79
Case 35	80
Compression Frac	81
Case 36	82
Transverse Process Fracture	83
Case 37	84
Two Column Fracture	85
Case 38	86
Epidural Hematoma	87
Chapter 4: Chest Ct	**89**
Chest	91
Case 39	92
Thoracic Aortic Dissection	93
Case 40	94
Thoracic Aortic Aneurysm	95
Case 41	96
Pulmonary Emboli	97
Case 42	98
Acute Traumatic Aortic Injury	99
Case 43	100
Pneumonia	101
Case 44	102
Usual Interstitial Pneumonia	103
Case 45	104
Lung Mass	105
Case 46	106
Pneumatocele	107
Case 47	108

Lymphoma	109
Case 48	110
Retrosternal Goiter	111
Case 49	112
Empyema	113
Case 50	114
Pneumothorax	115
Case 51	116
Pericardial Effusion	117
Case 52	118
Pulmonary Abscess	119
Case 53	120
Sternal Fracture	121
Case 54	122
Septic Emboli	123
Case 55	124
Left Ventricular Aneurysm	125
Case 56	126
Pneumomediastinum	127
Case 57	128
Nonspecific Interstitial Pneumonia	129
Case 58	130
Angioinvasive Aspergillosis	131
Case 59, Pediatric	132
Cystic Fibrosis Exacerbation	133
Case 60	134
Covid Pneumonia	135
Chapter 5: Abdominal And Pelvic Ct	**137**
Abdomen	139
Case 61	140
Liver Laceration	141
Case 62	142
Pancreatic Laceration	143
Case 63	144
Splenic Laceration	145
Case 64	146
Adrenal Hematoma	147
Case 65	148

Renal Laceration	149
Case 66	150
Shattered Kidney	151
Case 67	152
Bowel Hematoma	153
Case 68	154
Nephrolithiasis	155
Case 69	156
Pyelonephritis	157
Case 70	158
Xanthogranulomatous Pyelonephritis (Xgp)	159
Case 71	160
Renal Infarct	161
Case 72	162
Renal Cell Carcinoma	163
Case 73	164
Wunderlich Syndrome	165
Case 74	166
Enteritis	167
Case 75	168
Epiploic Appendagitis	169
Case 76	170
Diverticulitis	171
Case 77	172
Diverticulitis With Pericolonic Abscess	173
Case 78	174
Ischemic Colitis	175
Case 79	176
Intussusception	177
Case 80	178
Colonic (Sigmoid) Volvulus	179
Case 81	180
Closed-Loop Small Bowel Obstruction	181
Case 82	182
Colonic Mass	183
Case 83	184
Colonic Pseudo-Obstruction (Ogilvie's)	185
Case 84	186

Large Bowel Obstruction	187
Case 85	188
Infectious Colitis	189
Case 86	190
Free Air, Pneumoperitoneum	191
Case 87	192
Diaphragmatic Rupture	193
Case 88	194
Cirrhosis	195
Case 89	196
Liver Mass, Hcc	197
Case 90	198
Choledocholithiasis	199
Case 91	200
Liver Infarction	201
Case 92	202
Fatty Liver	203
Case 93	204
Acute Hepatitis	205
Case 94	206
Cholecystitis	207
Case 95	208
Cholelithiasis	209
Case 96	210
Gallbladder Carcinoma	211
Case 97	212
Emphysematous Cholecystitis	213
Case 98	214
Pancreatic Abscess	215
Case 99	216
Acute Pancreatitis	217
Case 100	218
Pancreatic Carcinoma	219
Case 101	220
Abdominal Aortic Dissection	221
Case 102	222
Abdominal Aortic Aneurysm	223
Case 103	224

Abdominal Aortic Aneurysm Rupture 225
Case 104 226
Retroperitoneal Hemorrhage 227
Case 105 228
Inferior Vena Cava Thrombosis 229
Case 106 230
Splenomegaly. 231
Case 107 232
Splenic Infarct 233
Case 108 234
Splenic Mass 235
Case 109 236
Shock Bowel 237
Case 110 238
Fournier's Gangrene. 239
Case 111 240
Urinary Bladder Rupture. 241
Case 112 242
Ovarian Dermoid 243
Case 113 244
Pelvic Inflammatory Disease 245
Case 114 246
Hemmorhagic Ovarian Cyst 247
Case 115 248
Urinary Bladder Carcinoma. 249
Case 116 250
Renal Abscess. 251
Case 117 252
Appendicitis. 253
Case 118 254
Ovarian Vein Thrombosis 255
Case 119 256
Perirectal Abscess. 257
Case 120 258
Stercoral Colitis. 259
Case 121 260
Morel-Lavallee Lesion 261
Case 122 Pediatrics 262

Neuroblastoma 263
Case 123 264
Omental Infarct. 265
Case 124 Pediatrics 266
Wilms Tumor 267

FORWARD

I would like to thank the department of radiology at Corewell Health East, Farmington Hills Hospital (formerly Botsford Hospital) for agreeing to contribute and help me put together this project. This includes my fellow staff Radiologists: Reehan Ali, Elias Antypas, Naveen Malay, Tim McKnight, and Andy Mizzi. Our prior graduates, now attending Radiologists who took time out of their practices to contribute: Raj Aravapalli, Tammam Beydoun, Lauren Corley, Zack Franks, Juliann Giese, Mike Legacy and Zophia Martinez. Also, special thanks to my current residents for their efforts: Colby Jones, Maqsood Khan, Ahmed Tahawi, Jordan Skrivanek, Jordan Verlare, and Matt Waldrop. Next, I would like to thank Dr. Greg Puthoff, my former resident and his prior fellow Madison Wulfeck, for finding the non-existing spare time in their busy lives to re-write the Chest Chapter 4. Thanks to all of you, I would not have been able to complete this 3rd Edition without your collaboration.

Lastly and most importantly, I would like to thank my loving family. I thank my brother Roland Saenz, and my father, Roque Saenz, who have provided me with enduring emotional support. My wife Blanca and sons, Rocky, Russell, Ronin, and Rex, for your understanding and patience watching me spend countless hours in my office to complete this book. I could not and would not be able to complete this academic project or any other without your love and support!

Rocky Saenz, DO, FAOCR
April 2023

INTRODUCTION

I was inspired to write this book because of the recurrent conversations that I have had with other non-Radiologist about various radiology topics. I have had innumerable encounters where I have been asked the same questions from my non-radiology physicians, medical residents, medical students, non-medical trained friends, and patients. It is their quest for basic Computed Tomography (CT) knowledge that initially inspired me to complete this work and now re-write and update this book for its 3rd edition.

My goal is to create a quick reference book for the non-Radiologist. This book is to aid in diagnosing frequent urgent conditions with Computed Tomography. Use this book for study, as each of the cases is presented as unknowns with a non-annotated image. Look at the non-annotated image and test yourself. If you cannot make the findings, then read the "key findings"… if you still don't know, then start reading the "facts" section which will give you more clues. Then, look at the next page for the diagnosis, the title of the case, and the annotated image (which is the most important part of the case). Each case highlights basic clinical information, radiographic findings, and basic anatomy.

Enjoy!

Rocky Saenz, DO, FAOCR
April 2023

CHAPTER 1
HEAD CT

HEAD

TO CONTRAST OR NOT TO CONTRAST?

Currently, computed tomography (CT) brain imaging is a useful tool in the emergent setting when patients present with risk factors, signs, or symptoms of acute intracranial pathology. In the setting of trauma, **NO** intravenous contrast should be used. The use of contrast may obscure acute hemorrhage and result in a false negative result. In addition, when attempting to exclude intracranial trauma, intravenous contrast could be a complicating factor with regards to renal status and allergic reactions to the contrast. Intravenous contrast should only be administered to exclude infection (meningitis, cerebritis, and brain abscess) and brain tumors (typically in patients with a known diagnosis of a primary carcinoma). At some institutions, contrast is administered to stroke patients in order to perform a CT "perfusion" study. Perfusion studies have shown improved accuracy in detecting acute ischemic stroke compared to non-contrast CT imaging. As it has been said, "Time is brain," and typically a non-contrast CT is utilized when the patient is within the window to receive tissue plasminogen activator (tPA).

CT VS. MRI

CT is not the gold standard for brain imaging. MRI has taken the place of CT as the best imaging modality for intracranial pathology. With this being said…Why not image all ER patients with MRI? There are too many reasons against this, so I will only discuss the most significant. First and most important is time (especially in the emergent setting)! With the advent of multi-slice CT, a CT scan of the brain (and whole body when needed) now only takes seconds. Typically, an MRI of the brain will take twenty to thirty minutes of imaging time (too long for unstable patients). In addition, the longer a patient is out of the ED can be crucial when providing care for a potentially unstable patient. So, an MRI would significantly delay treatment. Secondly, MRI safety must be considered. A patient must be deemed "MRI safe" before entering the magnetic environment. This means a thorough history must be obtained to exclude potentially unsafe implants. If an MRI is performed on a patient with an unsafe coil or hardware, it could be dislodged and be harmful or even fatal! In the emergent setting, an accurate history is usually not able to be elicited (i.e., patients may be unconscious or confused). Lastly, MRI availability is a limiting factor. Not all EDs have access to an MRI unit. For those institutions that do have the MRI capability, they may only have a single unit, which can increase patient delays to obtain imaging (delaying treatment further).

IMAGE INTERPRETATION

When attempting to interpret CT brain studies, it is easy to get lost in the detailed neuroanatomy. Therefore, the advice I give to a non-radiologist is to not worry about the anatomy. Instead, first look at each image evaluating the supratentorial and infratentorial brain for symmetry. The brain on every CT image should look symmetrical to the opposing side (i.e., a mirror image). When an area of asymmetry is noted, you now know where the pathology is located (easy)!. Now figure out the anatomy where the abnormality is located.

An important CT concept is "attenuation," specifically when a structure is hyper- or hypo-attenuated. This simply means the structure is brighter or darker than its surroundings. So, when you are trying to exclude brain hemorrhage, remember that acute blood is hyperattenuated (brighter than the brain and white in color). Just look for the white spots! Remember, that any structure can be measured on a PACS (picture archiving computer system) to obtain a value/unit based on its density; this is quantified in Hounsfield units (HU). This is helpful with diagnosing acute hemorrhage, which usually measures 35-45 HU. So, HU can help you decipher if a hyperattenuated focus is acute blood, an enhancing vessel, or calcium/mineralization since all are white on CT. Acute blood has the opposite appearance to a cerebral infarction/ischemic stroke. Infarction is hypoattenuated (dark) when compared to normal brain parenchyma.

I hope you learn from the cases in this chapter! For each case, look at the first image (non-annotated) and try to find the abnormality. Then, come up with a diagnosis. If you can't figure out a diagnosis, look at the "facts" section for diagnostic hints (wish my daily work cases came with hints). Next review the second page of the case, which has the diagnosis at the top with full annotations along with relevant anatomy, take-home points and tips for learning. Also, references for each case are provided for additional study.

Enjoy!

R Saenz DO, FAOCR

CASE 1

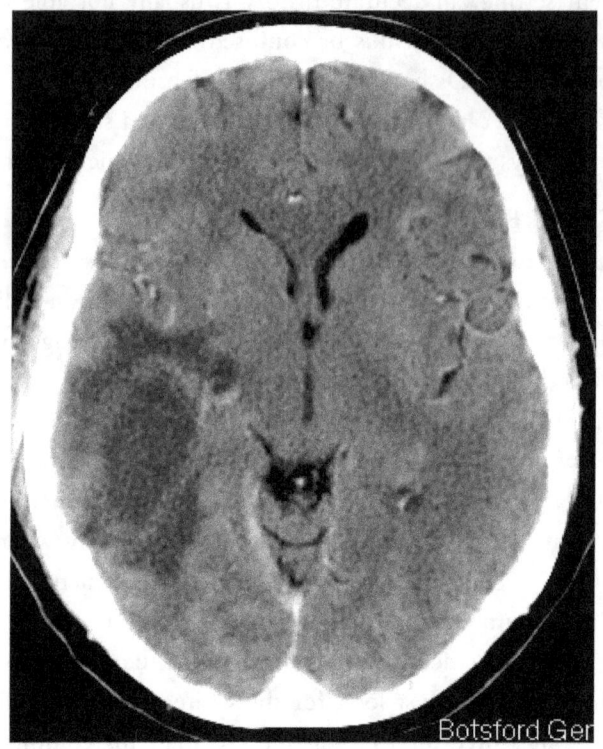

Best CT Study for Diagnosis:
CT Brain with IV contrast

Key to DX
Ring enhancing lesion with low central attenuation.

Facts
Most common bugs are *Streptococcus* and *Staphylococcus*.
Common with immunocompromised patients.
Most common source is bacterial endocarditis.
May also be secondary to sinus infections.
Realize that "ring" enhancing lesions have a broad differential. Most common etiologies are tumor, infection, or trauma. Therefore, history is essential for your radiologist!

TX
CSF analysis is important to identify the underlying pathogen and treat it.
Extreme cases may require surgery.

ABSCESS

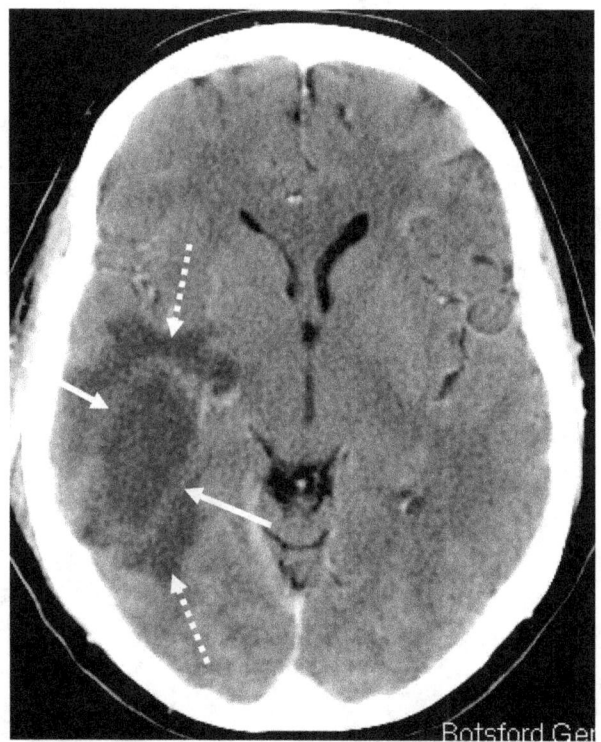

Study Above:
CT Brain with IV contrast at the level of the basal ganglia.

Radiographic findings:
A ring enhancing lesion is present with central low attenuation involving the deep white matter of the right temporal lobe (arrows). The lesion is causing surrounding vasogenic edema (dashed arrows). Early midline shift is present.

Tips
Decide if the lesion is truly intra-axial (within the brain parenchyma).
Extra-axial lesions are not within the brain parenchyma.
The most common extra-axial lesion is a meningioma.
A vasogenic edema pattern involves only white matter and spares the gray matter.
Check the septum pellucidum for displacement; when it is displaced this signifies midline shift (subfalcine herniation).

Further Reading
Villanueva-Meyer J.E., Soonmee C. From Shades of Gray to Microbiologic Imaging: A Historical Review of Brain Abscess Imaging. *RadioGraphics*. Volume 35, Issue 5 Jul 24, 2015.

CASE 2

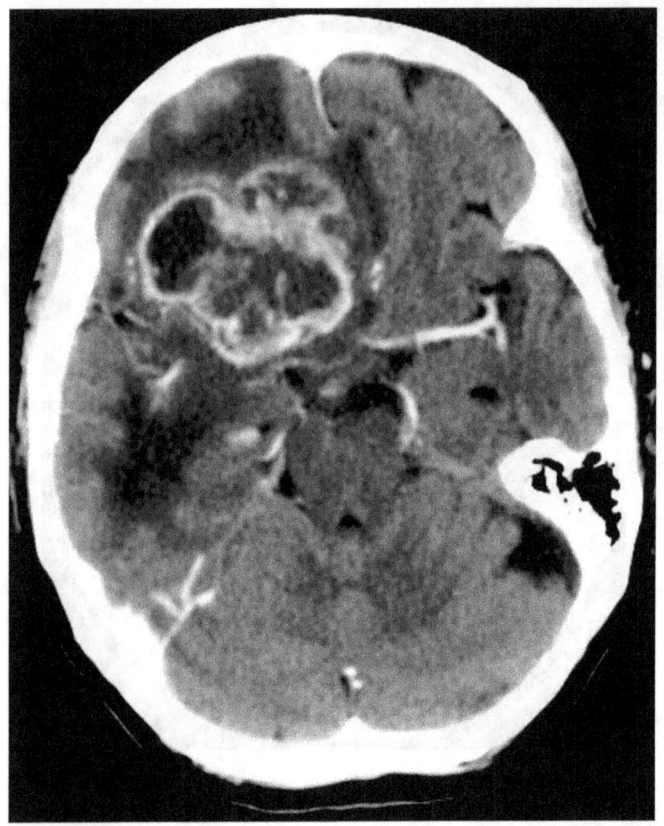

Best CT Study for Diagnosis:
CT Brain with IV contrast

Key to DX
Contrast enhancing, heterogeneous intra-axial lesion.

Facts
Most common primary brain tumor in an adult is a glioblastoma multiforme (GBM).
GBM patients typically are older than 50.
Most adult primary tumors are supratentorial, while pediatric tumors are infratentorial.
Realize that this appearance could represent a metastatic lesion, infection, or tumefactive demyelination. Therefore, please provide history for your radiologist!

TX
Typically a combination of surgery and chemotherapy.
IV steroids are useful in the acute setting to control intracranial pressure.

GILOBLASTOMA MULTIFORME

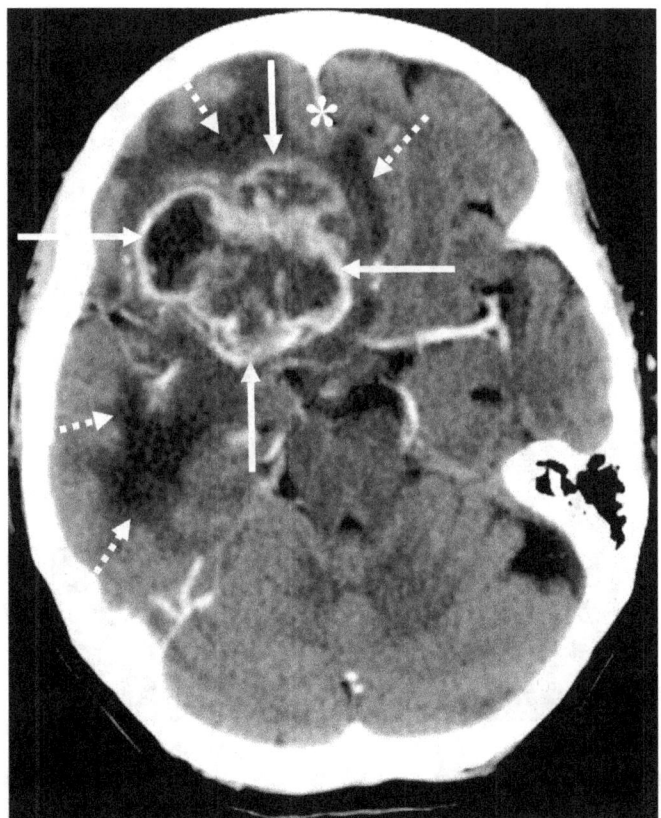

Study Above:
CT Brain with IV contrast at the level of the lower frontal lobes.

Radiographic findings:
A heterogeneous contrast enhancing lesion is present within the right frontal lobe (arrow). The lesion is causing regional vasogenic edema (dashed arrows) which is dark, hypoattenuated. This results in subfalcine herniation (midline shift) from right to left with displacement of the falx (asterisk).

Tips
Intra-axial lesions are surrounded by brain parenchyma.
An edema pattern that involves gray and white matter indicates an infarction (cytotoxic edema, see Case 3).
Multiple intra-axial lesions favor metastatic disease.
Check the septum pellucidum relationship with the falx for alignment (when not aligned with each other this signifies midline shift).

Further Reading
Villanueva-Meyer J.E., et al. MRI Features and IDH Mutational Status of Grade II Diffuse Gliomas: Impact on Diagnosis and Prognosis. *AJR*. 210: 621-628, 2018.

CASE 3

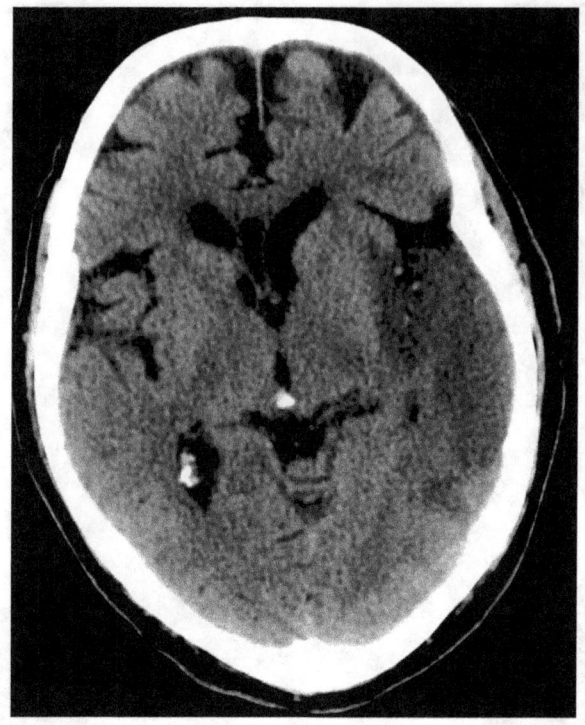

Best CT Study for Diagnosis:
CT Brain without contrast

Key to DX
Focal or wedge shaped hypoattenuated area involving both the gray and white matter.

Facts
Most common vascular territory involved is the middle cerebral artery.
In the first 24 hours, about 50% of ischemic strokes are not visible on CT.
MRI diffusion weighted imaging is sensitive in detecting ischemia (positive in minutes).
Maximum cytotoxic edema occurs about 72 hours after the ischemic insult.
About 15% of strokes are hemorrhagic.

TX
Supportive when neurologic deficit present beyond therapeutic window of intervention.
IV tPA if symptoms are determined within the window and the stroke is not hemorrhagic.

CEREBROVASCULAR ACCIDENT

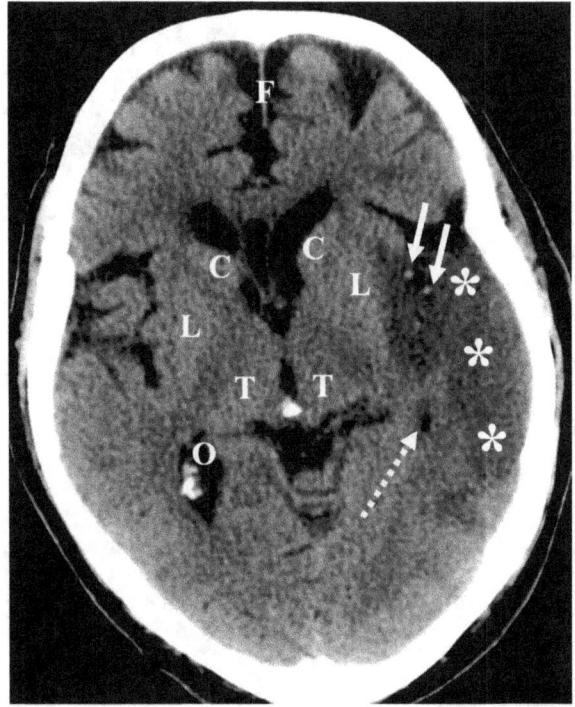

Study Above:
CT Brain without contrast at the level of the basal ganglia.

Radiographic findings:
A wedge-shaped area of hypoattenuation is seen within the left temporal lobe (asterisks). Within the Sylvian fissure are two high density dots (AKA "MCA DOT" sign), which is indicative of thrombus causing the infarct (arrows). The low attenuation represents cytotoxic edema and results in mass effect with effacement of the occipital horn of the left lateral ventricle (dashed arrow) compared to the contralateral right (O).

Tips
Cytotoxic edema is always indicative of an ischemic event (cytotoxic refers to cell death).
Cytotoxic edema patterns classically include both gray and white matter.
Cytotoxic edema always results in mass effect but not always midline shift.

Normal Anatomy
C – Caudate nucleus, L - Lentiform nucleus, T - Thalamus, O – Occipital horn, F - Falx

Further Reading
Kuner, A,D., and Rowley, H,A. Should Perfusion CT and CTA Be Performed in All Patients With Suspected Stroke? Point—Yes, for Fast and Accurate Stroke Triage and Treatment. *AJR.* 1-2. 10.2214/.20.25256, 2021.

CASE 4

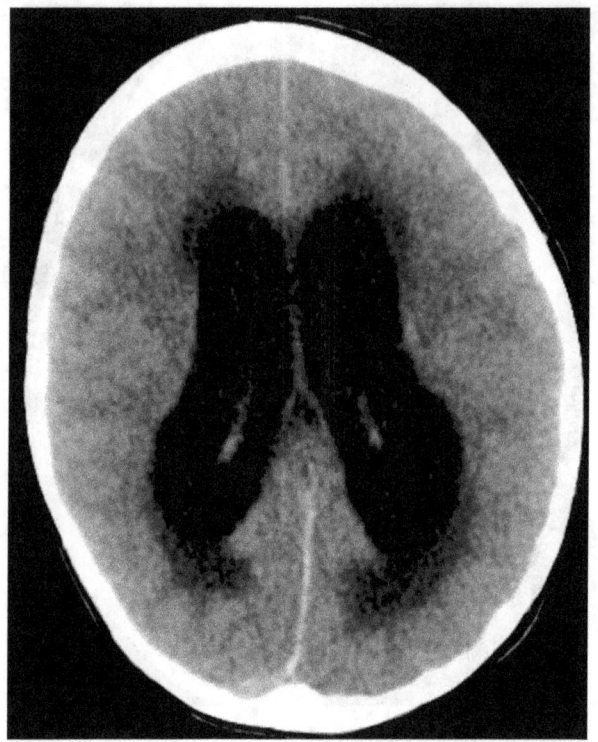

Best CT Study for Diagnosis:
CT Brain without contrast

Key to DX
Enlarged ventricles.

Facts
Consider normal pressure hydrocephalus (NPH) when dementia, gait disturbance, and incontinence are present.
In children, ventriculomegaly is most commonly related to congenital anomalies.
In adults, ventriculomegaly is usually related to hemorrhage, tumor, or normal pressure hydrocephalus.

TX
May require decompression with intraventricular shunt placement depending on the severity.

HYDROCEPHALUS

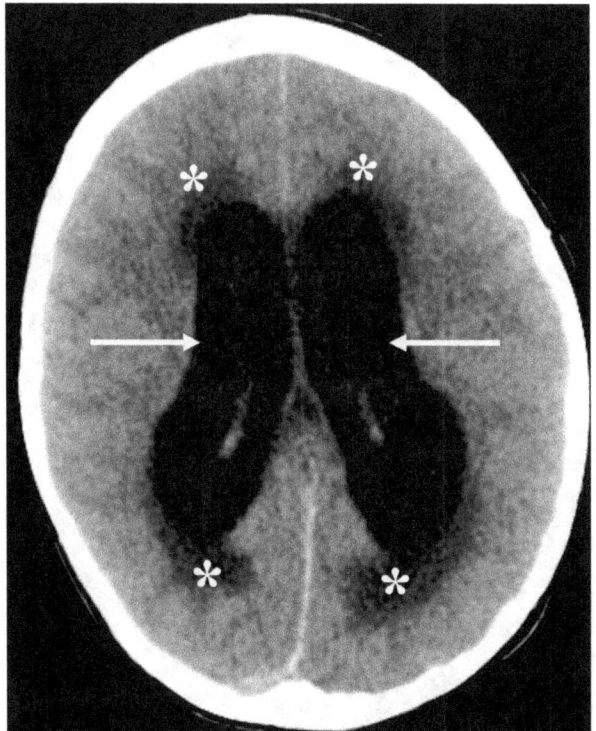

Study Above:
CT Brain without contrast at the level of the lateral ventricles.

Radiographic findings:
Marked enlargement is noted of the lateral ventricles (arrows). Notice that very few peripheral sulci are present (indicates increased intracranial pressure). Also, the periventricular white matter is dark (asterisks) meaning this hydrocephalus is acute with CSF leaking into the ventricular lining (subependymal cells).

Tips
Comparison with prior studies is key to deciphering acuity.
Acute hydrocephalus typically has a halo of periventricular low attenuation (edema).
Compare the size of all the ventricles.
Enlargement of all the ventricles implies "communicating hydrocephalus" AKA "extraventricular obstructive hydrocephalus."
Check the cerebral aqueduct for occlusion.

Further Reading
Huang BY, Castillo M. Hypoxic-ischemic brain injury: imaging findings from birth to adulthood. Radiographics. Apr;28(2):417-39; 2014.

CASE 5

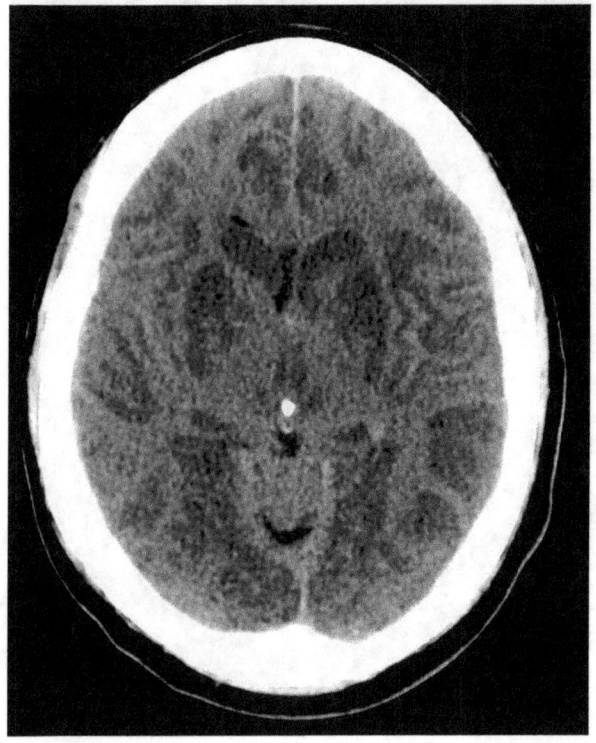

Best CT Study for Diagnosis:
CT Brain without contrast

Key to DX
Low attenuated appearance of the basal ganglia with bright white matter.

Facts
Any significant hypoxic event can lead to this entity.
Etiologies include asphyxiation, cardiac arrest, near drowning, and cerebrovascular disease.
One of the most important variables is the severity and duration of the event.
This condition is secondary to diminished cerebral blood flow and blood oxygenation.

TX
Supportive care.

HYPOXIC ISCHEMIC INJURY

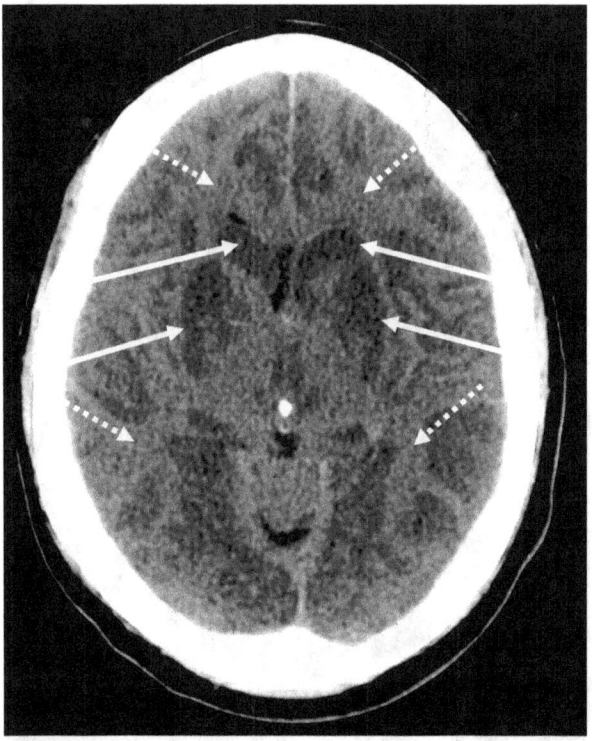

Study Above:
CT Brain without contrast at the level of the basal ganglia.

Radiographic findings:
The basal ganglia, including the caudate heads and lentiform nuclei, demonstrate abnormal low attenuation (arrows). No peripheral sulci are present. Abnormal high attenuation of the cerebral white matter (dashed arrows).

Tips
Global hypoxic events have a variable appearance and may be asymmetric.
Basal ganglia should be hyperattenuated compared to white matter (Cases 3 & 10).
The white matter should never be the brightest portion of the brain!
The "reversal sign" (white matter brighter than gray) is indicative of severe ischemia and a poor neurological outcome (as in this case).
No brain sulci indicates significant increased intracranial pressure!

Further Reading
Huang BY, Castillo M. Hypoxic-ischemic brain injury: imaging findings from birth to adulthood. Radiographics. Apr;28(2):417-39; 2014

CASE 6

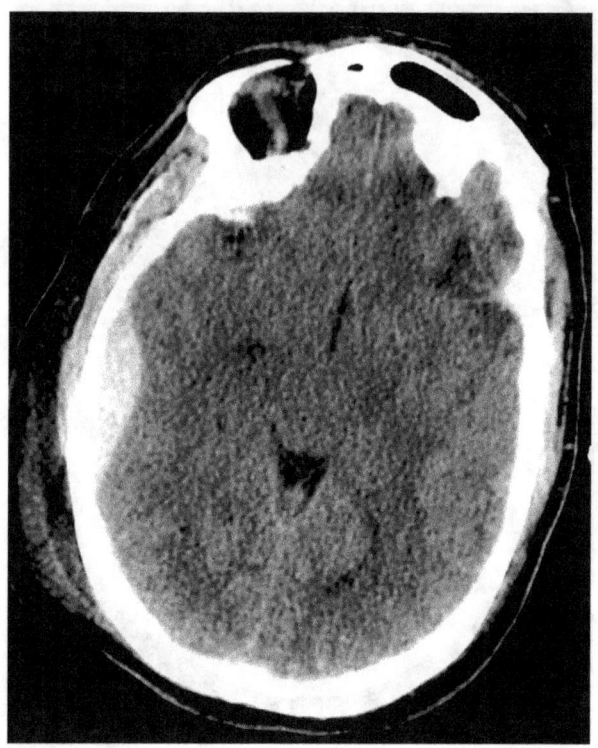

Best CT Study for Diagnosis:
CT Brain without contrast

Key to DX
Hyperattenuated, convex, extra-axial collection.

Facts
Most common etiology is trauma (direct blow AKA coup injury).
Most commonly seen in young adult males.
95% are associated with skull fractures and represent arterial bleeds.
Patients may have a lucid interval followed by a loss of consciousness.

TX
Close supervision with serial CT scans to assess hematoma stability is necessary. Neurosurgical decompression is considered when midline shift is greater than 5 mm.

EPIDURAL HEMATOMA

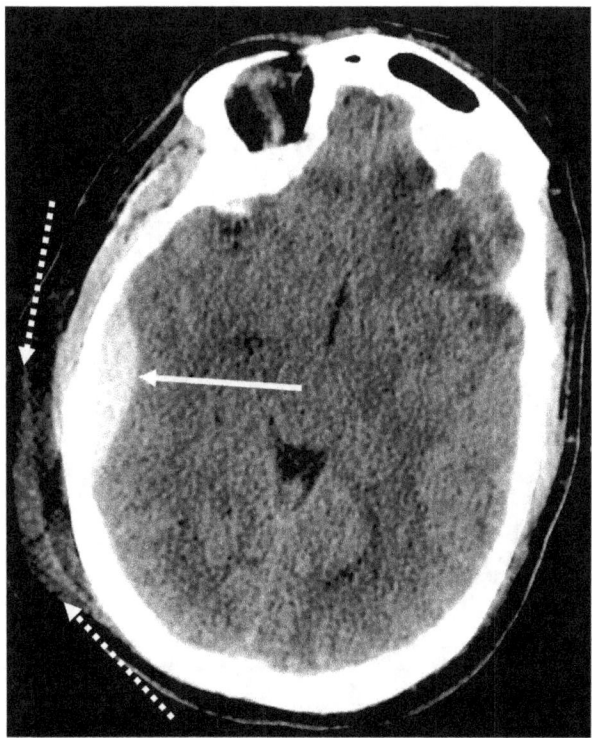

Study Above:
CT Brain without contrast at the level of the third ventricle.

Radiographic findings:
Hyperattenuated, lenticular, extra-axial fluid collection layering adjacent to the right temporal lobe (arrow). Soft tissue hematoma with edema is noted (dashed arrows). Notice that very few peripheral sulci are present which indicates cerebral edema.

Tips
Epidural hematomas are lenticular in shape (bulging, convex inner margin).
Use the hematoma inner margin to distinguish between subdural and epidural bleeds.
Epidural collections cannot cross suture lines but can cross midline.
Since they are bound by sutures, epidurals are more focal and enlarge transversely.
You must exclude an underlying fracture (check bone windows)!

Further Reading
Wright, J.N., Review. CNS Injuries in Abusive Head Trauma. *AJR.* 208:991-1001, 2017.

CASE 7

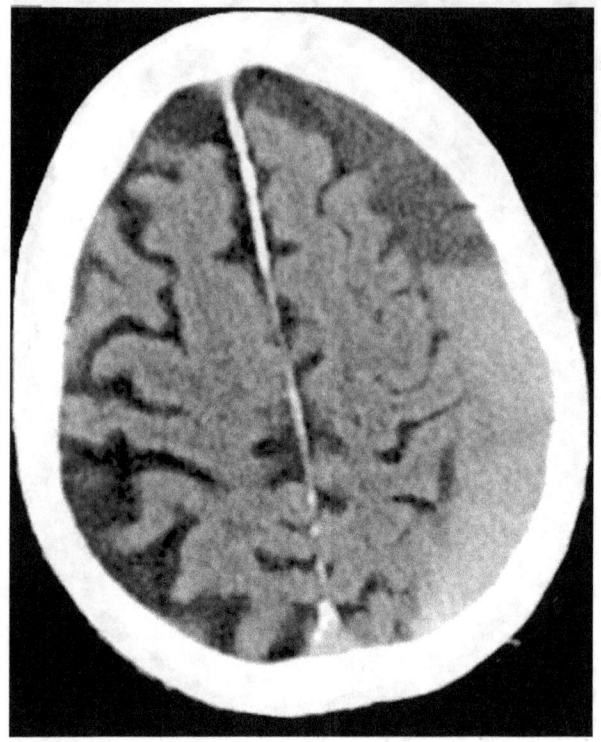

Best CT Study for Diagnosis:
CT Brain without contrast

Key to DX
Hyperattenuated, crescentic, concave, extra-axial fluid collection.

Facts
Most common etiology is trauma (MVAs and falls).
Most commonly seen in elderly women and infants (shaken baby syndrome).
The majority are related to venous hemorrhage (bridging veins).
Typically, the collections are contrecoup (opposite the side of trauma).
TX
Supportive care for small collections.
Neurosurgical decompression is considered when midline shift is greater than 5 mm.

SUBDURAL HEMATOMA

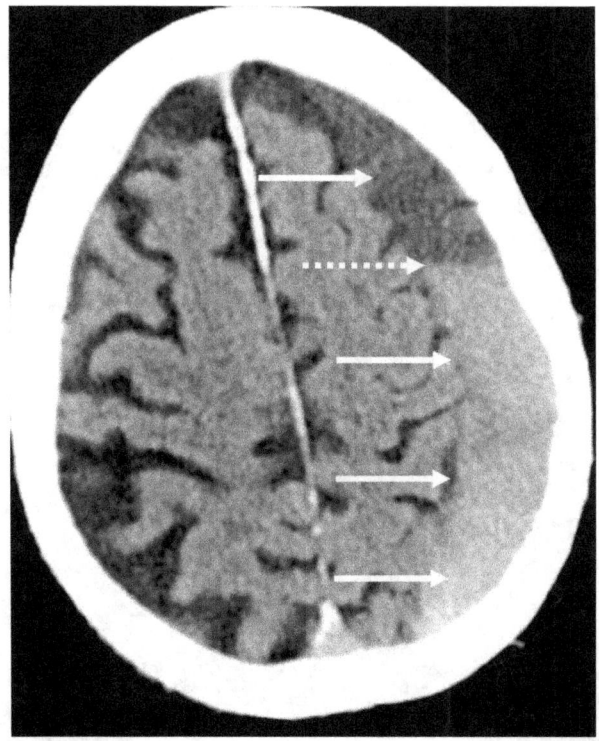

Study Above:
CT Brain without contrast at the supraventricular level.

Radiographic findings:
A crescentic, extra-axial fluid collection is seen layering adjacent to the left cerebral hemisphere (arrows). The large collection is creating significant mass effect upon the left hemisphere. The fluid collection is layering with increased density dependently representing clotted blood with a fluid-fluid level (dashed arrow). All the left sulci are significantly smaller than the right sulci and displaced which is the result of mass effect (indicates intracranial pressure).

Tips
Subdurals are crescent shaped (concave inner margin).
Subdurals usually have a longer AP dimension than transverse dimension.
Use the hematoma inner margin to distinguish between subdural and epidural bleeds.
Subdural collections cannot pass midline, but they can cross suture lines.
Subdurals may layer along the falx cerebri.

Further Reading
Aiken AH, Gean AD. Imaging of head trauma. Semin Roentgenol. Apr;45 (2):63-79, 2010.

CASE 8

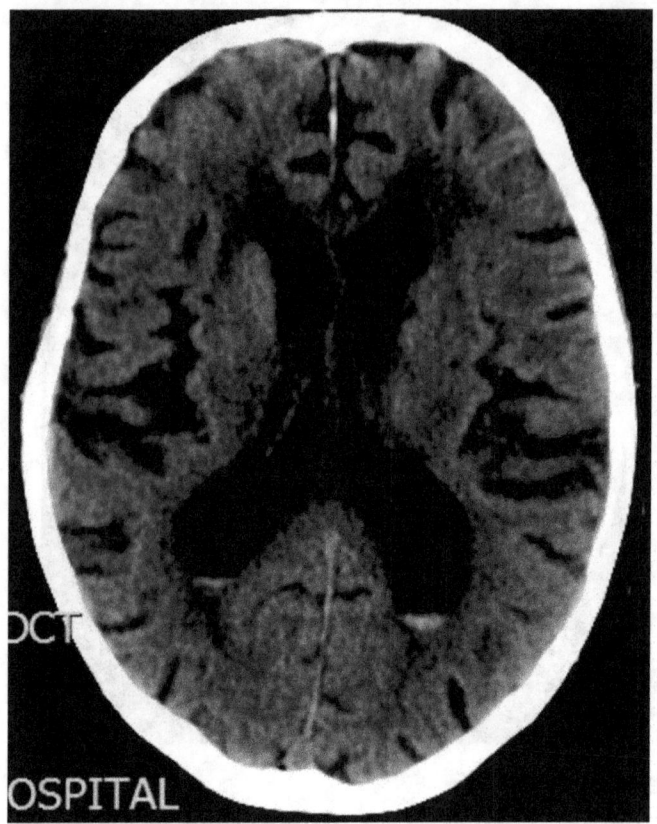

Best CT Study for Diagnosis:
CT Brain without contrast

Key to DX
Hyperattenuated collections within the ventricular system.

Facts
Common etiologies include hypertension, trauma, tumor, and coagulopathy.
In premature infants, it is related to germinal matrix development.
May lead to acute obstructive hydrocephalus when clots obstruct the cerebral aqueduct or the foramen of Monro.

TX
The etiology of the hemorrhage must be addressed.
Neurosurgical shunting may be needed with acute ventricular obstruction.

INTRAVENTRICULAR HEMORRHAGE

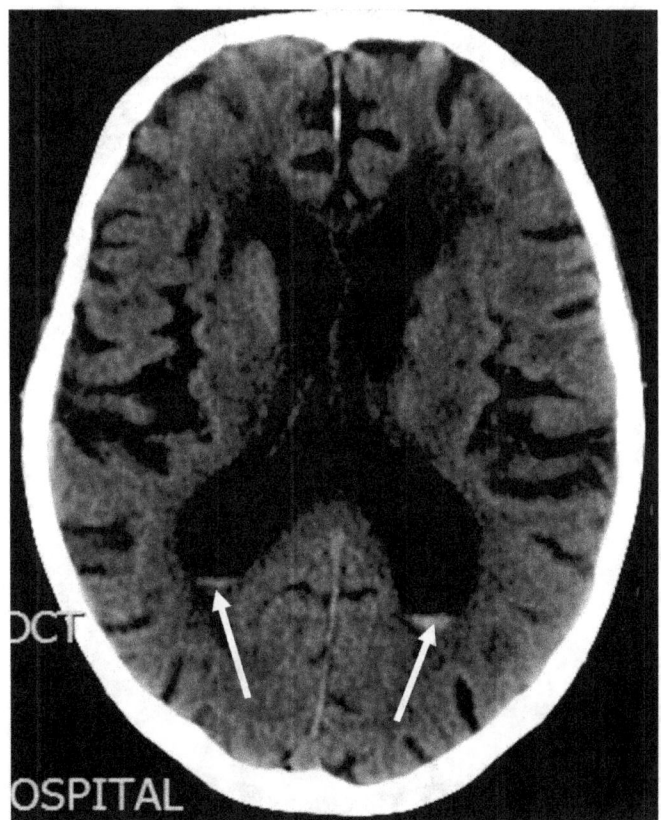

Study Above:
CT Brain without contrast at the level of the lateral ventricles.

Radiographic finding:
Hyperattenuated intraventricular collections layering within the lateral ventricles posteriorly (arrows). The periventricular white matter has low attenuation. This may represent pre-existing gliosis/small vessel ischemic disease vs acute edema (from transependymal flow of CSF like Case 4).

Tips

Check the cerebral aqueduct and foramen of Monro for blood as this can lead to ventricular obstruction.

Acute hydrocephalus has a halo of periventricular low attenuation (edema, like Case 4).

Do not confuse calcified choroid with blood; calcium is much brighter (HU in 100s).

Remember blood will be in the dependent portion of the ventricles and sulci.

Further Reading
Wright, J.N., Review. CNS Injuries in Abusive Head Trauma. *AJR*. 208:991-1001, 2017.

CASE 9

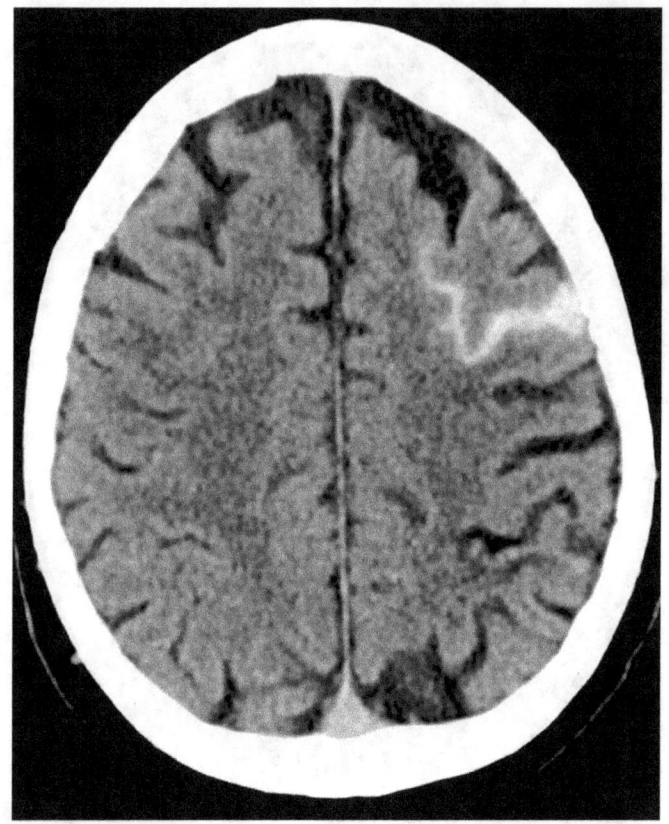

Best CT Study for Diagnosis:
CT Brain without contrast

Key to DX
Hyperattenuated collection within the CSF space.

Facts
Hemorrhage can layer in any sulcus or cistern.
Common etiologies include trauma and aneurysm.
Consider spinal tap if subarachnoid hemorrhage is suspected and CT is negative.
Patients present with classic history of "worst headache of their life."

TX
The etiology of the hemorrhage must be addressed.
Neurosurgical shunting may be needed with acute ventricular obstruction.
Consider nifedipine for vasoconstriction.

SUBARACHNOID HEMORRHAGE

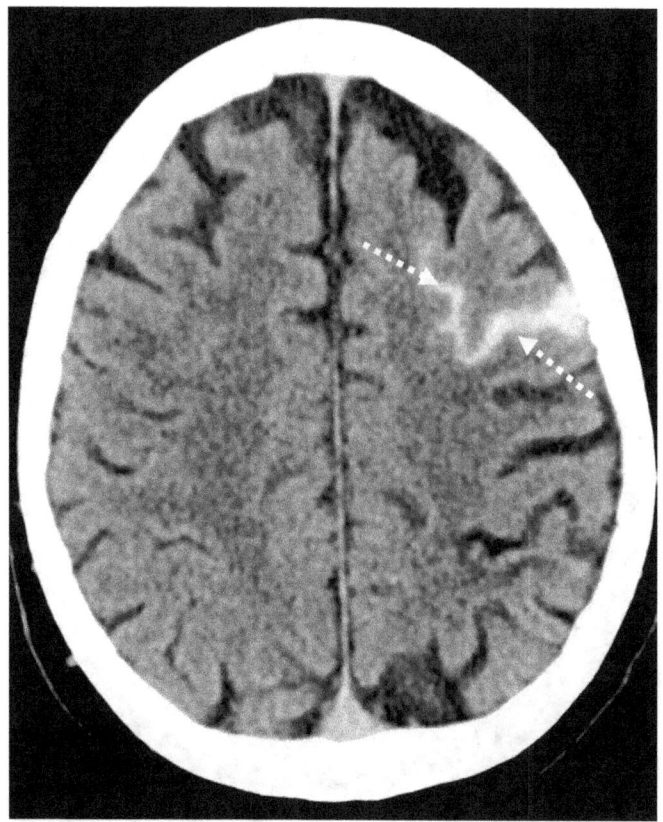

Study Above:
CT Brain without contrast at the supraventricular level.

Radiographic findings:
Hyperattenuated appearance involving a left frontal lobe sulcus consistent with subarachnoid hemorrhage (dashed arrows).

Tips
Anywhere CSF lives defines the subarachnoid space. Therefore, any CSF space with increased attenuation represents subarachnoid hemorrhage.
Blood will have Hounsfield units of 35 to 45.
Check the cerebral aqueduct and foramen of Monro for blood. Blood in these locations may lead to obstructive hydrocephalus (Case 4).
Remember, all CSF spaces should be dark on non-contrast CT!

Further Reading
Wright, J.N., Review. CNS Injuries in Abusive Head Trauma. *AJR.* 208:991-1001, 2017.

CASE 10

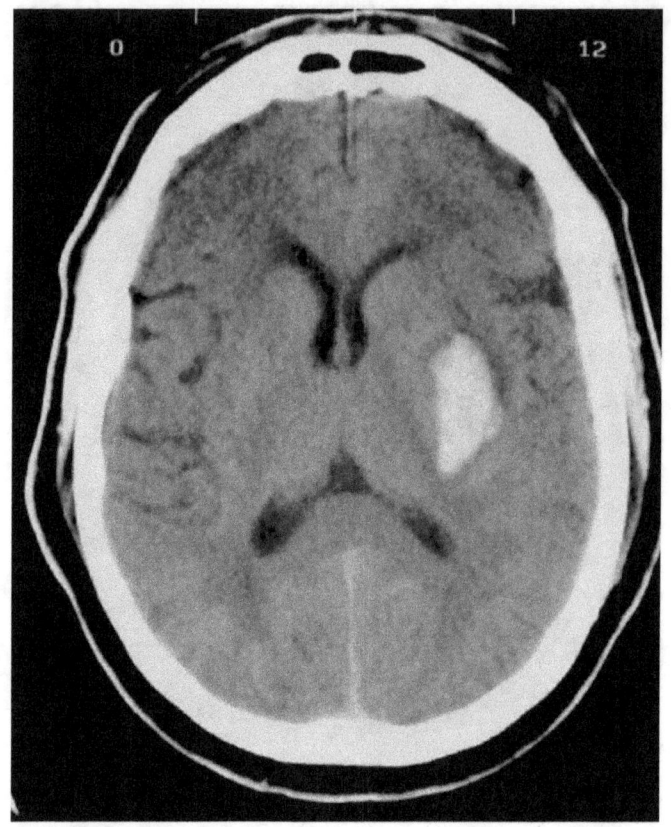

Best CT Study for Diagnosis:
CT Brain without contrast

Key to DX
Hyperattenuated collection within the basal ganglia.

Facts
Most common location for hemorrhagic stroke is the basal ganglia.
Basal ganglia hemorrhage in young patients may be related to cocaine use.
The majority of intraparenchymal hemorrhage is related to trauma and hypertension.
Most common demographic is elderly males.

TX
Supportive care with control of hypertensive crisis.

HYPERTENSIVE BLEED

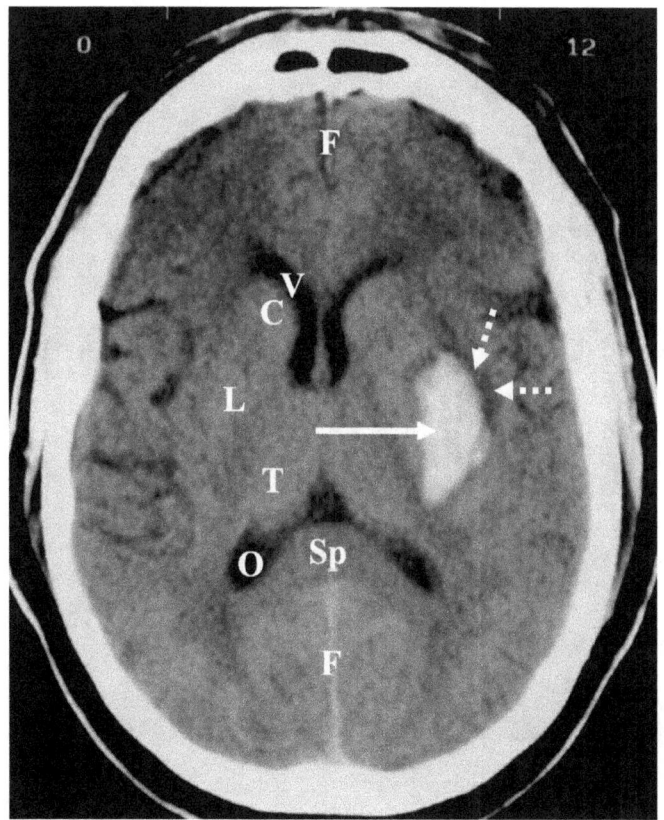

Study Above:
CT Brain without contrast at the level of the basal ganglia.

Radiographic findings:
Hyperattenuated, intra-axial collection centered in the left lentiform nucleus (arrow). This collection is associated with regional mass effect as evidenced by a halo of low attenuation, vasogenic edema (dashed arrows).

Tips
Follow-up imaging may help to exclude an underling mass causing the bleed.
Vasogenic edema spares cortical gray matter.
Look for blood (white or high density) in occipital horns to exclude ventricular extension (Case 8).

Normal Anatomy
V - Ventricle anterior horn, C – Caudate nucleus, L - Lentiform nucleus, T - Thalamus, Sp - Splenium of corpus callosum, O – Occipital horn, F - Falx

Further Reading
Wright, J.N., Review. CNS Injuries in Abusive Head Trauma. *AJR*. 208:991-1001, 2017.

CASE 11

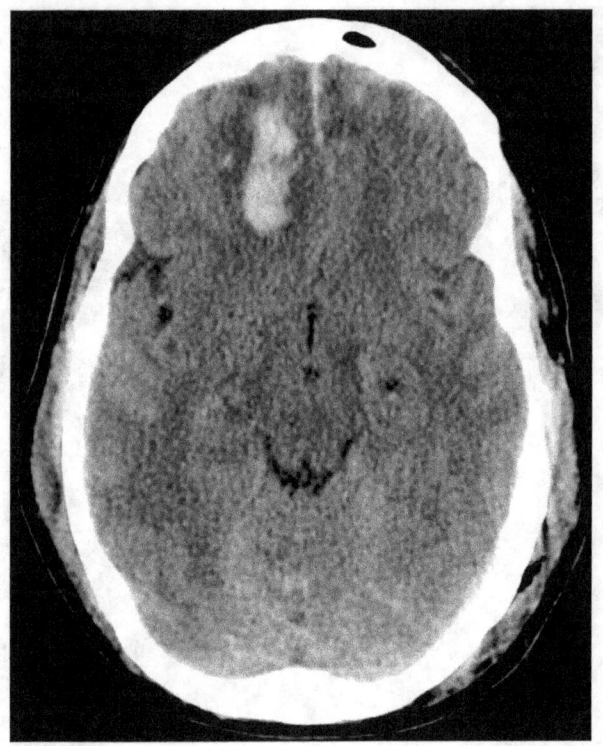

Best CT Study for Diagnosis:
CT Brain without contrast

Key to DX
Hyperattenuated, round focus located at the gray white junction.

Facts
Occurs when the brain parenchyma impacts the inner table of the skull.
Most common location at the coup site (site of impact).
Most common locations are the frontal lobes and temporal lobes.
Contusions are not classically associated with a loss of consciousness.

TX
Supportive care and close follow-up to monitor contusion size.

CEREBRAL CONTUSION

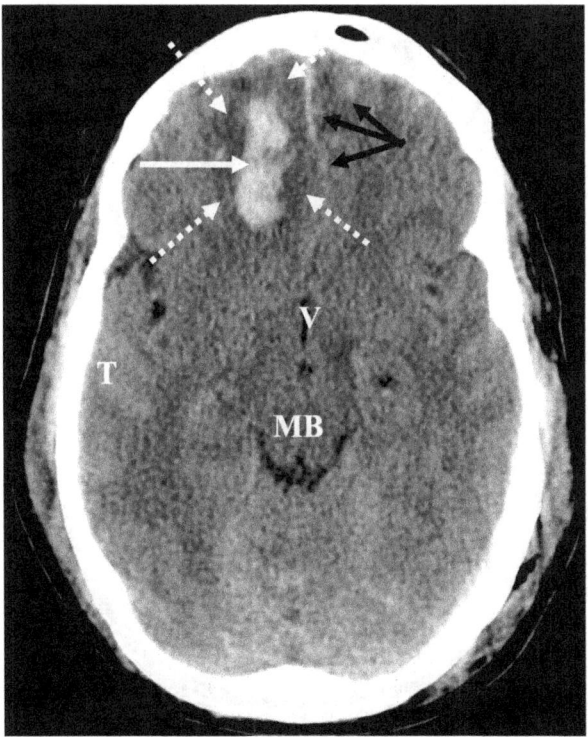

Study Above:
CT Brain without contrast at the level of the third ventricle.

Radiographic findings:
Hyperattenuated, oval, intra-axial collection within the right frontal lobe (arrow). A halo of low density consistent with vasogenic edema is surrounding the hematoma (dashed arrows). Also seen is a small amount of subarachnoid hemorrhage along the falx and left frontal sulci (black arrows).

Tips
Contusions are typically located adjacent to bone centered at the gray white junction.
Soft tissue or scalp edema is a clue where to look.
Always check the contrecoup site for injury (another bleed may be present: contusion, subarachnoid, or subdural).

Normal Anatomy
V – Third ventricle, MB – Midbrain, T – Temporal lobe

Further Reading
Wright, J.N. Review. CNS Injuries in Abusive Head Trauma. *AJR*. 208:991-1001, 2017.

CASE 12

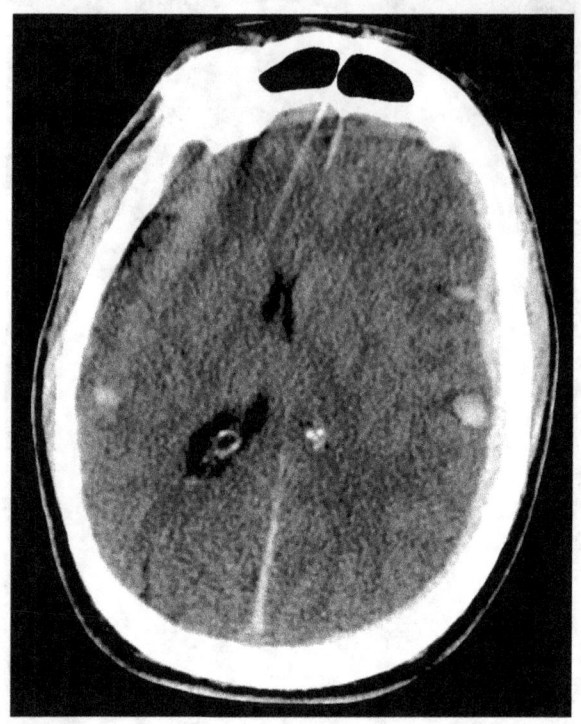

Best CT Study for Diagnosis:
CT Brain without contrast

Key to DX
Multiple, small, hyperattenuated, intra-axial foci.

Facts
Initial CT is commonly negative in the first 24 hours.
Best clue is round high density foci involving the basal ganglia, corpus callosum, and/or deep white matter.
Most commonly due to acceleration/deceleration accident results in shearing of axons.
The patients will have a low Glasgow-Coma Scale (GCS).

TX
Supportive care with attention to other body injuries.
Poor patient prognosis.

DIFFUSE AXONAL INJURY

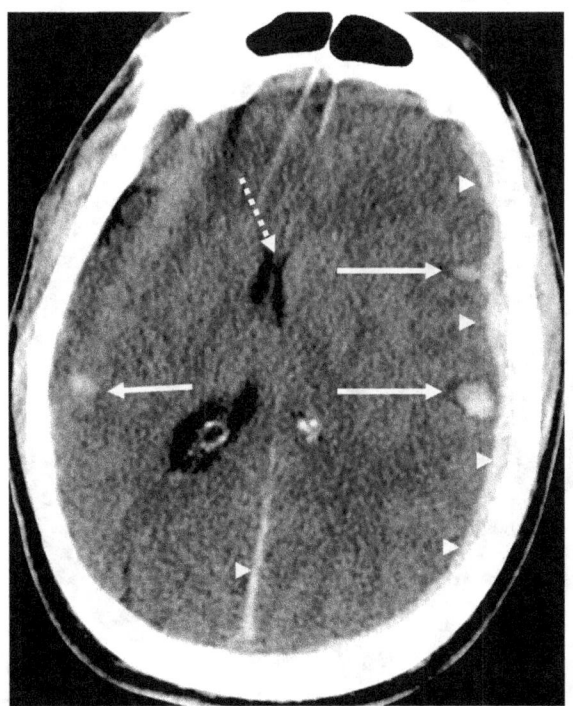

Study Above:
CT Brain without contrast at the level of the basal ganglia.

Radiographic findings:
Hyperattenuated, small, oval, intra-axial foci seen in the subcortical white matter of the left frontal lobe, left temporal lobe, and right temporal lobe (arrows). Along the left hemisphere is a crescentic hyperattenuated extra-axial collection which extends along the falx posteriorly consistent with a subdural hematoma (arrowheads). Notice there is significant mass effect with effacement of the left lateral ventricle and a midline shift from left to right (dashed arrow). Also, only a few sulci are seen which is reflective of increased intracranial pressure.

Tips
Think DAI in a trauma patient with multiple intra-axial deep contusions and a low GCS.
Most reliable finding is a contusion involving the basal ganglia or corpus collosum.
Suspect the diagnosis when CT findings do not correlate with the clinical picture.
MRI gradient echo or SWI sequences can be diagnostic 2-3 days post injury.

Further Reading
Wright, J.N. Review. CNS Injuries in Abusive Head Trauma. AJR. 208:991-1001, 2017.

CASE 13

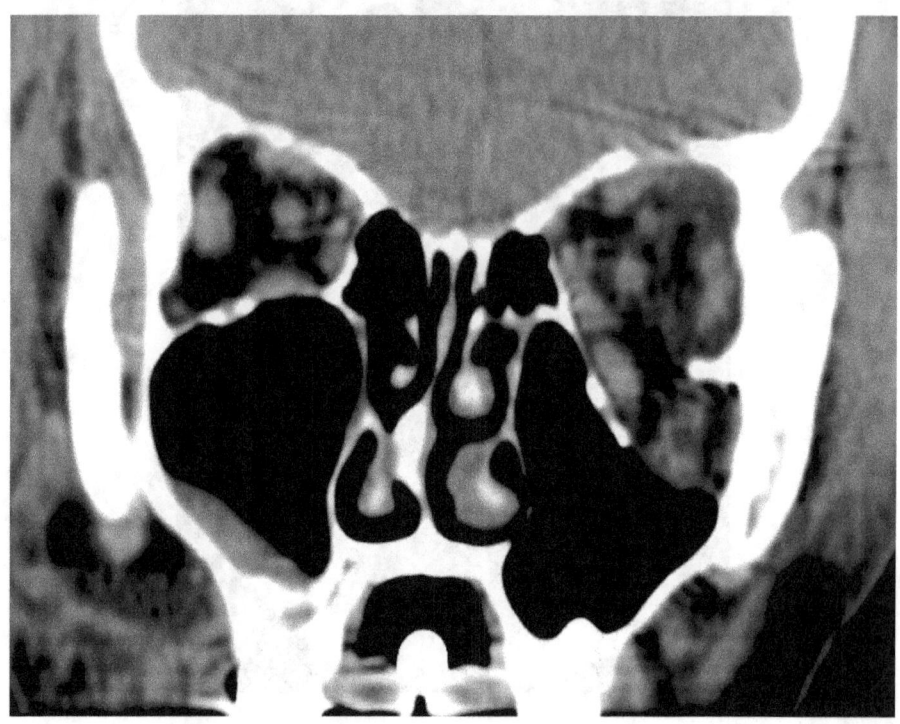

Best CT Study for Diagnosis:
CT Face without contrast

Key to DX
Orbital wall discontinuity.

Facts
Most common etiology is a direct blow to the eye.
Force is translated through the periorbital fat to the orbital wall.
The inferior wall is the most commonly injured.
Diplopia is caused by inferior rectus muscle entrapment within the fracture.
Orbital wall fractures are commonly associated with orbital emphysema.

TX
Diplopia that does not resolve in 2-4 weeks requires surgery for muscle entrapment.
Superior orbital fractures are usually surgical because of the increased risk of meningitis, potential dural tear with CSF leak, and potential for brain herniation.

ORBITAL FRACTURE

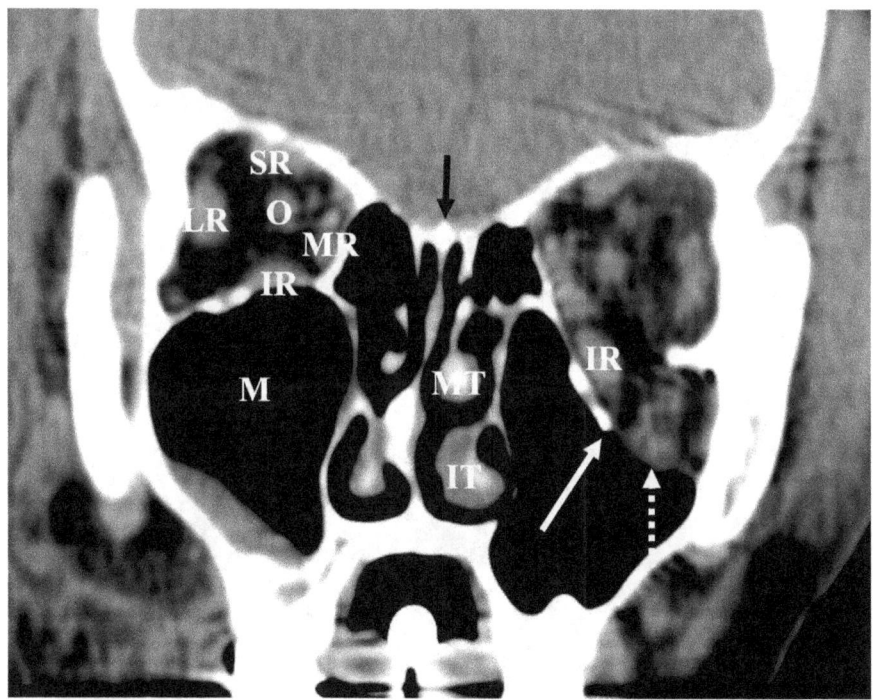

Study Above:
CT Face without contrast, coronal reformat through the mid orbits.

Radiographic findings:
Displacement of the inferior orbital wall (white arrow). Orbital hematoma with fat herniating into the left maxillary sinus (dashed arrow). Also, notice the increased attenuation of the left orbital fat compared to the right orbit.

Tips
Opacification of the neighboring sinus is a clue to the fracture site.
Air in the orbital fat (orbital emphysema) means fracture, so find it!
Always check the ocular muscles for entrapment or displacement.
When pneumocephalus is seen, a fracture is almost always present!

Normal Anatomy
IR - Inferior rectus, MR - Medial rectus, LR - Lateral rectus, SR - Superior rectus,
O - Optic nerve, MT - Middle turbinate, IT - Inferior turbinate, M - Maxillary sinus, Black Arrow - Crista galli

Further Reading
Reiter M.J., Schwope R.B.,. Theler J.M. Postoperative CT of the Orbital Skeleton After Trauma: Review of Normal Appearances and Common Complications. *AJR*. 206: 1276-1285, 2016.

CASE 14

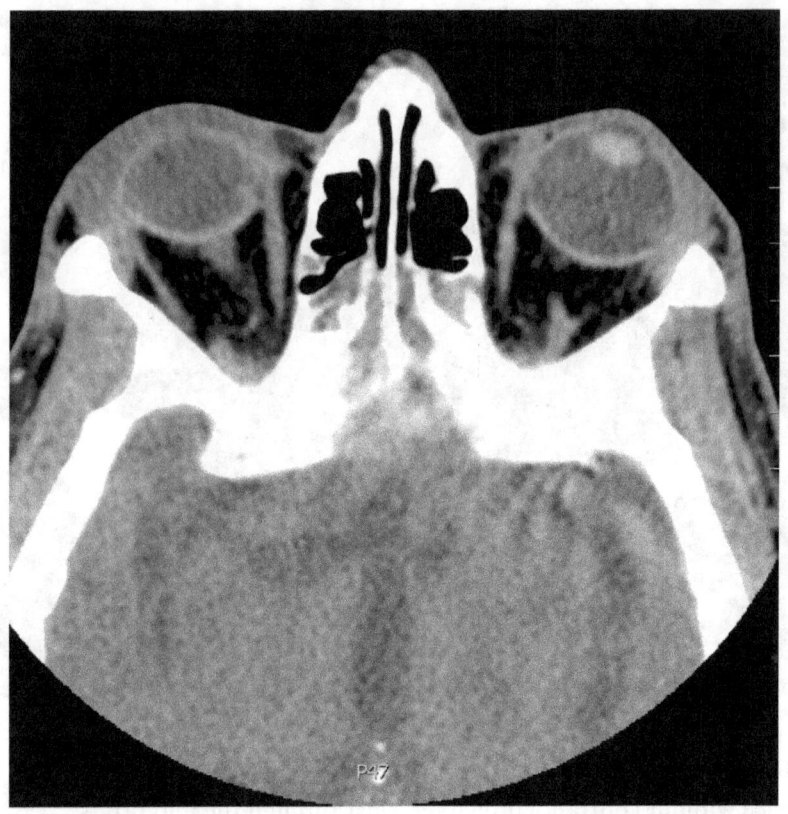

Best CT Study for Diagnosis:
CT Orbit without contrast

Key to DX
Non-spherical, asymmetric shape of the globe.

Facts
Most common cause is blunt or penetrating trauma resulting in laceration or perforation of the globe.
Loss of globe contour is due to decreased intraocular pressure.
May have unilateral exophthalmos or enophthalmos. Chronic sequela is a shrunken calcified globe called phthisis bulbi.

TX
Eye shield, avoid eye manipulation, administer anti-nausea and pain medications.
Immediate referral to an ophthalmologist for potential surgical repair.

GLOBE RUPTURE

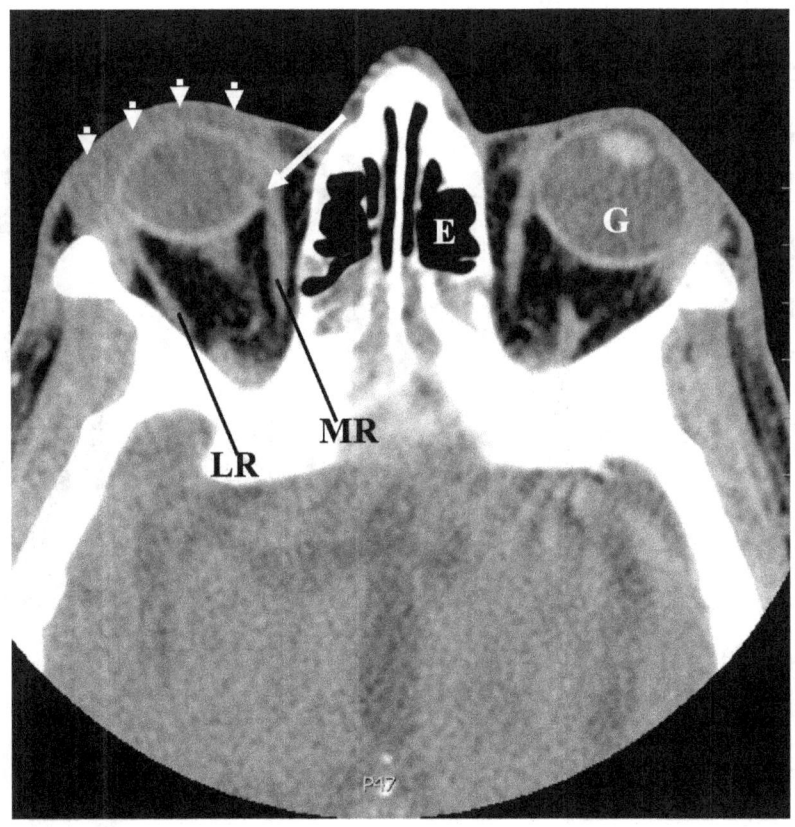

Study Above:
CT Orbits without contrast.

Radiographic findings:
Irregular contour of the right globe with buckling of the contour (arrow). The left globe is normal (G). Extensive preseptal edema is present (arrowheads).

Tips
Compare globes to each other to identify asymmetry.
Intraconal fat stranding is commonly seen with a globe injury.
Always check the posterior and anterior chambers for blood (hyperattenuation).
Air in orbital fat is highly sensitive for an associated fracture.
Rupture is common at the attachment of the intraocular muscles where the sclera is the thinnest.

Normal Anatomy
G – Globe, LR - Lateral rectus, MR - Medial rectus, E - Ethmoid sinus

Further Reading
Gad K., Singman E.L,., Nadgir R.N., et al. CT in the Evaluation of Acute Injuries of the Anterior Eye Segment. *AJR*.17.18279. 209:1353-1359, 2017.

CASE 15

CASE AUTHOR: Gregory D. Puthoff

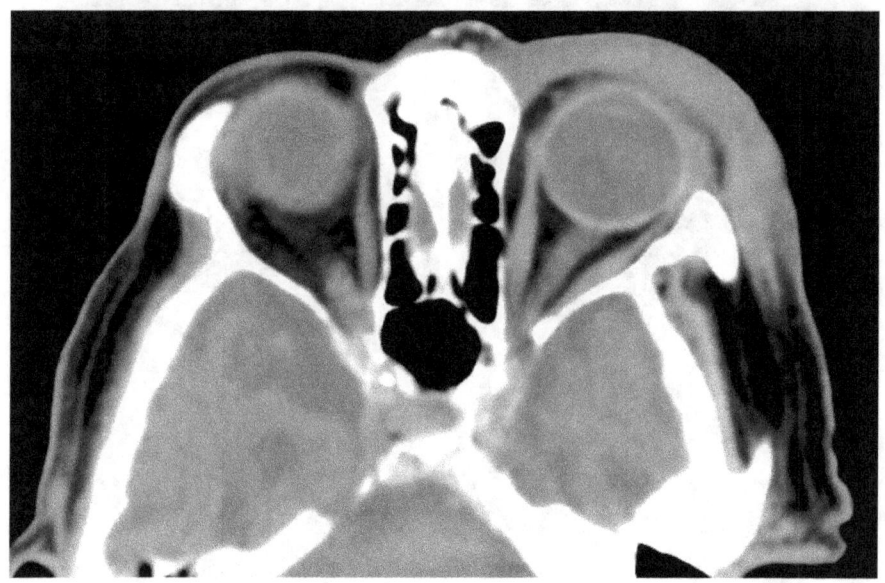

Best CT Study for Diagnosis:
CT Orbit or Face with IV contrast

Key to DX
Thickening and fat stranding of the preseptal soft tissues.

Facts
Also known as periorbital cellulitis.
The orbital septum separates the anterior facial soft tissues from the orbit.
Infection anterior to the orbital septum is preseptal cellulitis.
Infection posterior to the orbital septum is orbital cellulitis. Orbital cellulitis has a much worse prognosis and requires IV antibiotics, therefore accurate diagnosis is important.
Typically arises from contiguous spread of adjacent infectious processes such as a dental or sinus infection.

TX
Oral antibiotics on an outpatient basis.

PRESEPTAL CELLULITIS

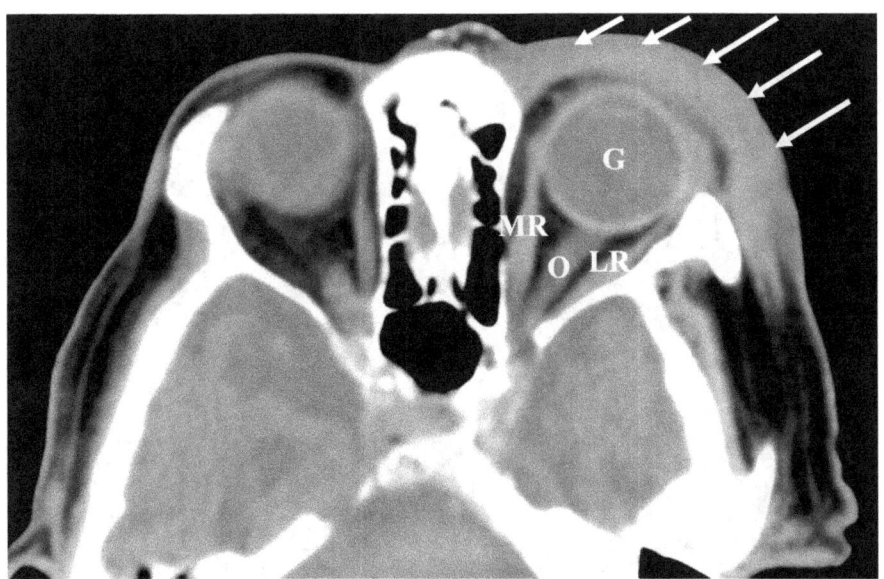

Study Above:
CT Orbit without IV contrast.

Radiographic Findings:
Single axial CT image enhanced with IV contrast demonstrates asymmetric soft tissue swelling involving the anterior soft tissues adjacent to the left orbit (arrows). Note that the orbital fat is well preserved posterior to the orbital septum (differentiating from orbital cellulitis).

Tips
Search for contrast enhancing fluid collections to exclude abscess.
Inspect the retrobulbar fat for fat stranding.
If postseptal or asymmetric scleral thickening is present, consider orbital cellulitis.
If there is enlargement of a single extraocular muscle, consider pseudotumor.

Normal Anatomy
G – Globe, LR - Lateral rectus, MR - Medial rectus, O - Optic nerve

Further Reading
Lebedis CA, et al. Nontraumatic Orbital Conditions: Diagnosis with CT and MR Imaging in the Emergent Setting. *Radiographics.* 28(6):1741-1753, 2008.

CASE 16

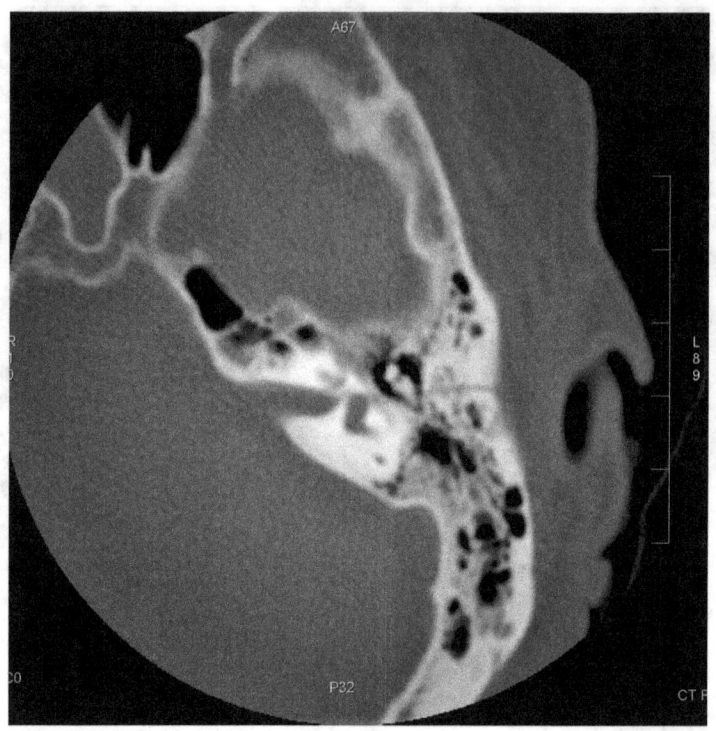

Best CT Study for Diagnosis:
CT Temporal Bone study without contrast

Key to DX
Linear low attenuation traversing the temporal bone.

Facts
Temporal bone fractures are categorized into longitudinal, transverse, and mixed.
Longitudinal fractures are more common.
Longitudinal fractures may be associated with ossicle chain disruption resulting in conductive hearing loss.

TX
Initially requires antibiotic therapy.
Surgical repair to address middle and inner ear damage.

TEMPORAL BONE FRACTURE

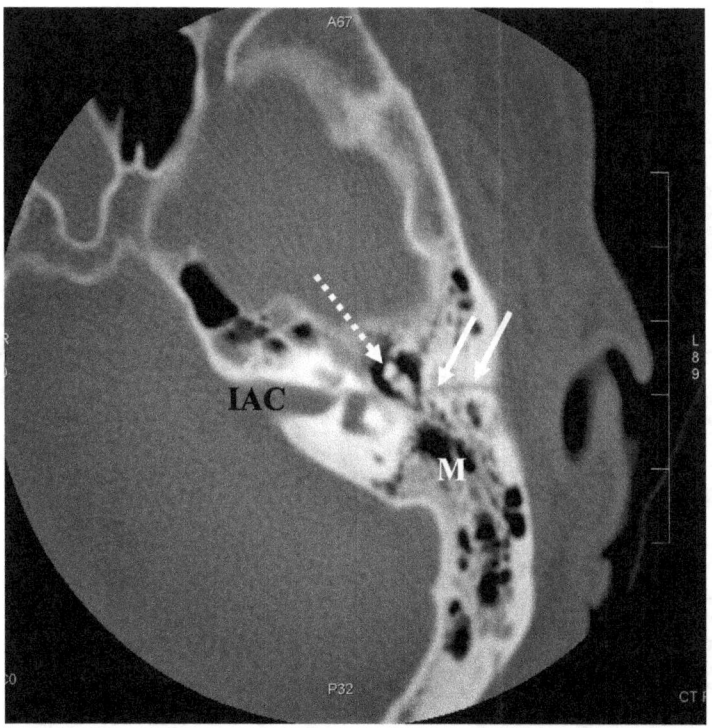

Study Above:
CT Temporal Bone study without contrast, left axial thin reformat.

Radiographic findings:
Linear low attenuation traversing the left temporal bone consistent with a fracture (arrows). Subtle widening noted of the incudomalleal joint consistent with ossicular dislocation (dashed arrow).

Tips
Temporal bone fractures are classically named with regards to the orientation of the fracture line to the long axis of the temporal bone. Other fracture classification systems are based on involvement of the otic capsule.
Otic capsule compromise is more likely to develop facial paralysis, CSF leak, and profound hearing loss.
Look for fracture extension into the jugular foramen which may cause thrombosis.
Normal Anatomy
IAC – Internal auditory canal, M - Mastoid

Further Reading
Kurihara Y.Y., et al. Temporal Bone Trauma: Typical CT and MRI Appearances and Important Points for Evaluation. *RadioGraphics*. Vol 40, Issue 4 May 2020.

CASE 17

CASE AUTHOR: Gregory D. Puthoff

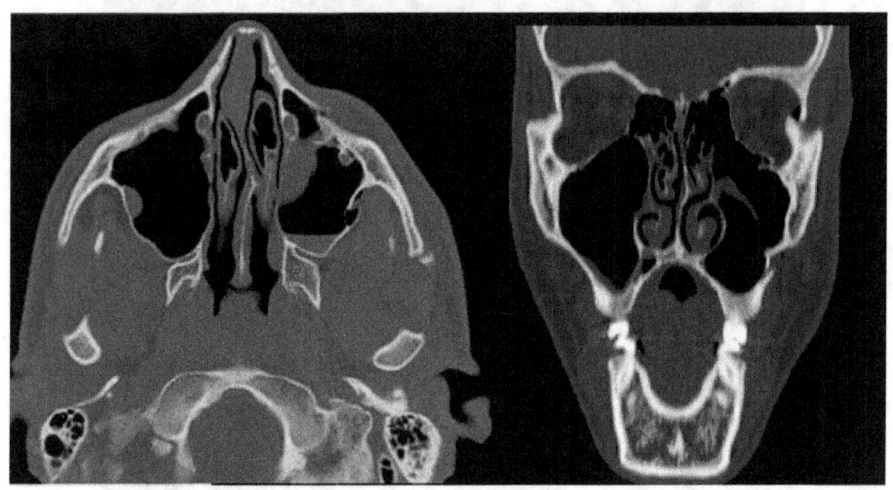

Best CT Study for Diagnosis:
CT Face without contrast

Key to DX
Fracture involving three articulations of the zygoma resulting in dissociation.

Facts
Three attachments of the zygoma are: temporal, orbital, and maxillary processes. Tripod means a three-legged stool. A tripod fracture involves three fractures of the zygoma (zygomaticofrontal, zygomaticomaxillary, and zygomaticotemporal sutures) resulting in dissociation of the zygoma from the skull (AKA floating zygoma).
Tripod fracture is also known as: zygomaticomaxillary fracture complex, zygomaticofacial fracture, or quadripod fracture.
Traditionally, the tripod fracture involved the three fracture sites above, but the increased use of CT has led to the discovery of a fourth component involving the zygomaticosphenoid suture, making the tripod fracture actually a quadripod fracture.
The fracture can impinge the muscles in the infratemporal fossa and result in difficulty with mastication.

TX
After pain control, surgical fixation is needed to re-approximate the zygoma.

TRIPOD FRACTURE

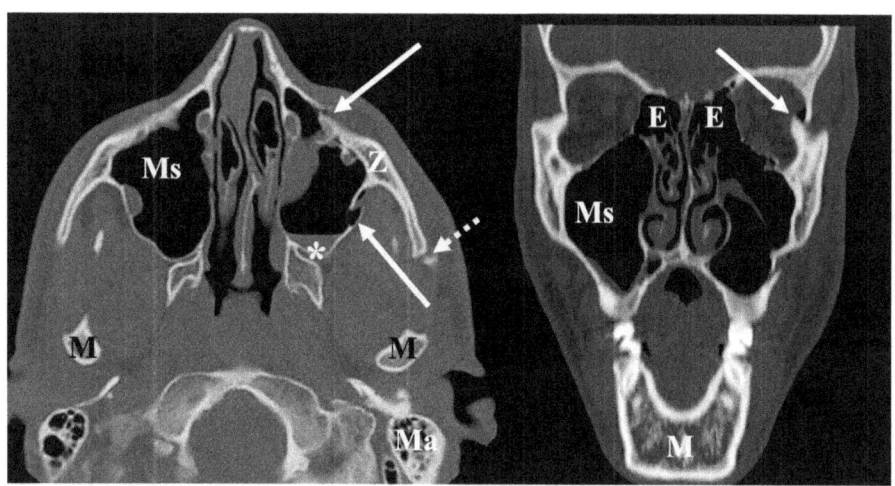

Study Above:
Ct Face without contrast, axial and coronal reformat.

Radiographic Findings:
Comminuted and displaced fractures are demonstrated of the left lateral orbit, left zygomatic arch, and left maxillary sinus (arrows). The fracture involves the left zygomaticomaxillary suture, left zygomatic arch (dashed arrow) and zygomaticofrontal suture. An associated air-fluid level is present in the left maxillary sinus (asterisk).

Tips
Displacement of fracture fragments is typically secondary to rotational forces applied by the masseter muscle.
Always look for other fractures.
Check the brain for a bleed (use non-contrast CT Brain).
Subcutaneous air is a clue for corresponding fracture from an adjacent sinus.

Normal Anatomy
M - Mandible, Z - Zygoma, Ma - Mastoid air cells,
E - Ethmoid air cells, Ms - Maxillary sinus

Further Reading
Reiter M.J., Schwope R.B.,. Theler J.M. Postoperative CT of the Orbital Skeleton After Trauma: Review of Normal Appearances and Common Complications. *AJR*. 206: 1276-1285, 2016.

CHAPTER 2
NECK CT

**Edited by
Naveen Malay, M.B.B.S**

NECK CT

TO CONTRAST OR NOT TO CONTRAST
In order to properly evaluate the neck for pathology with CT, IV contrast is a must! The neck anatomy is complex and packed into a small space. Therefore, IV contrast helps discriminate vessels from glands and soft tissues. Almost all diagnoses require IV contrast. If necrotizing fasciitis is of clinical concern, this would not require contrast.

CT VS. MRI
CT remains the "work horse" for neck imaging. MRI may provide additional information for soft tissue lesions but is not commonly used. Typically, most lesions and pathology can be accurately diagnosed with CT. Remember that MRI is not ideal in the emergent setting secondary to long imaging time, MRI safety issues, and availability (see discussion in Chapter 1, CT vs. MRI).

IMAGE INTERPRETATION
When attempting to interpret CT neck studies, it is easy to get lost in the detailed anatomy. Therefore, I recommend a non-radiologist to not initially focus on anatomy. Instead, simply evaluate each image for symmetry. The neck on every CT image should look symmetrical to the opposite side. When you detect an area of asymmetry, now you know where the pathology is located! At this point, you can now work through the anatomy to specifically localize the pathology (which narrows the differential diagnosis). Do not forget to interrogate the airway for patency. When trying to exclude an abscess, remember it will have a typical appearance of a fluid attenuated collection with a contrast enhancing border. This has a similar appearance to a mass in morphology, but

a mass is typically soft tissue attenuation with homogeneous or heterogeneous enhancement.

I hope you learn from the cases in this chapter! For each case, look at the first image (non-annotated) and try to find the abnormality. Then, come up with a diagnosis. If you can't figure out a diagnosis, look at the "facts" section for diagnostic hints (wish my daily work cases came with hints). Next review the second page of the case, which has the diagnosis at the top with full annotations along with relevant anatomy, take-home points and tips for learning. Also, references for each case are provided for additional study.

R Saenz DO, FAOCR

CASE 18

CASE AUTHOR: Naveen Malay

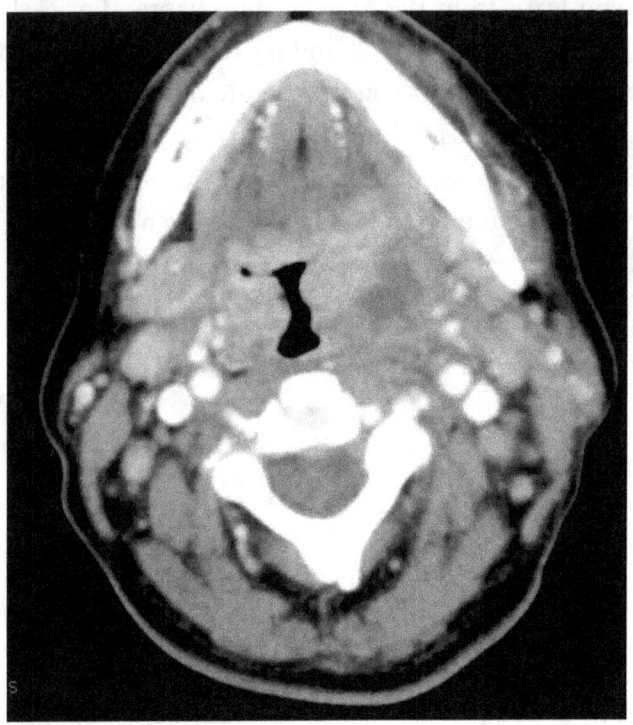

Best CT Study for Diagnosis:
CT Neck with IV contrast

Key to DX
Focal fluid collection within the oropharynx in the region of the palatine tonsil.

Facts
Most common bugs are *Streptococcus, Staphylococcus* and *H. influenzae*.
Also known as quinsy or quinsy abscess.
Present with fever, sore throat, trismus, halitosis and "hot potato" voice.
Peritonsillar abscesses tend to recur.
Do not confuse it with Ludwig angina, which is a cellulitis (not a focal abscess) with potential life-threatening complications.

TX
Incision and drainage with oral antibiotics is needed. Recurrence may require tonsillectomy.

PERITONSILLAR ABSCESS

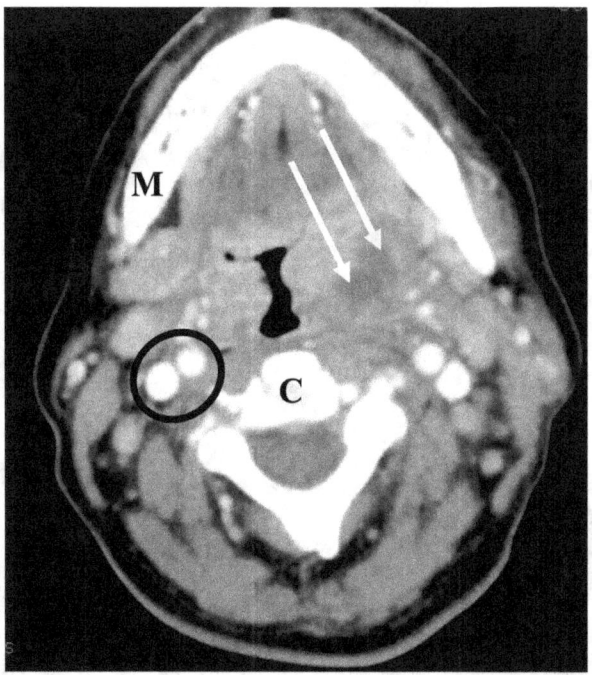

Study Above:
CT Neck with IV contrast at the level of the palatine tonsils.

Radiographic findings:
Enlargement of the left tonsil with focal areas of low attenuation consistent with abscess (arrows). The abscess creates mass effect resulting in narrowing the oropharynx.

Tips
Without IV contrast, small abscesses less than 1.5 cm may not be visible.
Look for odontogenic etiology when an abscess is near the mandible.
Assess airway for mass effect because narrowing may require airway management.
It is important to differentiate acute tonsillitis from tonsillar abscess. CT findings of tonsillitis include a "tiger stripe pattern" with enlargement and no focal fluid collection.
Reactive adenopathy is usually present.
Don't forget to check the retropharyngeal space as its involvement can extend into the mediastinum (descending necrotizing mediastinitis).

Normal Anatomy
M – Mandible, C - Cervical vertebral body, Circle - Carotid sheath

Further Reading
Finnila, T.L. & Sherman, P.M. At-the-viewbox-tonsillitis-versus-tonsillar-peritonsillar-absces. JAOCR..

CASE 19

CASE AUTHOR: Naveen Malay

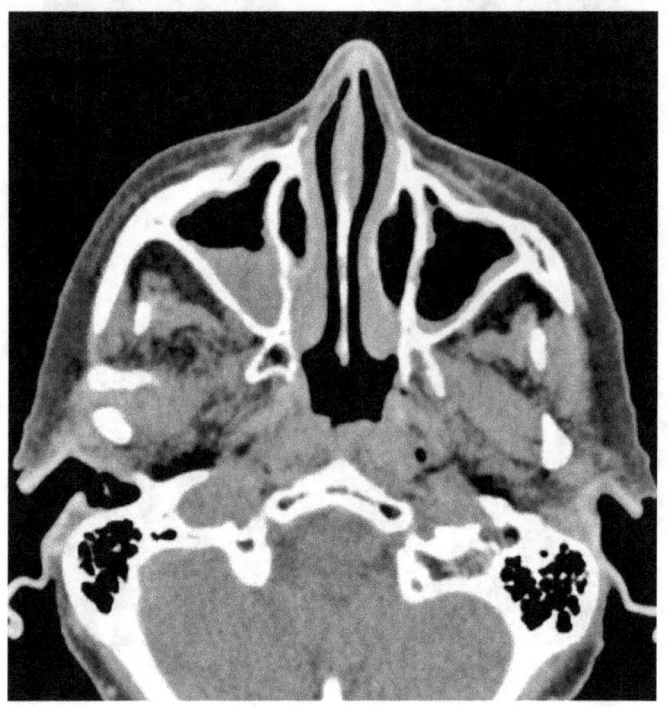

Best CT Study for Diagnosis:
CT Sinus without contrast

Key to DX
Air-fluid level in a sinus.

Facts
Most common pathogens are *Streptococcus pneumoniae*, *Haemophilus influenzae*, and *Moraxella catarrhalis*.
Consider a fungal etiology in immunocompromised patients.
Patients present with congestion, purulent rhinorrhea, cough, facial pain, malaise, and occasionally fever.
May be preceded by an upper respiratory infection.

TX
Oral antibiotic treatment and decongestants.

SINUSITIS

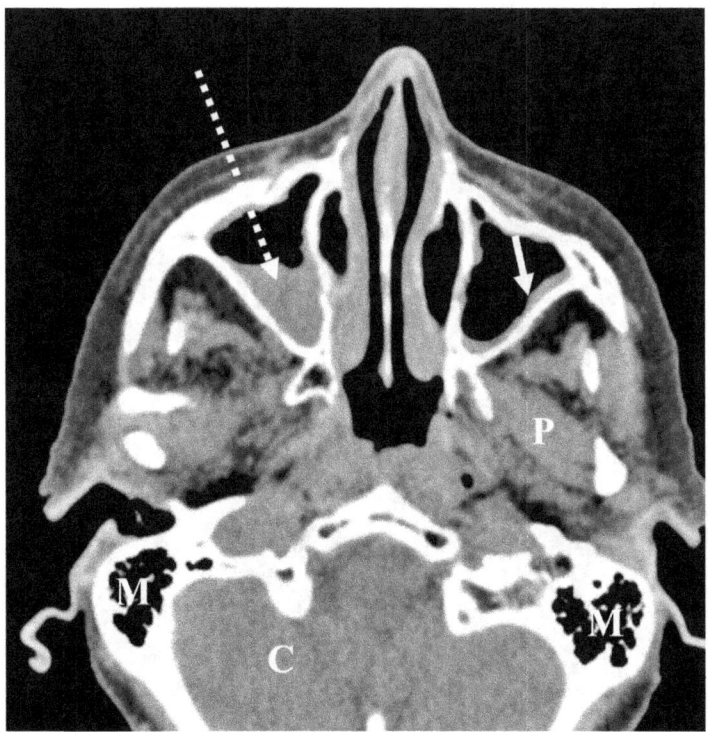

Study Above:
CT Sinus non-contrast image at the level of the maxillary sinuses.

Radiographic findings:
An air-fluid level is seen within the right maxillary sinus consistent with acute sinusitis (dashed arrow). The left maxillary sinus has mild mucosal thickening (arrow).

Tips
True air-fluid levels are orientated with the air on the non-dependent side.
The coronal plane is important to evaluate for ostiomeatal complex patency.
Beware of high attenuation within the sinus which may represent blood (related to trauma) or fungal disease (in immunocompromised from aspergillosis or mucormycosis).
Chronic sinus disease is suggested when the sinus demonstrates bone thickening.

Normal Anatomy
C - Cerebellum, P - Pterygoid, M - Mastoid

Further Reading
Poyiadji N, et al.. Imaging Findings in Non-Neoplastic Sinonasal Disease: Review of Imaging Features With Endoscopic Correlates. Current Problems in Diagnostic Radiology 2020;

CASE 20

CASE AUTHOR: Naveen Malay

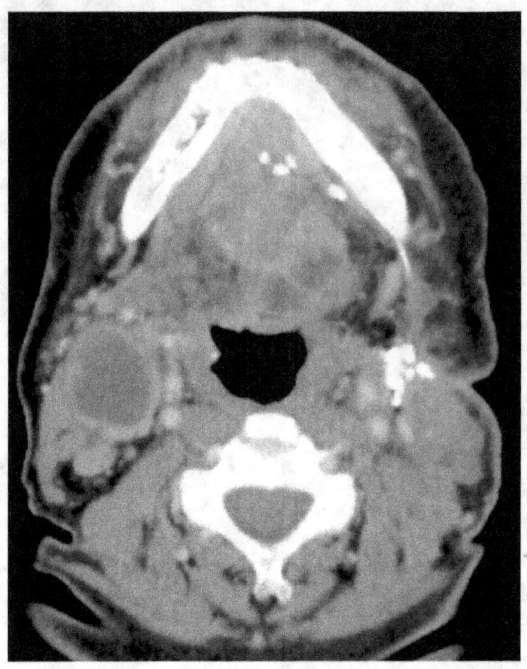

Best CT Study for Diagnosis:
CT Neck with IV contrast

Key to DX
Partially necrotic, heterogeneously enhancing mass in the neck.

Facts
Most common carcinoma of the neck is squamous cell carcinoma (SCC).
A heterogeneous neck mass in this location could represent squamous cell carcinoma, lymphoma (usually presents with multiple large solid lesions), necrotic lymph node (such as scrofula or other infection), and abscess.
Risk factors for head and neck SCC: tobacco, alcohol, and chemical exposure.
Infected branchial cleft cyst can appear similar but is more common in younger patients.
Lymphoma is the second most common cause of neck carcinoma.

TX
Soft tissue biopsy is needed for diagnosis.
Treatment depends on the stage of the disease and includes surgery, radiation therapy, and chemotherapy.

METASTATIC SQUAMOUS CELL CARCINOMA

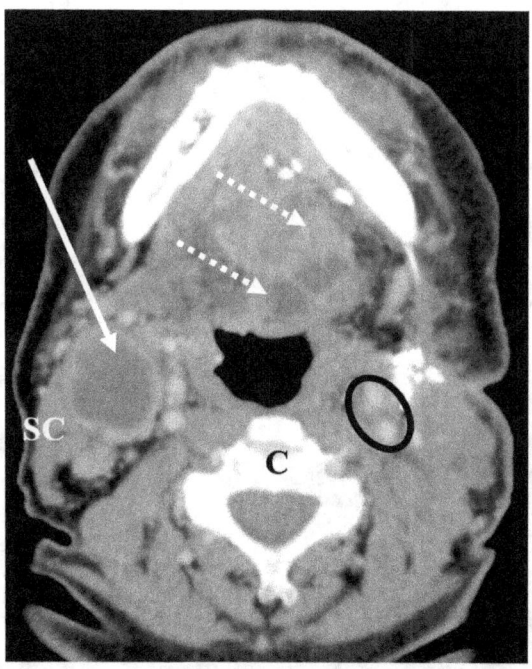

Study Above:
CT Neck with IV contrast at the level of the mandible.

Radiographic findings:
A round, heterogeneously enhancing mass is seen in the right neck with partial necrosis (arrow). The primary malignancy is seen at the base of the tongue as a necrotic mass (dashed arrows).

Tips
Look for a possible primary malignant mass in the neck.
The absence of fat-stranding helps exclude an abscess.
Consider a metastatic lymph node if the patient has a primary carcinoma.
Check for contralateral adenopathy and bone involvement.

Normal Anatomy
SC – Sternocliedomastoid muscle, C - Cervical vertebral body, Circle - Carotid sheath

Further Reading
Chung M.S., Choi Y.J., Kim S.O., et al. A Scoring System for Prediction of Cervical Lymph Node Metastasis in Patients with Head and Neck Squamous Cell Carcinoma. *American Journal of Neuroradiology*. 40 (6) 1049-1054; 2019.

CASE 21

CASE AUTHOR: Naveen Malay

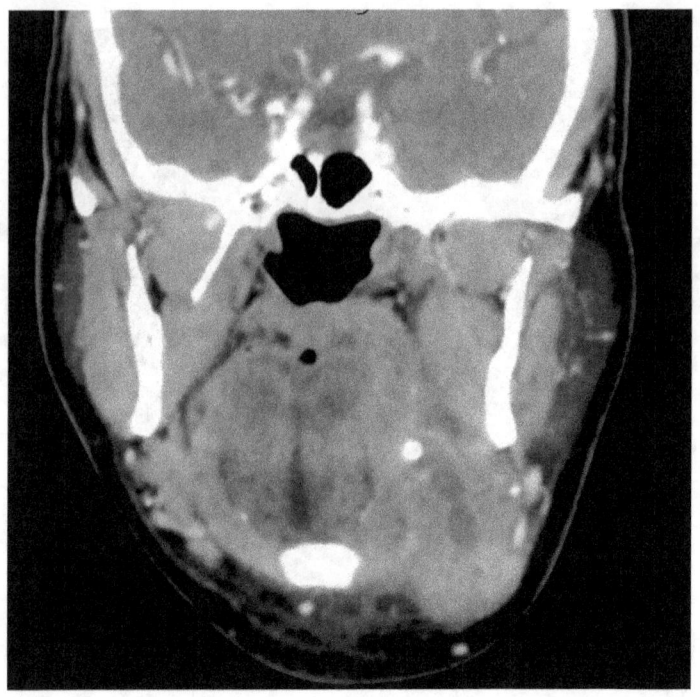

Best CT Study for Diagnosis:
CT Neck with IV contrast

Radiographic findings:
Calcified focus in the floor of the mouth with an associated tubular structure.

Facts
Patients present with postprandial pain and facial edema.
Sialoliths (salivary stones) most commonly occur in the submandibular gland.
Etiology is not known but believed to be related to gland stagnation.
There may be multiple stones.
More common in males.

TX
Surgical removal of the stone is definitive. Manual extraction may be possible.

SIALOLITHIASIS

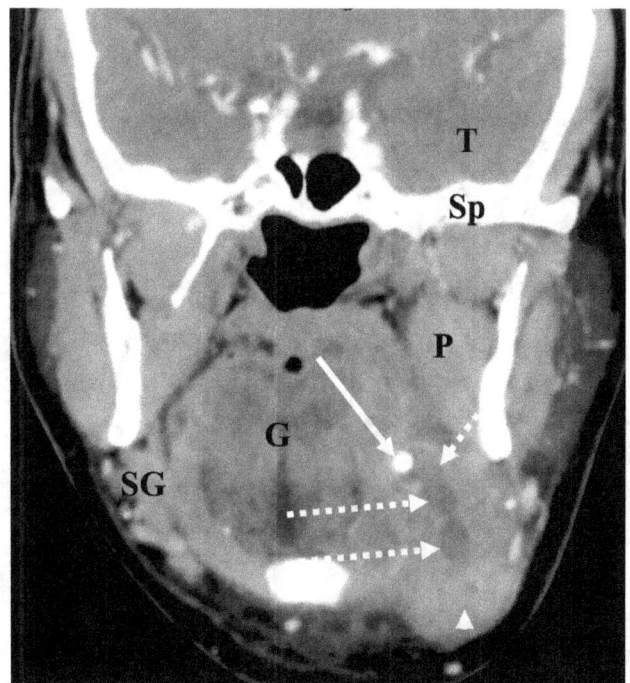

Study Above:
CT face with IV contrast, coronal reformat.

Radiographic findings:
A calcified, oval structure is seen in the left floor of the mouth consistent with a sialolith (arrow). In addition, a tubular structure is noted inferior to the sialolith, representing a dilated submandibular duct, AKA Wharton's duct (dashed arrows). The left submandibular gland is enlarged from inflammation (arrowhead).

Tips
Bone windows may be helpful to visualize small stones.
Review multiple planes because stones can be difficult to see when artifacts from dental amalgam are present.
Remember, more than one stone may be present.
Sialadenitis may be seen as an enlarged, hyperemic gland.

Normal Anatomy
SG - Submandibular gland, T - Temporal lobe, Sp - Sphenoid bone, G - Genioglossus

Further Reading
Purcell Y.M. The Diagnostic Accuracy of Contrast-Enhanced CT of the Neck for the Investigation of Sialolithiasis. *AJNR*. 38:2161–66, 2017.

CASE 22

CASE AUTHOR: Naveen Malay

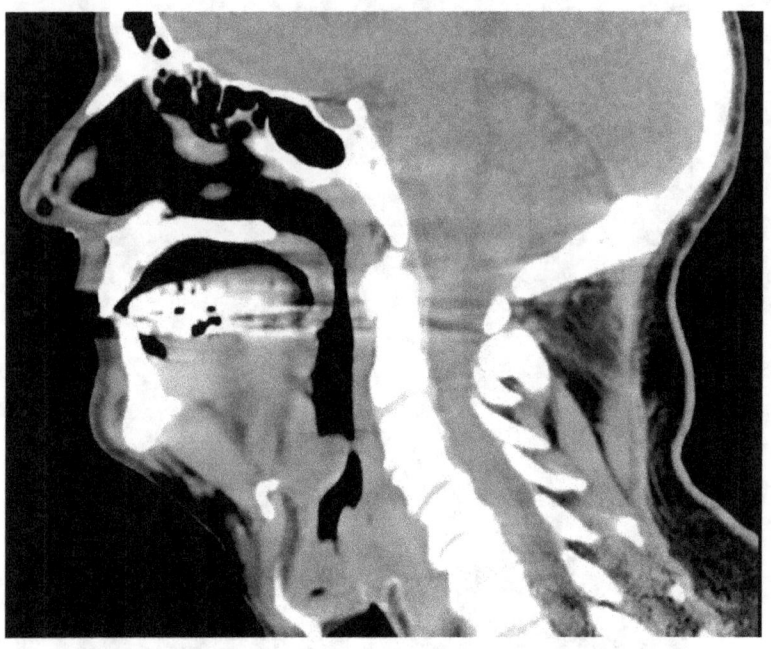

Best CT Study for Diagnosis:
CT Neck with IV contrast

Key to DX
Enlarged epiglottis.

Facts
Most common etiology is *Haemophilus influenzae*.
Also known as supraglottitis (since the epiglottis is part of the supraglottic airway).
Most commonly seen in children.
Clinical triad includes dysphagia, distress, and drooling.
Significantly reduced incidence due to widespread vaccination.
Similar appearance can be seen in angioedema.

TX
Antibiotic therapy and steroids.
Emergency intubation may be required.

EPIGLOTITIS

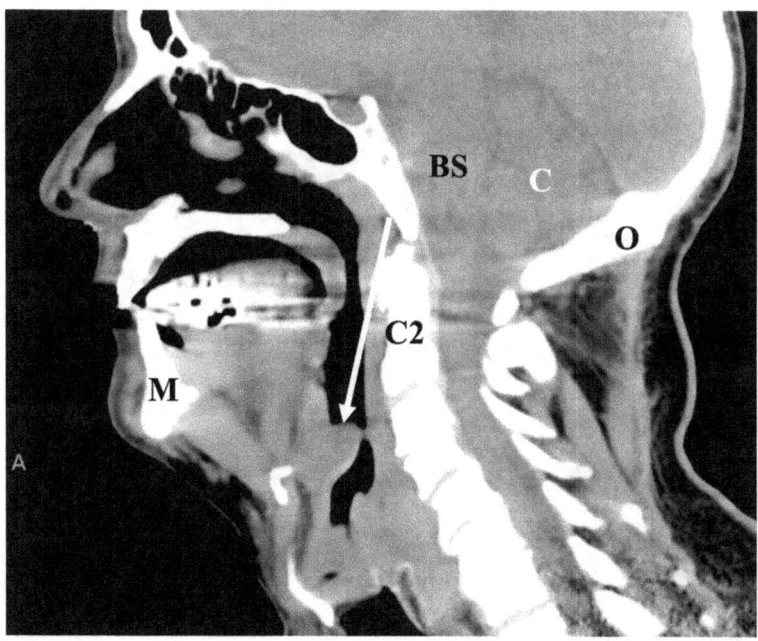

Study Above:
CT Neck without contrast, sagittal reconstruction.

Radiographic findings:
The epiglottis is enlarged from diffuse edema consistent with epiglottitis (arrow).

Tips
Enlarged aryepiglottic folds are more reliable than an enlarged epiglottis.
Edema should be diffuse. Consider another etiology if edema is focal.
If any fluid collection is present, consider abscess (not in this case).
Always evaluate the airway for patency.
On lateral neck radiograph, look for an enlarged epiglottis: the "thumb sign."

Normal Anatomy
BS -Brain stem, C - Cerebellum, O- Occiput, C2- C2 vertebra, M- Mandible

Further Reading
Darras KE, Roston, AT, & Yewchuk, LK. Imaging Acute Airway Obstruction in Infants and Children. *RadioGraphics*. 35:2064–2079; 2015.

CASE 23

CASE AUTHOR: Naveen Malay

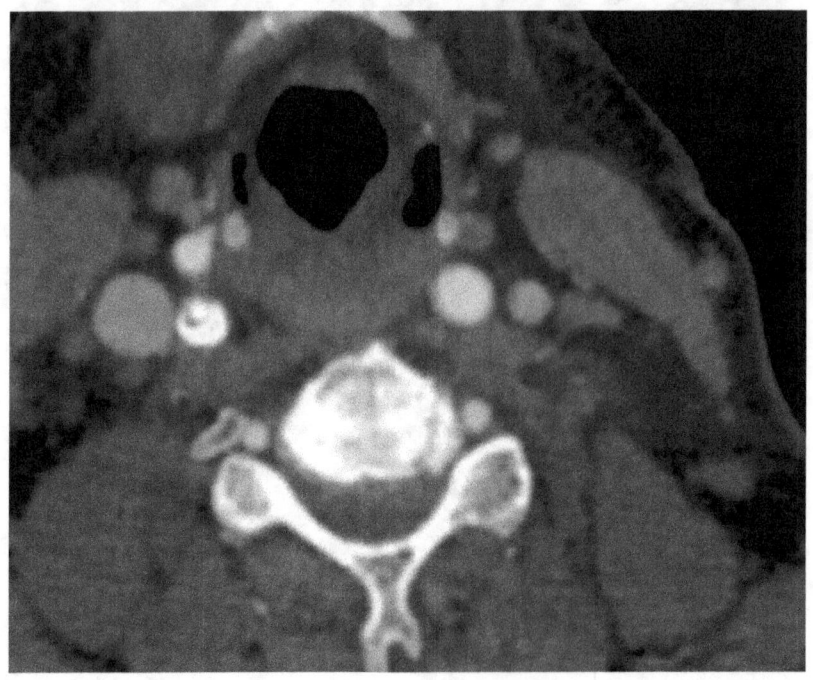

Best CT Study for Diagnosis:
CT Neck with IV contrast

Key to DX
Carotid artery lumen narrowing.

Facts
Patients may present with vertigo, syncope, or neurological deficit.
Carotid bruit may be auscultated.
The gold standard for arterial evaluation is catheter angiography.
CTA is a reliable non-invasive means of diagnosis.
As luminal stenosis increases, the risk of stroke also increases.
Smoking is a significant risk factor.

TX
Carotid stenosis greater than 70% requires surgical treatment.
Complete vascular occlusion is not treated.

CAROTID ARTERY STENOSIS

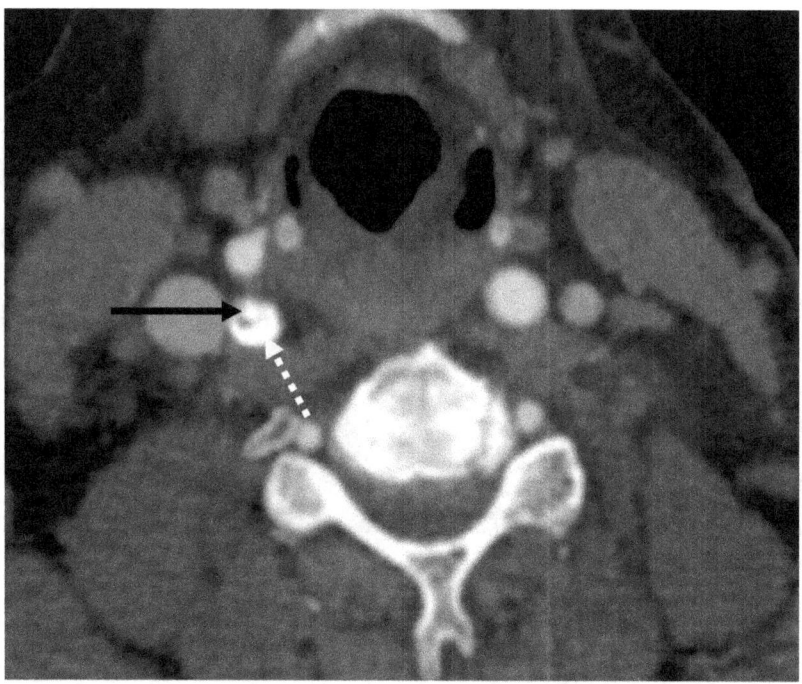

Study Above:
CTA Neck with IV contrast above the carotid bifurcation.

Radiographic findings:
Hypoattenuating soft plaque within the right internal carotid artery surrounds the opacified lumen resulting in stenosis (arrow). Calcified plaque is seen along the posterior aspect of the right internal carotid artery (dashed arrow).

Tips
CTA is preferred and has higher resolution than MRA.
To accurately diagnose carotid stenosis, a CTA technique is needed with thin 1 millimeter (or submillimeter) slice images with multi-plane reconstruction.
To distinguish the internal from external carotid arteries, remember that the internal does not branch in the neck
For CTA confirmation, a conventional catheter angiogram may be necessary but is usually reserved for treatment.
Reviewing reconstructed images in the coronal and sagittal planes is helpful.
Percent Stenosis = (1 - [smallest diameter/ normal distal diameter]) x 100
Normal diameter should be measured distally, not immediately after the stenosis, because post stenotic dilatation can give inaccurate results of narrowing.

Further Reading
Samaržija K., Milošević,P., Jurjević Z., et al. Comparison Of Carotid Stenosis Grading By CT Angiography And Doppler Ultrasonography: *Acta Clin Croat*. Sep; 60(3): 457–466; 2021.

CASE 24

CASE AUTHOR: Rocky Saenz

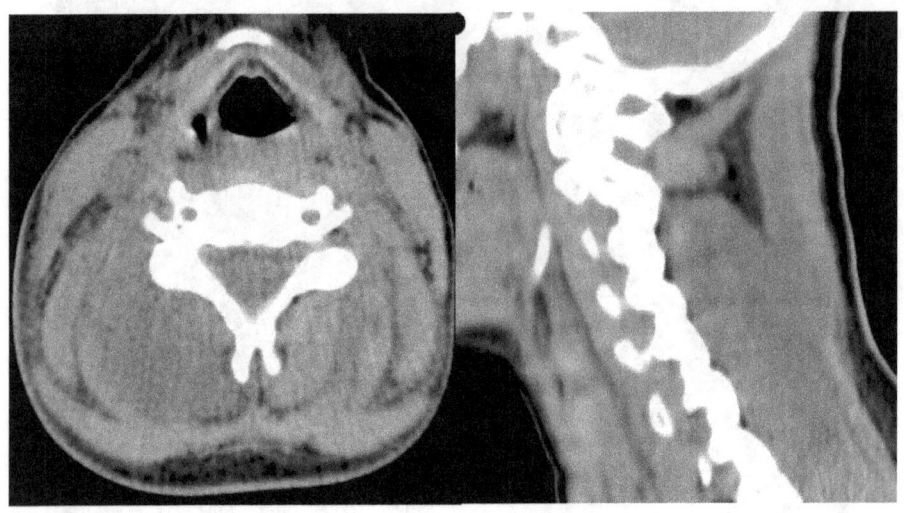

Best CT Study for Diagnosis:
CT Cervical spine without contrast

Key to DX
Hypoattenuated area centered in the soft tissue with loss of fat planes.

Facts
Patients will present with focal pain and edema at site.
Common etiologies include blunt trauma.
May be associated with a fracture.
CT is superior to MRI in the diagnosis of fracture.

TX
The etiology of the hematoma must be addressed. Usually, treatment is conservative with NSAIDs for pain.

SOFT TISSUE HEMATOMA

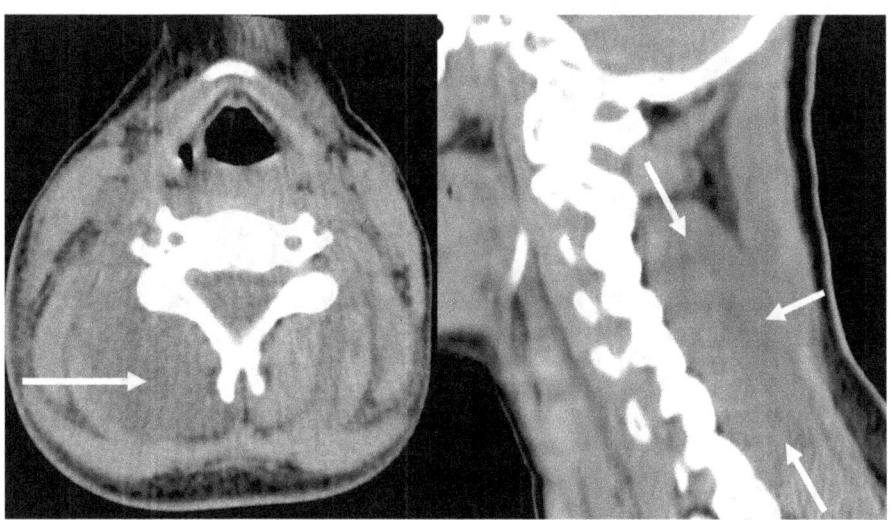

Study Above:
CT Cervical spine without contrast axial image at the mid cervical spine (left image). The right image is a sagittal reformat of the right neck.

Radiographic findings:
A hypoattenuated area is seen involving the right paraspinal muscle (arrows). Notice the loss of the fat planes on the right compared to the contralateral side.

Tips
Evaluate closely for an associated fracture.
Contrast is useful in the setting of infection to exclude an abscess or tumor.
MRI non-contrast may be helpful in a patient with a negative CT to exclude soft tissue injury, disc pathology, or cord injury.
Whiplash injuries typically have no CT findings.
One of the most important findings for neck trauma is enlargement of the pre-vertebral soft tissues… so make sure it is normal! Use the sagittal midline image to measure AP dimension (should be less than 7 mm at C3 and 21 mm at C7).

Further Reading
Kamalian S., Avery L., Lev M.H., et al. Nontraumatic Head and Neck Emergencies. *Radiogrpahics*. Published Online:Oct 7 2019.

CASE 25

CASE AUTHOR: Gregory D. Puthoff

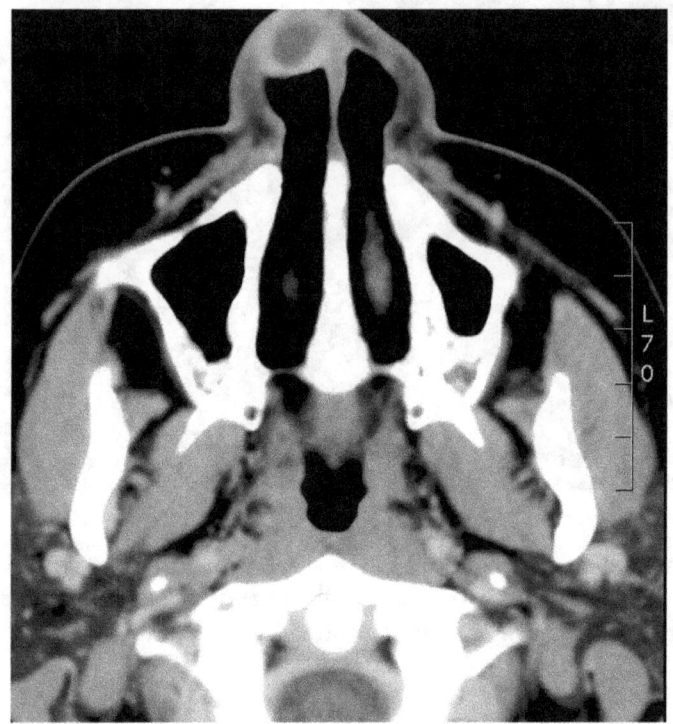

Best CT Study for Diagnosis:
CT Face with IV contrast

Key to DX
Contrast enhancing fluid collection involving the nasal vestibule.

Facts
The nasal vestibule is the most anterior cartilaginous part of the nose and is lined by stratified squamous skin epithelium (the remaining nasal structures are lined with respiratory epithelium).
Typically arise from accidental or iatrogenic trauma.
May also be seen in immunocompromised patients or as a result of direct extension from dental infection.
Also known as nasal septal abscess.

TX
Surgical incision and drainage with antibiotic therapy.

VESTIBULAR ABSCESS

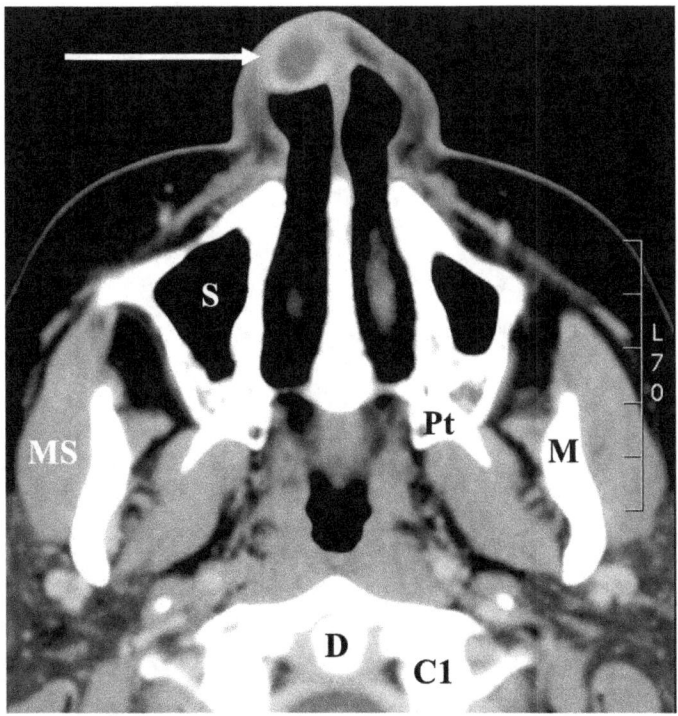

Study Above:
CT Face with IV contrast at the level of the nasal vestibule.

Radiographic Findings:
A peripherally enhancing fluid collection with mild surrounding inflammatory fat-stranding is identified with the right nasal vestibule (arrow).

Tips
Abscess should always be the diagnosis of exclusion when a contrast enhancing fluid collection is seen.
Always evaluate the nasal septum and vestibule for fluid collections as these lesions are not always detectable on physical examination.
Evaluate for the presence of nasal foreign bodies, especially in the pediatric population.

Normal Anatomy
D - Dens, C1 - C1 vertebra, MS - Masseter, Pt - Pterygoid, S – Maxillary sinus, M - Mandible

Further Reading
Guakil-Haber A. , Kuri-García A., Espinosa-Mancilla A.E., et al. Nasal Tip Abscess: A Rare Infection of the Head and Neck: *International Journal of Contemporary Medicine Surgery and Radiology.* Vol 4;Issue 4, October-December 2019.

CHAPTER 3
SPINE CT

Edited by

Timothy McKnight, D.O.

SPINE

TO CONTRAST OR NOT TO CONTRAST?

CT spine imaging does not require IV contrast when done for trauma or disc degeneration. IV contrast should be used only to exclude tumor or infection. Epidural abscess can be diagnosed with CT when large or significant osteomyelitis is present with vertebral endplate advanced erosions. Otherwise, it can only be completely excluded with MRI (as small abscesses and early osteomyelitis may not be visualized on CT).

CT VS. MRI

CT and MRI share complementary roles in spine imaging. CT is the best for imaging cortical bone in the setting of trauma and has exquisite bone detail with higher resolution than MRI. MRI is the gold standard for spinal cord and disc imaging. Both MRI and CT are complementary for bone tumor imaging. In the setting of epidural abscess, MRI is more accurate than CT. MRI can detect discitis and osteomyelitis earlier and with greater accuracy than CT. With CT, the diagnosis is usually made when vertebral body endplate erosion is seen which occurs with advanced disease (see Case 29). In the setting of trauma, MRI should never be done before CT! This puts the patient at risk because of the possibility of an unstable spinal fracture. CT can also provide useful reformats in the coronal and sagittal planes (these are not actual scans but are post processed and can be produced minutes or even days after the initial study). Three-dimensional or 3D images may also be reformatted from the CT images which are helpful for surgical planning.

IMAGE INTERPRETATION

The key to interpreting spine studies is to have a methodical approach. I suggest an "**A, B, C, D**" approach. Do this pattern to evaluate for **A**lignment, **B**one morphology, spinal **C**anal patency, and **D**isc integrity. Coronal and sagittal reformats are very important to evaluate the spinal alignment and subtle compression fractures. The posterior vertebral line is the most reliable to rule out spinal malalignment. When there is malalignment, this usually results in a component of spinal canal stenosis. The sagittal images are crucial to evaluate for loss of vertebral body height. When evaluating discs, you must carefully evaluate the posterior contour. If the disc focally protrudes posteriorly, then it is a disc herniation (see Case 27). The relationship of the intervertebral disc to the spinal canal is critical to determine if significant spinal canal stenosis exists. In addition, inspect the neural foramen as disc material and/or bone impingement may create significant neural foraminal stenosis. Do not forget to evaluate the paraspinal muscles and other soft tissues on the scan (for example, renal stones can present with back pain without hematuria mimicking disc disease).

R Saenz.DO, FAOCR

CASE 26

CASE AUTHOR: Tim McKnight

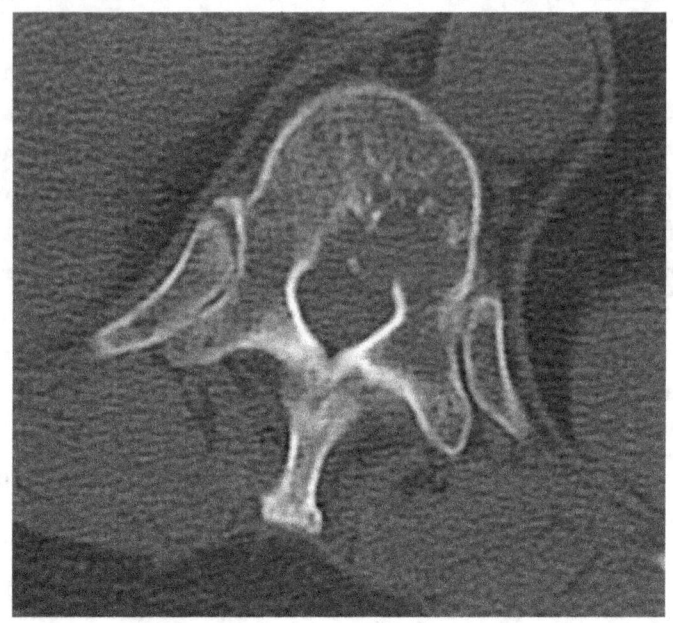

Best CT Study for Diagnosis:
CT Thoracic spine without contrast

Key to DX
Lytic lesion within the vertebral body.

Facts
Multiple myeloma is the most common primary malignant bone tumor (1% of all cancers) and the second most common hematologic malignancy (10%).
A lytic spine lesion is non-specific and the differential diagnosis includes a metastatic lesion, infection, or multiple myeloma.
Multiple myeloma bone involvement is usually multifocal.
Median age of onset is 69 with 10% of patients 50 years old or younger.
M-protein produced by the malignant plasma cells is IgG in the majority of patients.
Diagnostic criteria include: hyper**c**alcemia, **r**enal failure, **a**nemia, **b**one lesions (CRAB criteria).

TX
Chemotherapy and bone marrow transplant increase survival but are not curative.

MULTIPLE MYELOMA

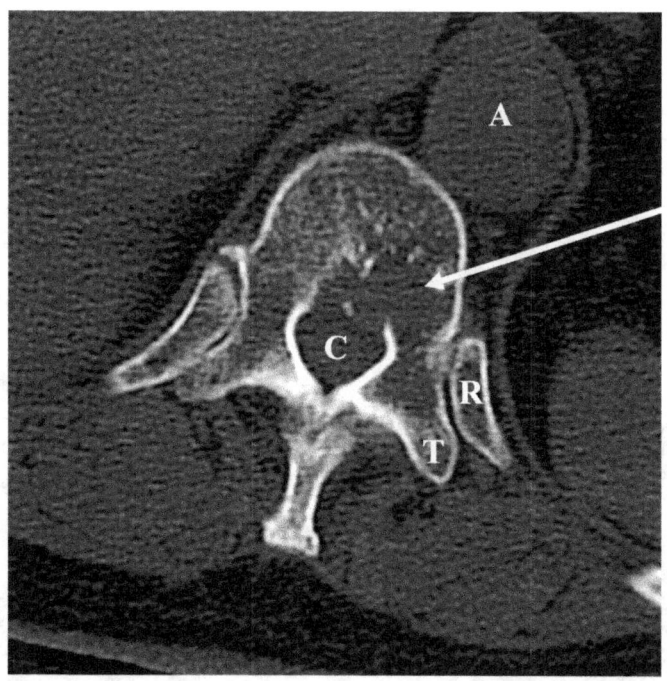

Study Above:
CT thoracic spine without contrast

Radiographic findings:
Irregular lytic lesion within the vertebral body (arrow). Notice that the spinal canal (C) anterior margin is eroded, which is concerning for disease extension into the spinal canal epidural space.

Tips
Check the relationship of the bone lesion to the spinal canal.
Look for other lesions!
Sagittal images are helpful to judge for loss of vertebral body height (pathologic fracture).
Scrutinize the posterior vertebral line for malalignment (use sagittal images).
Best imaging for staging is low dose whole body CT or PET/CT. Skeletal radiograph surveys were the traditional imaging modality, but now have limited role due to poor sensitivity.

Normal Anatomy
R- Rib, T - Transverse process, A – Aorta, C – Spinal canal

Further Reading
AG. Ormond Filho, MD, et al Whole-Body Imaging of Multiple Myeloma: Diagnostic Criteria. *RadioGraphics*. 39:1077–1097, 2019.

CASE 27

CASE AUTHOR: Tim McKnight

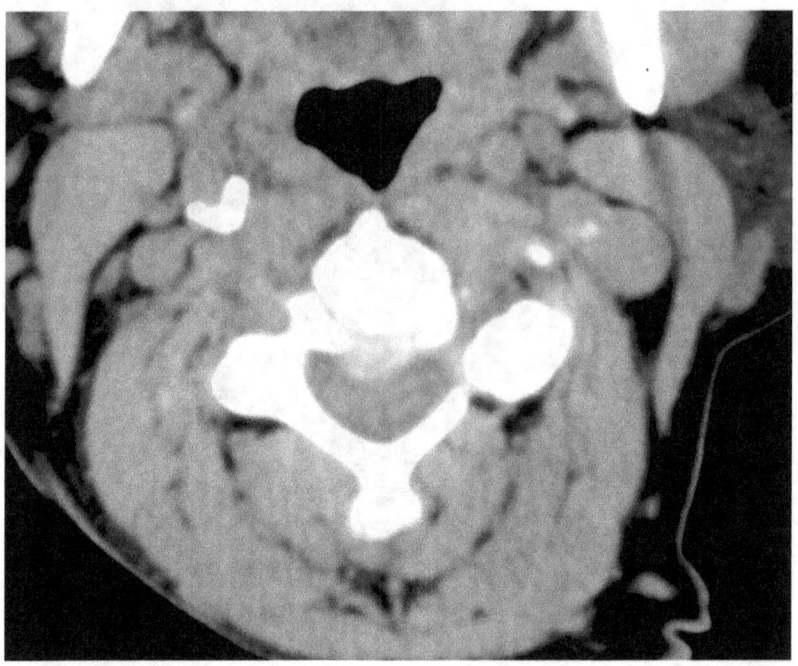

Best CT Study for Diagnosis:
CT cervical spine without contrast

Key to DX
Focal protrusion of the intervertebral disc.

Facts
Patients present with neck pain that typically radiates down the extremity (radiculopathy).
Herniations are caused by breakdown of the annulus fibrosus.
The most common disc herniations are in the lower lumbar spine (L4-L5 and L5-S1).
The most common location for thoracic herniations are at the lower levels.
The most common herniations within the cervical spine are at C5-C6 and C6-C7.

TX
Conservative therapy initially with steroids and analgesics.
Surgical therapy may be necessary when conservative therapy fails.

CERVICAL DISC HERNIATION

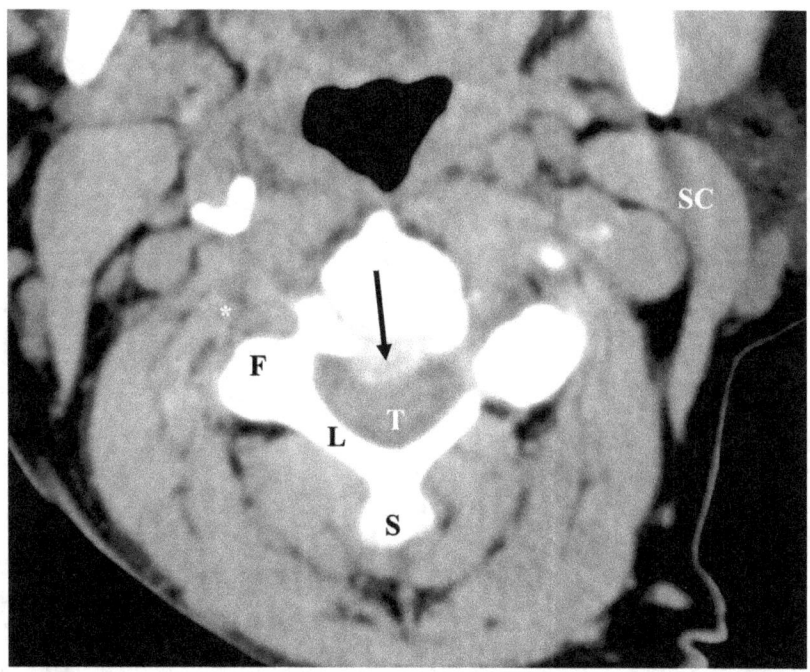

Study Above:
CT cervical spine without contrast

Radiographic findings:
Focal protrusion of the intervertebral disk centrally (arrow). Note the mass effect on the thecal sac (T), which is no longer circular in shape. Therefore, the disc material is creating significant spinal canal stenosis.

Tips
Disk bulges are non-focal (>25% disc circumference) and herniations are focal (<25%).
Disk herniations may be protrusions (wider than tall) or extrusions (taller than wide) and can even break away from the parent disc (free fragment or sequestration).
MRI may be confirmatory if CT findings are equivocal.

Normal Anatomy
SC - Sternocleidomastoid muscle, T - Thecal sac, F - Facet joint, L - Lamina, S - Spinous process, Asterisk - Exiting spinal nerves.

Further Reading
Fardon D.F., Williams A.L. Lumbar disc nomenclature: version 2.0. Recommendations of the combined task forces of NASS, ASSR and ASNR. *The Spine Journal.* vol. 14(11), 2525-2545, 2014.

CASE 28

CASE AUTHOR: Tim McKnight

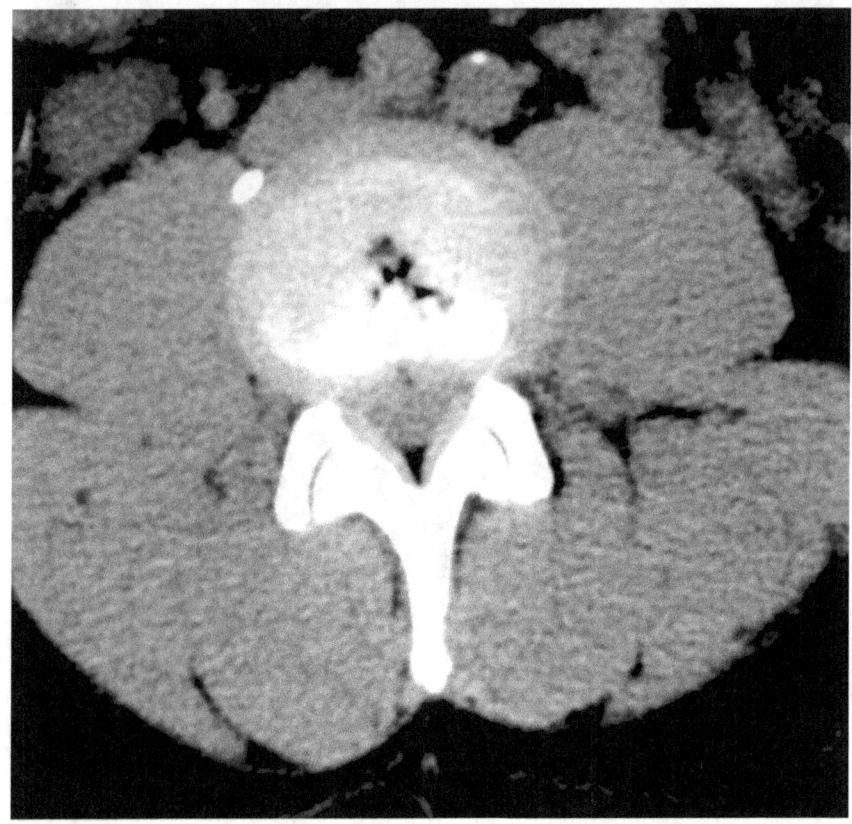

Best CT Study for Diagnosis:
CT lumbar spine without contrast

Key to DX
Disc extending beyond the margin of the bone with a symmetric shape (greater than 25% of disc circumference).

Facts
Patients may present with back pain.
Disc bulges may lead to spinal canal stenosis and neurologic deficits.
An MRI may be necessary for surgical planning to better delineate the disc.
Similar to disc herniations, bulges are more common in the lower lumbar spine.

TX
Rest, NSAIDs, and occasionally narcotics to relieve neuropathic pain.
When disc bulges are associated with significant spinal canal stenosis and cannot be controlled medically, surgical decompression may be needed.

DISC BULGE

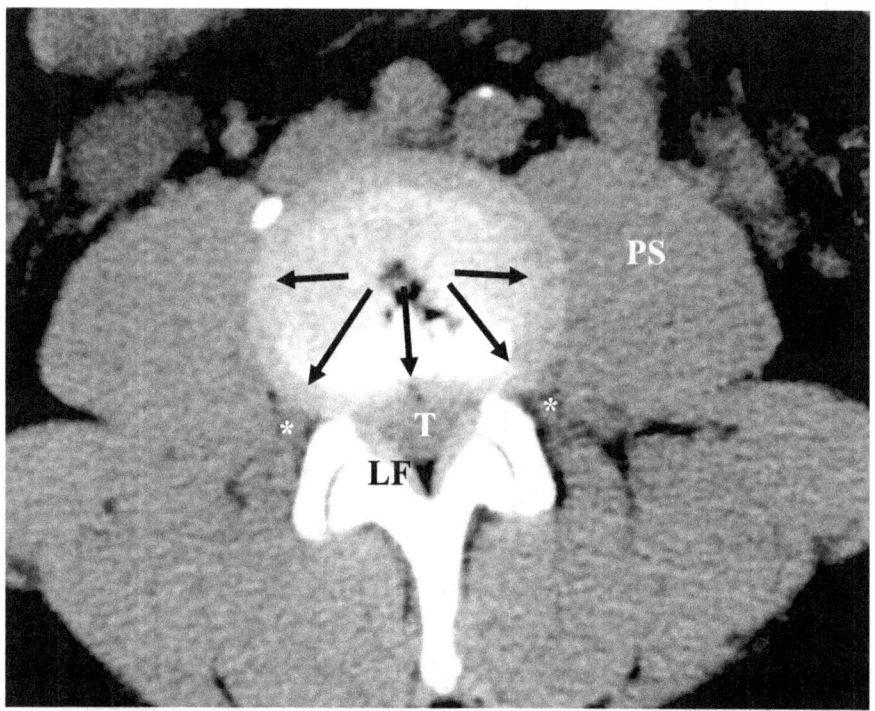

Study Above:
CT lumbar spine without contrast

Radiographic findings:
The disc extends beyond the margin of the posterior vertebral body and is without focality, consistent with a disc bulge (arrows).

Tips
Bulges may create significant spinal canal and/or neural foraminal narrowing. Spinal canal stenosis can be exacerbated by bony productive changes (osteophytes and facet arthropathy), ligamentum flavum, and disc disease.

Normal Anatomy
Asterisks – Exiting spinal nerves, LF - Ligamentum flavum, T - Thecal sac, PS – Psoas muscle

Further Reading
Fardon D.F., Williams A.L.. Lumbar disc nomenclature: version 2.0. Recommendations of the combined task forces of the North American Spine Society, the American Society of Spine Radiology and the American Society of Neuroradiology. *The Spine Journal*. vol. 14(11), pp 2525-2545, 2014.

CASE 29

CASE AUTHOR: Tim McKnight

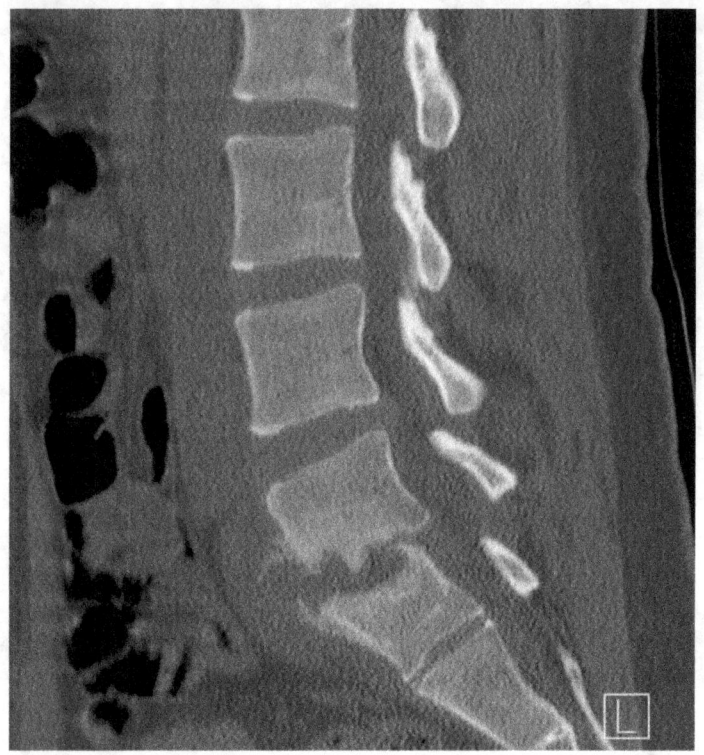

Best CT Study for Diagnosis:
CT with IV contrast in the absence of MRI (see chapter introduction)

Key to DX
Widening of the disc space with erosion of the endplates.

Facts
Patients usually present with back pain and fever.
The most common organism is *Staphylococcus aureus*.
Risk factors include diabetes, IV drug use, immunosuppression, and recent instrumentation.
The lumbar spine is most commonly involved followed by the thoracic spine.

TX
IV antibiotics are used. Surgical decompression may also be needed.
CT guided biopsy may be of benefit to identify an organism (low yield).

DISCITIS OSTEOMYELITIS

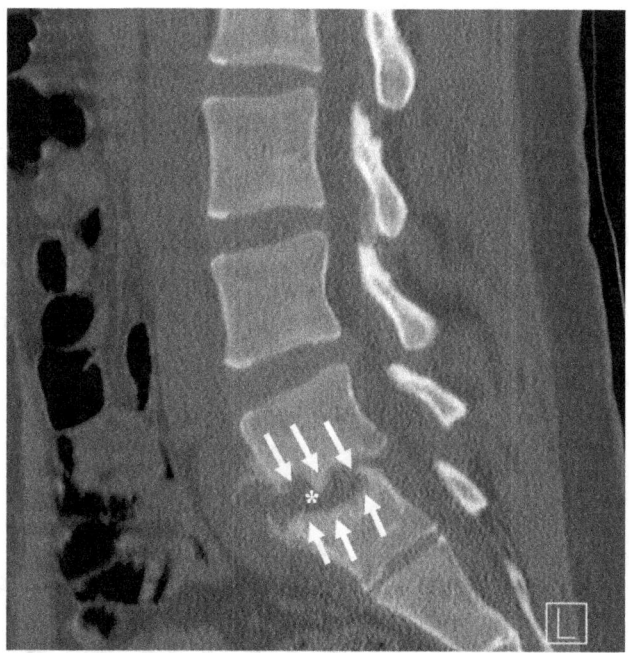

Study Above:
CT lumbar spine without contrast, sagittal reformat of lower levels.

Radiographic findings:
Widening of the disc space (asterisk) with an undulating appearance to the corresponding endplates (arrows). There is frank destruction of the endplates at the infected level which is obvious when compared to the remaining normal levels.

Tips
Narrow windows (similar to liver windows) are helpful for visualizing epidural abscess.
If epidural abscess is not seen on CT, it cannot be excluded without an MRI.
On CT, IV contrast may help visualize epidural involvement.
Sagittal and coronal reformats are helpful to evaluate the disc spaces and endplates.
If correlation with MRI is needed, IV gadolinium should be utilized.
Neoplastic processes should not be considered when the pathology is centered at the disc.
Mimics can include severe disc degeneration and chronic neuropathic spine. Review prior imaging to confirm.

Further Reading
Talbott J.F., Shah V.N., Uzelac A., et al. Imaging-Based Approach to Extradural Infections of the Spine. *Semin Ultrasound CT MR.* 39(6):570-586, 2018.

CASE 30

CASE AUTHOR: Tim McKnight

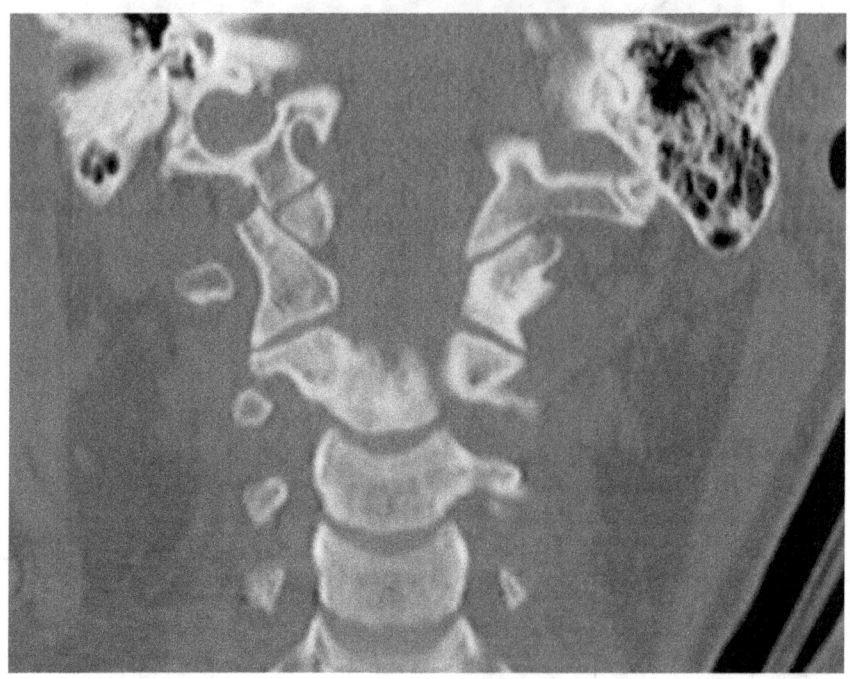

Best CT Study for Diagnosis:
CT cervical spine without contrast

Key to DX
Lucency traversing the occipital condyle.

Facts
Present with high cervical pain or occasionally neurological deficits (cranial nerves 9-12).
High energy trauma.
Anderson and Montesano classification by mechanism: type 1 - axial loading, type 2- extension of skull base fracture, type 3 - avulsion and distraction injury.
Tuli classification by imaging appearance on x-ray, CT or MR: type 1 - non-displaced stable, type 2A displaced and stable, type 2B – displaced with occipi-toatlantoaxial instability or ligament disruption (bony separation between structures >2mm).
Increased likelihood of additional cervical spine injuries >30%.

TX
Typically treated with reduction and external stabilization.
Complex cases or cases with neurological deficits may require surgical fixation.

OCCIPITAL CONDYLE FRACTURE

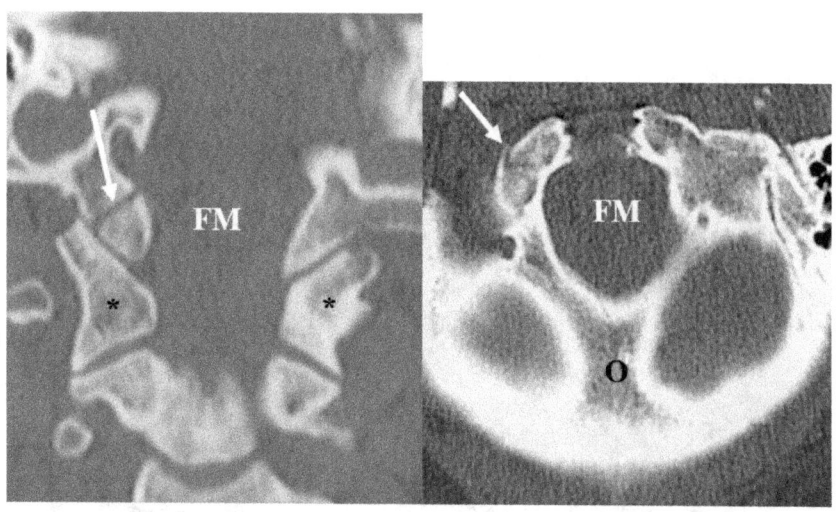

Study Above:
CT cervical spine without contrast, coronal and axial images at the level of the occiput.

Radiographic findings:
A fracture line is seen traversing the right occipital condyle (arrow).

Tips
Look for fragments displaced into the spinal canal.
Fragments into the foramen magnum signify a potentially unstable injury.
Check the hypoglossal canal and jugular foramen for fracture extension.
If the fracture extends into the jugular foramen, CTV should be done to exclude vascular thrombosis.
Fracture may also extend into the skull base or temporal bone.

Normal Anatomy
FM - Foramen magnum, O - Occiput, Asterisks - C1 lateral masses

Further Reading
Hanson JA, Deliganis AV. Radiologic and Clinical Spectrum of Occipital Condyle Fractures. *AJR.* 178:5, 1261-1268, 2002.

CASE 31

CASE AUTHOR: Tim McKnight

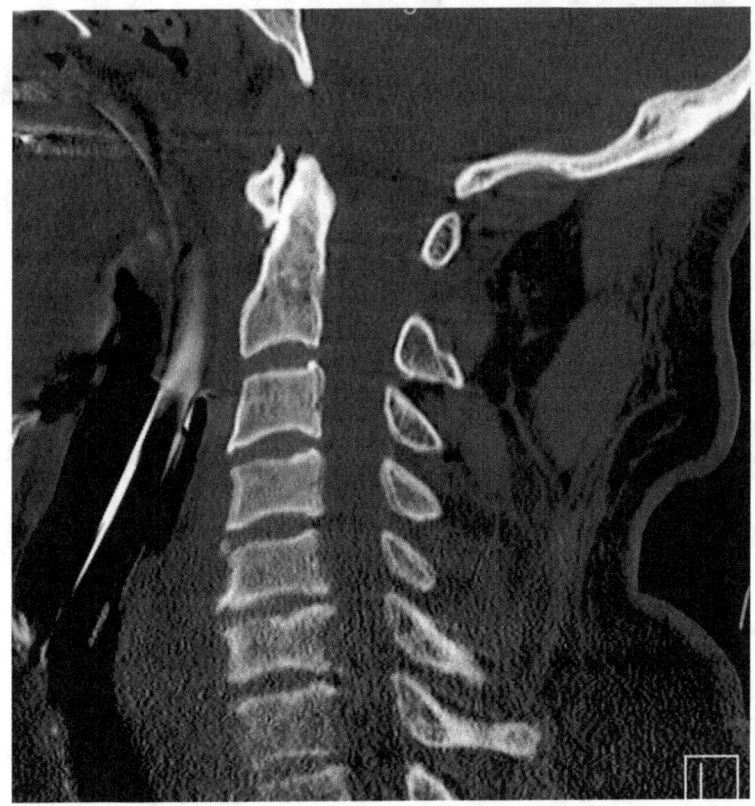

Best CT Study for Diagnosis:
CT cervical spine without contrast

Key to DX
Increased distance between the basion and the dens (>12 mm).
Widening between the occipital condyles and the atlas.

Facts
Life-threatening emergency!
Unstable craniocervical junction injury with widespread ligamentous disruption.
Most commonly due to high-energy trauma and often results in death at the scene.
Predisposing factors include rheumatoid arthritis and Down syndrome.

TX
Emergent external halo immobilization initially, followed by internal occipito-cervical fixation and fusion.

ATLANTO-OCCIPITAL DISSOCIATION, AOD

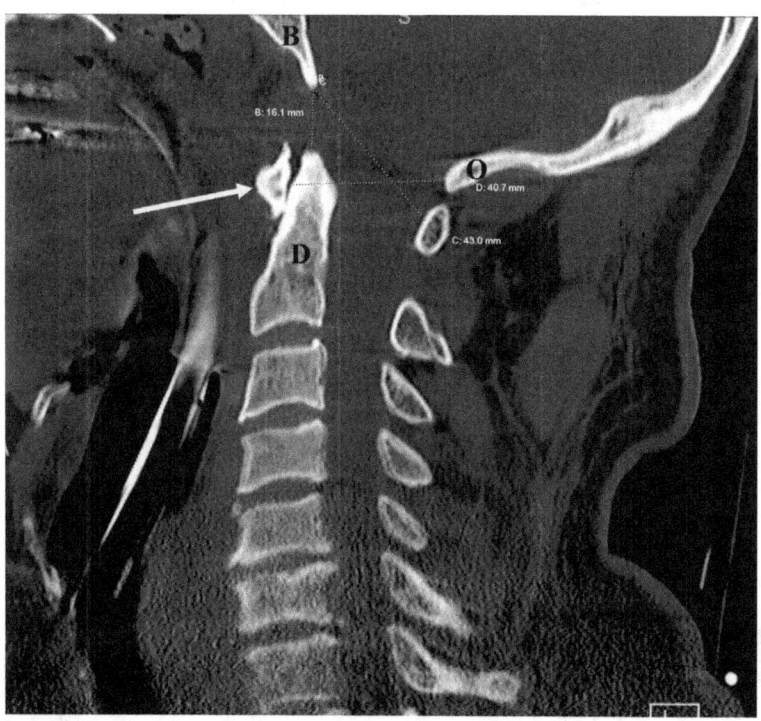

Study Above:
CT cervical spine without contrast, sagittal reformat.

Radiographic findings:
Sagittal reformat image demonstrates a widened Basion-Dens Interval (BDI) of 16 mm (arrow). Also, the Powers Ratio is elevated at 1.0 (normal is <0.9).

Tips
Various measurements exist to aid in assessment of AOD (BDI and Powers Ratio).

BDI: Distance from basion to tip of the dens is measured. If > 12 mm, suspect AOD.

Powers Ratio: Distance from basion (B) to the midpoint of the anterior posterior arch of C1. The distance from the opisthion (O) to the midpoint of the posterior anterior arch of C1 (A) is measured. If BxC/OxA >1, then AOD should be suspected. Look for other fractures of the occipital condyles or the tip of the dens.

Further Reading
Riascos R., Bonfante E. Imaging of Atlanto-Occipital and Atlantoaxial Traumatic Injuries: What the Radiologist Needs to Know. *RadioGraphics* 35:7, 2121-2134, 2015.

CASE 32

CASE AUTHOR: Tim McKnight

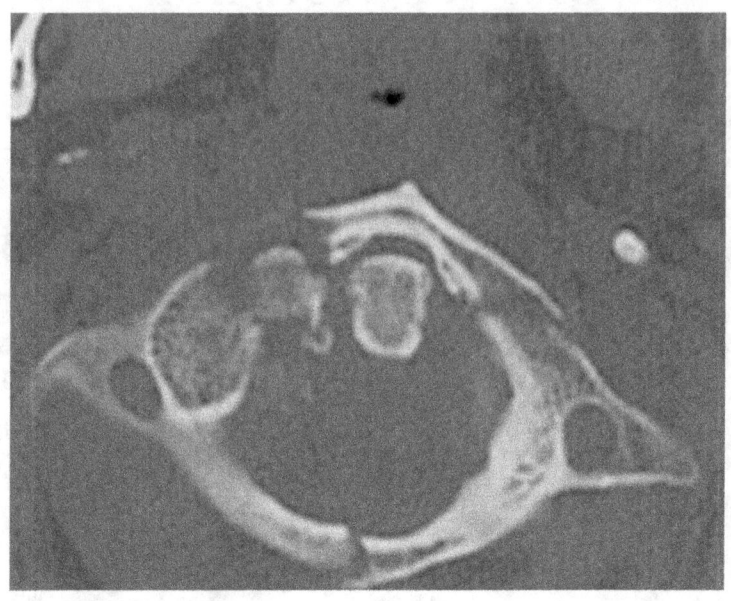

Best CT Study for Diagnosis:
CT cervical spine without contrast

Key to DX
Lucency traversing the C1 arch.

Facts
Mechanism of injury is usually axial loading (direct blow to head).
Also known as Jefferson burst fracture and are unstable.
On dens view radiograph, there will be displacement of the lateral masses of C1 secondary to transverse ligament rupture.
Classification: Type 1- isolated anterior or posterior arch fracture, Type 2- anterior and posterior arch fractures, Type 3- arch fractures including lateral mass.

TX
Halo fixation for 3 months.

C1 FRACTURE (JEFFERSON)

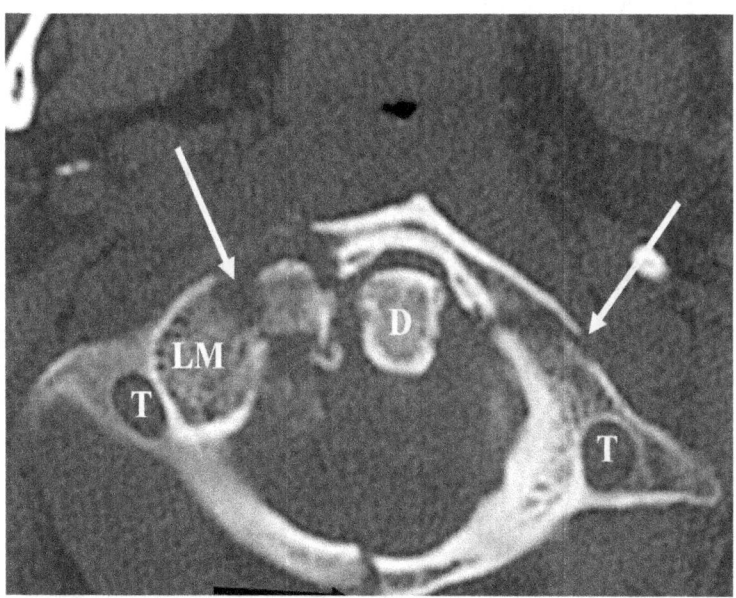

Study Above:
CT cervical spine without contrast at the level of C1.

Radiographic findings:
An axial CT of C1 shows fracture lines extending through the anterior arch of C1 (white arrows) bilaterally and the involved right lateral mass. Additional fracture line in the mid posterior arch of C1 is present (black arrow). This is a type 3 fracture pattern.

Tips
Check the posterior arch of C1 since both arches are typically fractured.
An isolated anterior arch fracture is usually secondary to hyperextension.
Typically, the spinal cord is not injured as the spinal canal is widened.
Beware of congenital non-union (non-ossified growth centers) which are well corticated (this means the bone is outlined by cortex, a white line).
If fracture extends into the transverse foramen, CTA is needed to exclude vertebral artery dissection.

Normal Anatomy
D - Dens of C2, LM - Lateral mass of C1, T - Transverse foramen (for vertebral artery)

Further Reading
Mead L.B., Millhouse P.W. C1 fractures: a review of diagnoses, management options, and outcomes. *Current Reviews in Musculoskeletal Medicine.* 9 (3): 255, 2016.

CASE 33

CASE AUTHOR: Tim McKnight

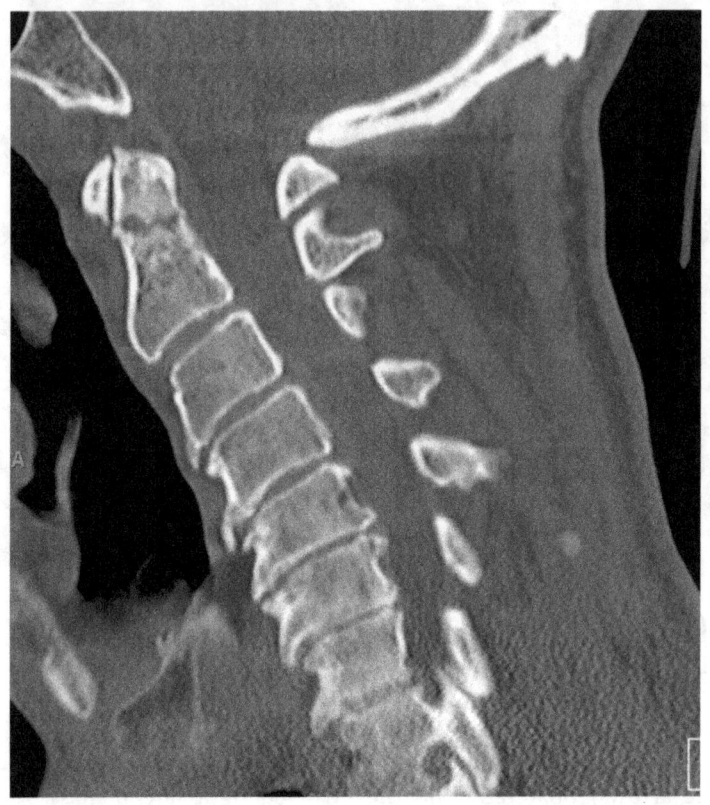

Best CT Study for Diagnosis:
CT cervical spine without contrast

Key to DX
Lucency traversing the dens (C2).

Facts
Mechanism of injury is complex, but hyperextension plays a major role.
C2 injuries account for 17-20% of cervical spine trauma.
Anderson/D'Alonzo classification: Type 1 (1-3%, stable)- odontoid tip, Type 2 (59%, unstable)- odontoid-body junction, Type 3 (40%, stable)- C2 body fracture into the dens.
Type 2 dens fracture: complication of non-union has increased incidence with age over 50, displacement > 6mm, and comminution.

TX
Surgical reduction is necessary for the majority of fractures.

DENS FRACTURE

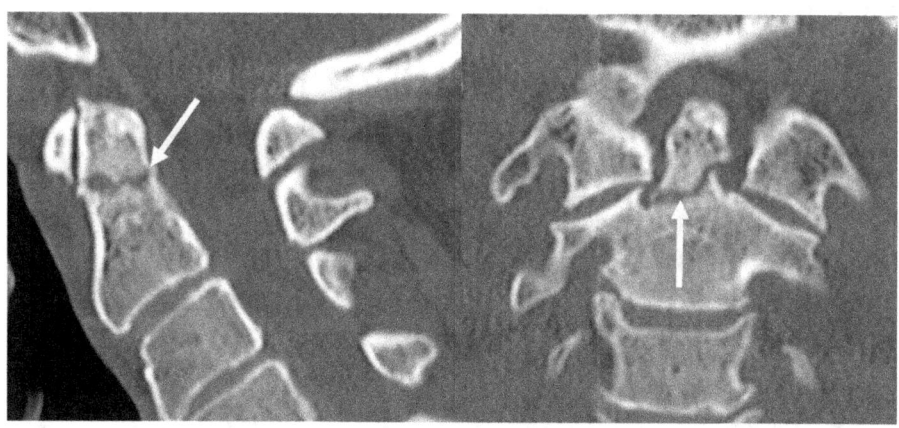

Study Above:
CT cervical spine without contrast, sagittal and coronal reformat.

Radiographic findings:
Lucency seen traversing the dens at its base (arrows). This is a Type II dens fracture.

Tips
Check the relationship of the fracture fragment to the thecal sac for canal stenosis.
MRI should be considered with neural deficits to exclude spinal cord injury.
Remember that MRI evaluation of the spinal cord does not require contrast.
CT coronal and sagittal reformats are valuable to delineate the exact path of the fracture line.
Interrogate the spine for other fractures.
If fracture extends into the transverse foramen, CTA is needed to exclude vertebral artery dissection.

Further Reading
Dreizin D., Letzing M. Multidetector CT of Blunt Cervical Spine Trauma in Adults. *RadioGraphics*. 34:7, 1842-1865, 2014.

CASE 34

CASE AUTHOR: Tim McKnight

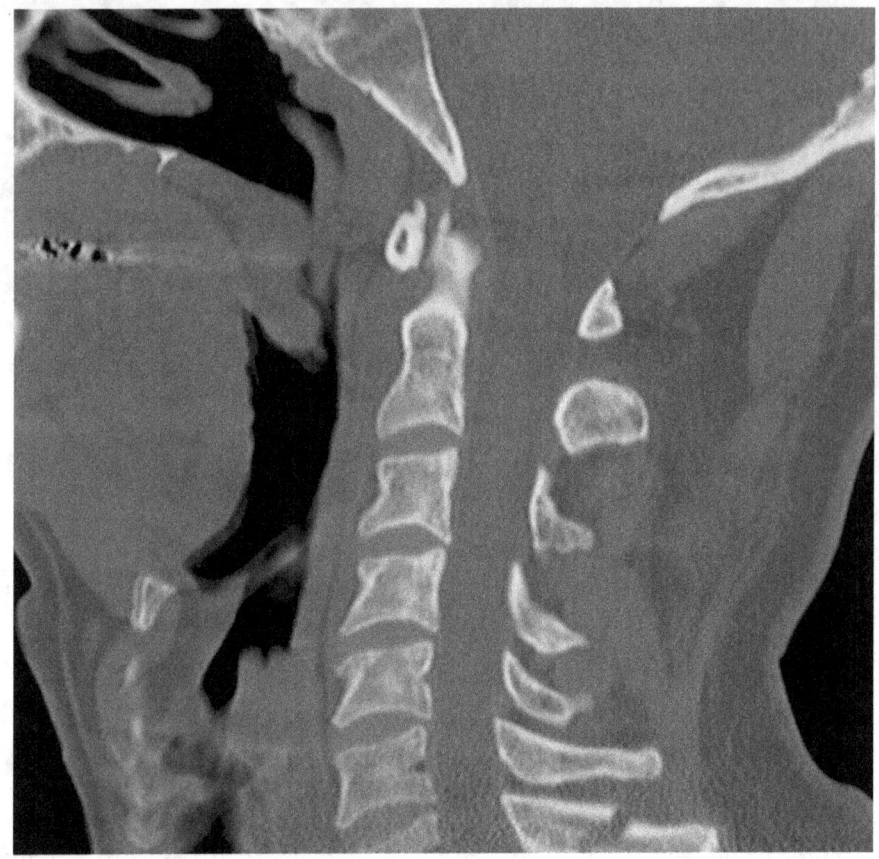

Best CT Study for Diagnosis:
CT cervical spine without contrast

Key to DX
Disruption of the spinous process of C7.

Facts
The mechanism of injury is typically hyperflexion and less commonly a direct blow.
These injuries are considered stable.
C7 is by far the most common, but this injury has also been reported at other cervical levels.
These injuries are named after workers who were injured while shoveling clay.
Radiographs are typically diagnostic.

TX
Analgesics for pain. Surgery is rarely needed unless there is debilitating pain.

CLAY SHOVELER FRACTURE

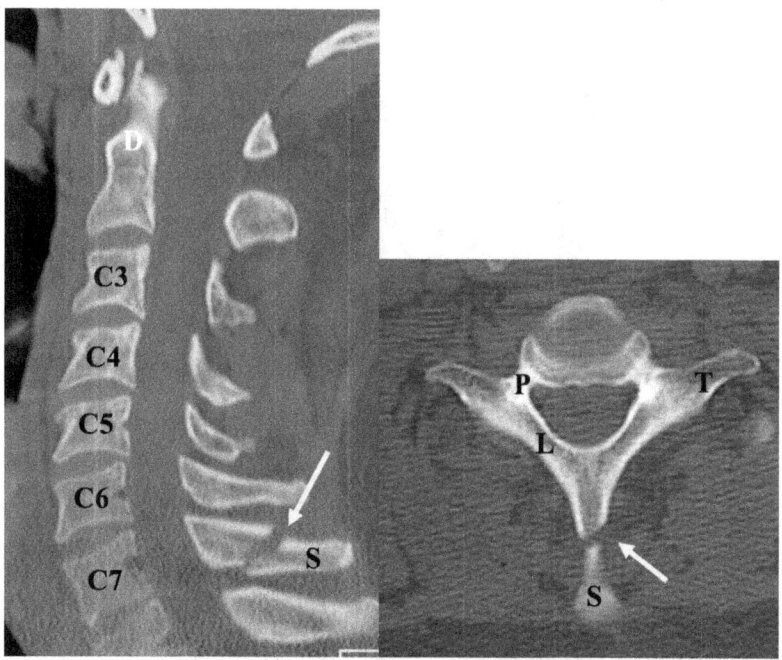

Study Above:
CT cervical spine without contrast, sagittal reformat and axial image.

Radiographic findings:
Fracture with displacement of the C7 spinous process (arrow).

Tips
These are typically avulsion injuries from the interspinous ligament.
Analyze the margins of the fracture. If it is well corticated, then it is a remote injury.
Appreciating the margins of the fracture is helpful as it may decipher if the fracture in question is acute or chronic.
Be sure to exclude other fractures that may be more clinically important.

Normal Anatomy
D - Dens of C2, L - Lamina, T- Transverse process, S - Spinous process, P - Pedicle

Further Reading
Berritto D., Pinto A. Trauma Imaging of the Acute Cervical Spine. *Semin Musculoskelet Radiol*, 21(03): 184-198, 2017.

CASE 35

CASE AUTHOR: Tim McKnight

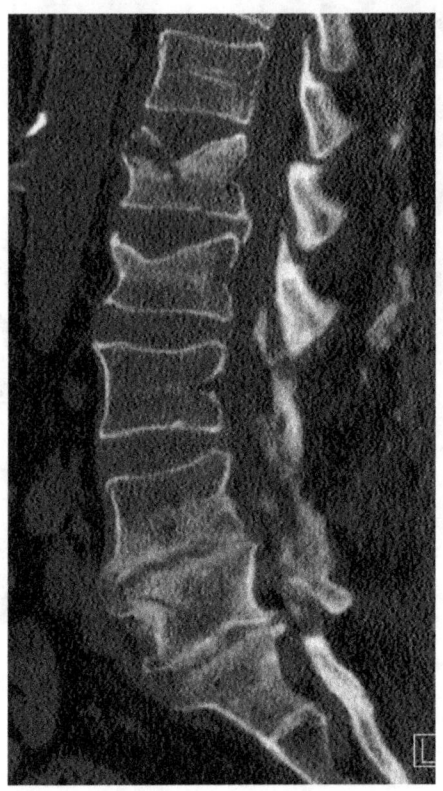

Best CT Study for Diagnosis:
CT lumbar spine without contrast

Key to DX
Loss of vertebral body height.

Facts
Patients usually present with focal back pain or radiculopathy if significant canal stenosis is present.
Most common level involved is L1 followed by T12 and T11.
Over 25% of postmenopausal women will experience a compression fracture.
Pathologic compression fractures from neoplasm or infection will often have additional abnormal epidural or paravertebral soft tissue density.

TX
Supportive care is the usual treatment.
If pain is refractory or fracture is potentially unstable, fixation or vertebroplasty may be indicated.

COMPRESSION FRACTURE

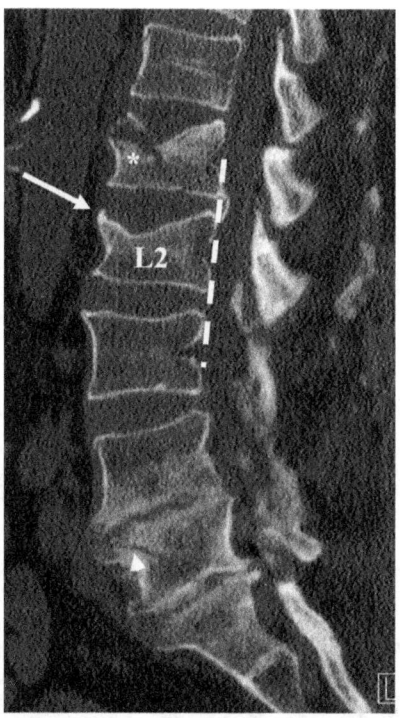

Study Above:
CT lumbar spine without contrast, sagittal reformat.

Radiographic findings:
Loss of vertebral body height involving the L2 vertebral body superior endplate is noted (arrow). Also, note a more complex L1 fracture involving both endplates (asterisk) and a subtle fracture at the anterior L5 vertebral body (arrowhead). There is also degenerative spondylosis of L4-L5 and L5-S1 with anterior osteophytes, endplate sclerosis, and severe disc space narrowing.

Tips
Check the posterior vertebral line (dotted line) for retropulsion of bony fragments (signifies significant spinal canal stenosis).
If fracture age is not known clinically, MRI or nuclear scan can detect acuity.
A soft tissue mass is a hint of a pathologic fracture related to malignancy.
MRI (non-contrast) can diagnose cervical and thoracic spinal cord damage.
Coronal and sagittal reformats are helpful to visualize subtle fractures.

Further Reading
Mauch JT. Review of the Imaging Features of Benign Osteoporotic and Malignant Vertebral Compression Fractures. *American Journal of Neuroradiology*, January 2018.

CASE 36

CASE AUTHOR: Tim McKnight

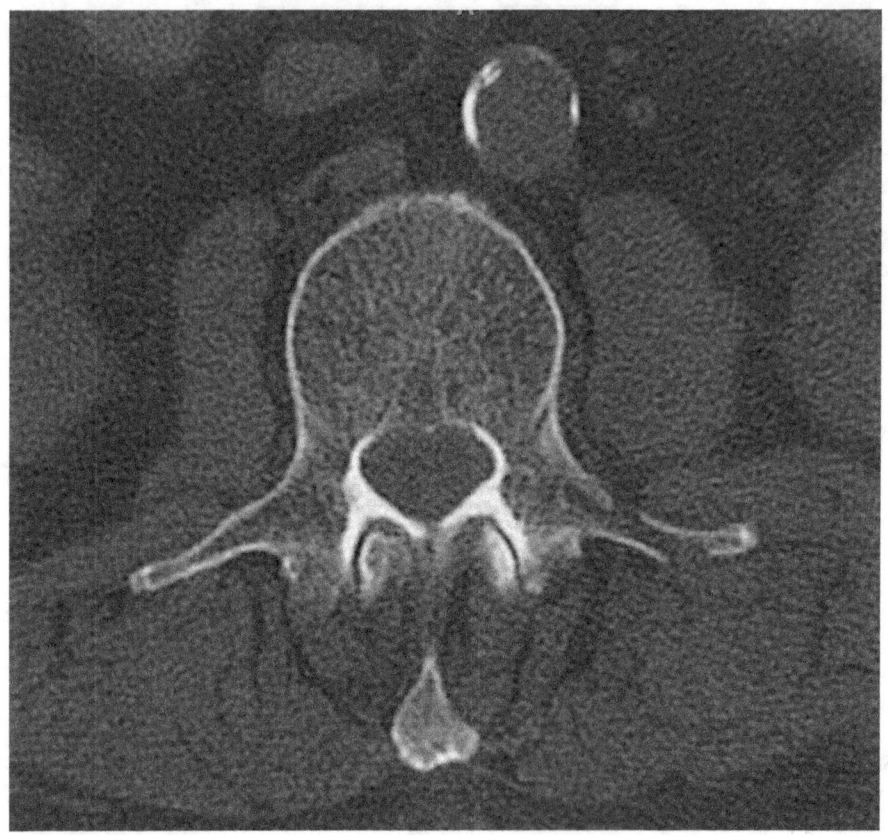

Best CT Study for Diagnosis:
CT lumbar spine without contrast

Key to DX
Fracture of the left transverse process.

Facts
Patients will usually have focal pain at the fracture site.
These fractures occur secondary to direct trauma at the site.
These injuries are considered stable.
The most common level is L3.
About 20% of these fractures are associated with abdominal injuries.

TX
Analgesics for pain without specific intervention for the fracture. Patients are usually treated for the associated intra-abdominal and pelvic injuries.

TRANSVERSE PROCESS FRACTURE

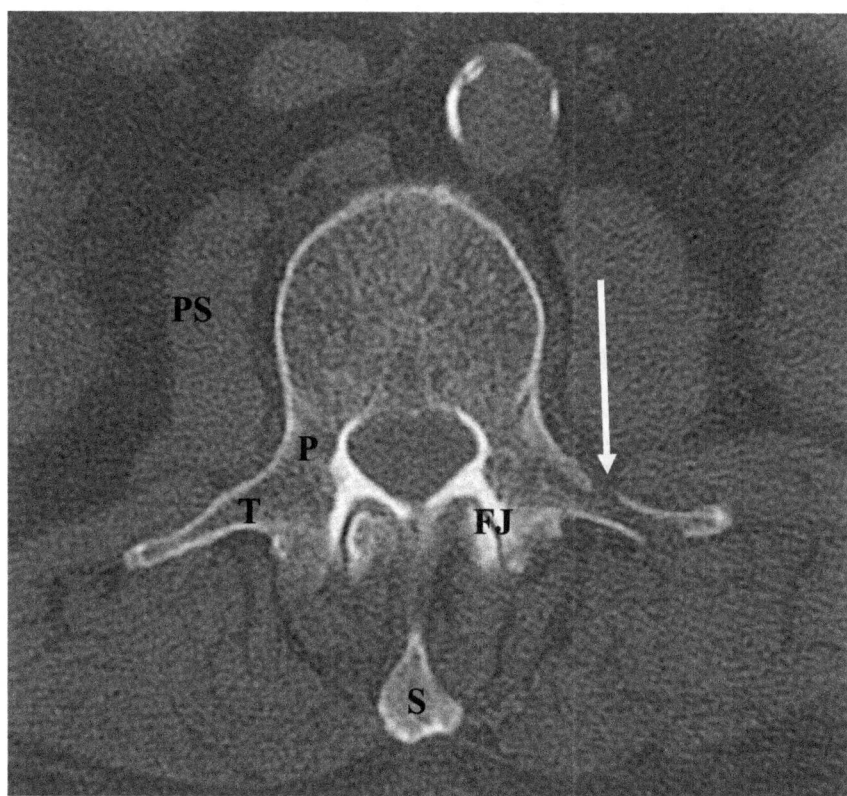

Study Above:
CT lumbar spine without contrast at the level of L2.

Radiographic findings:
Displaced left transverse process (arrow).

Tips
Check the abdomen and pelvis for other injuries.
Consider delayed imaging of the abdomen in order to evaluate for expanding hematoma (active extravasation).
Make sure no other spinal fractures are present.
Coronal and sagittal reformats may be helpful in search of other fractures.

Normal Anatomy
P - Pedicle, T - Transverse process, FJ – Facet joint, S - Spinous process, PS - Psoas muscle

Further Reading
Gray M,, Catterson P. Multilevel lumbar transverse process fractures in a professional association football player: a case report.. *Oxf Med Case Reports*. May;2015(5):288-91, 2015.

CASE 37

CASE AUTHOR: Tim McKnight

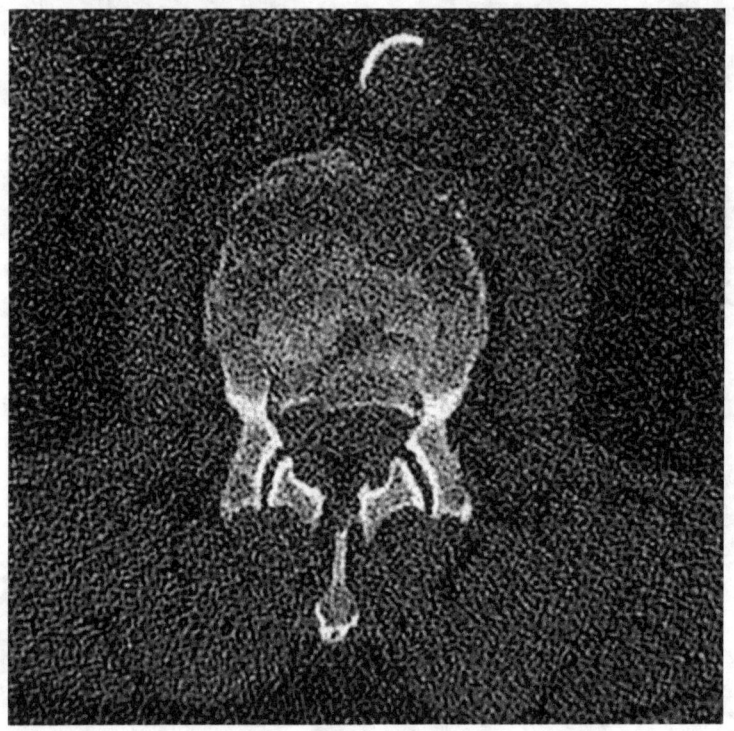

Best CT Study for Diagnosis:
CT lumbar spine without contrast

Key to DX
Multiple linear lucencies seen traversing the vertebral body.

Facts
The mechanism of injury is typically hyperflexion from a high velocity trauma.
This injury is unstable and neurological deficits may be present.
The retropulsion of bone indicates disruption of the posterior longitudinal ligament.
These fractures typically occur from T12 to L2.
If the posterior vertebral body is involved or pedicles are widened, then it is a "burst fracture."
Classification with the Thoracolumbar Injury Classification and Severity Score (TLICS) guides management.

TX
Surgical decompression is needed to preserve the spinal canal patency and ensure stability of the vertebral body.

TWO COLUMN FRACTURE

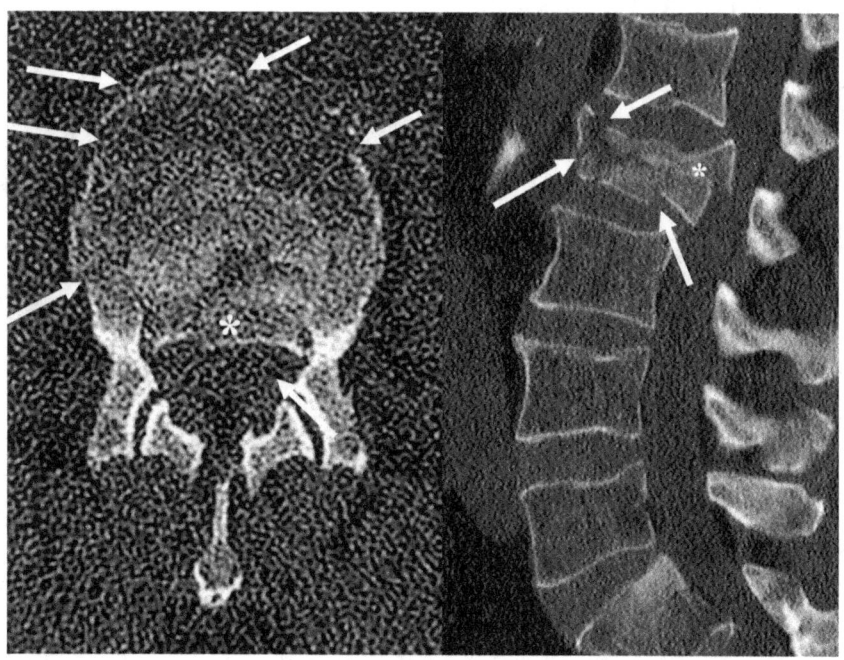

Study Above:
CT lumbar spine without contrast, axial and sagittal reformat.

Radiographic findings:
Comminuted fracture involving the L2 vertebral body with disruption of the posterior endplate (arrows). There is retropulsion of the posterior superior portion of the vertebral body (asterisk).

Tips
If the anterior and posterior halves of the vertebral body are fractured, then a 2-column injury is present. When the posterior elements are involved (pedicles, lamina, or spinous process), it is a 3-column fracture.
Check for retropulsion of bone which indicates spinal canal stenosis and instability. This is usually surgical (as in this case).
Check coronals for horizontal displacement/translational injury, which is a higher grade injury with increased complications.
MRI (non-contrast) is warranted in this case to evaluate for spinal cord injury.

Further Reading
Khurana B., Sheehan S.E., Sodickson A. Traumatic Thoracolumbar Spine Injuries: What the Spine Surgeon Wants to Know. *RadioGraphics*. 33:7, 2031-2046, 2013.

CASE 38

CASE AUTHOR: Tim McKnight

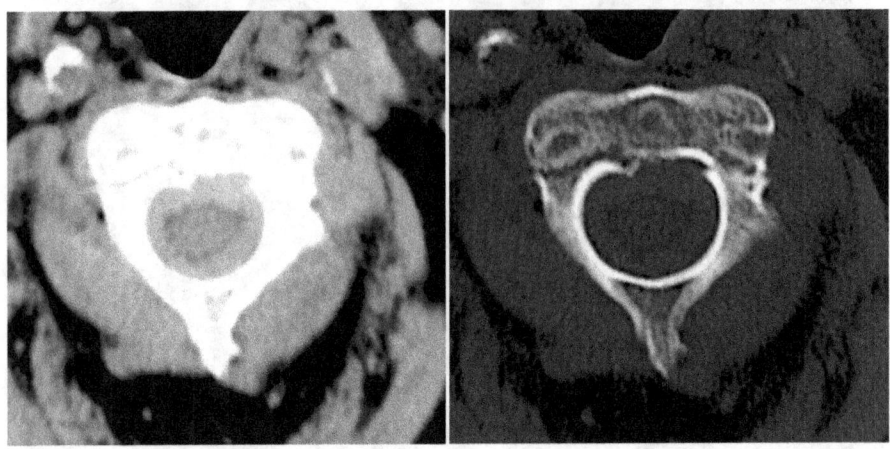

Best CT Study for Diagnosis:
CT spine with and without IV contrast in the absence of MRI (see chapter introduction)

Key to DX
High density in the epidural space.

Facts
70% of spinal canal hematomas are epidural.
Patients present with neck pain and neurological deficits.
Realize that an epidural collection is non-specific, and the differential diagnosis includes hematoma, infection, and tumor. Therefore, history for these patients is essential.
Radiographs are typically negative.
MRI with contrast helps to narrow the differential.

TX
If signs of spinal compression are present, emergent decompression and evacuation is indicated.
Severity of the neurologic deficit at time of surgical treatment is the most important factor in determining prognosis, long-term outcomes, and recovery of function.

EPIDURAL HEMATOMA

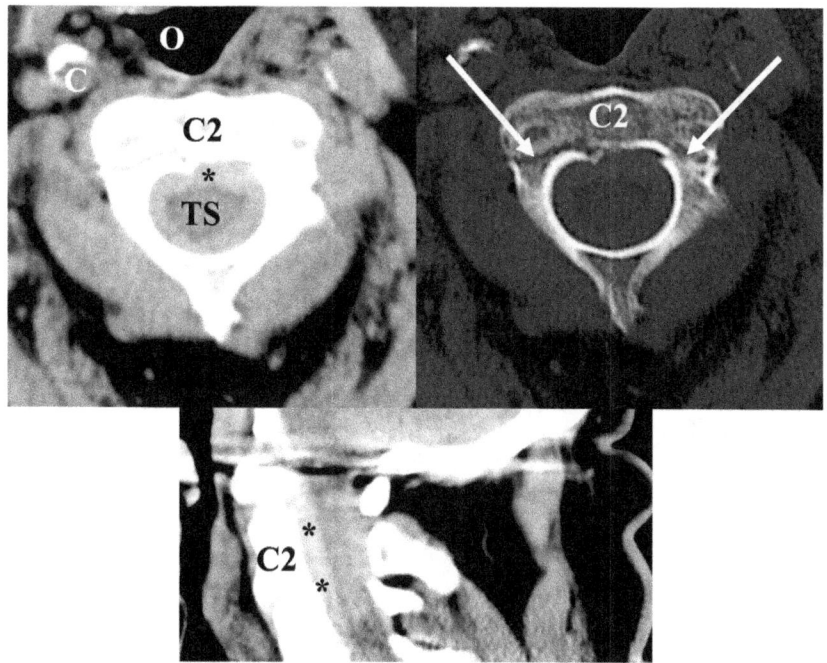

Study Above:
CT cervical spine without contrast, axial soft tissue and bone windows, coronal reformat.

Radiographic findings:
Hyperattenuation is seen circumferentially within the spinal canal (asterisk). This is creating significant mass effect upon the thecal sac (TS). Also, note the presence of a fracture across the base of C2 including the pedicles (arrows).

Tips
Look for effacement of the epidural fat, displacement of the dura mater, and compression of the thecal sac.
If there is a history of trauma, look for a spinal fracture.
MRI (non-contrast) is needed to diagnose spinal cord compression or edema.

Normal Anatomy
C2 - C2 Vertebral body, O - Oropharynx, C - Internal carotid artery
TURE

Further Reading
Pierce J.L., Donahue J.H. Spinal Hematomas: What a Radiologist Needs to Know *RadioGraphics*. 38:5, 1516-1535, 2018.

CHAPTER 4
CHEST CT

Edited by

Gregory D. Puthoff, D.O.

CHEST

As an ordering physician, the question of utilizing IV contrast for an examination is often a misunderstood topic. There are a multitude of indications to use IV contrast and many indications in which contrast is not required. IV contrast is required when considering vascular pathology, such as vascular dissection, thrombus or embolism. Entities such as pneumothorax, fractures (ribs, sternum, and clavicles), pleural effusion or pneumonia do not require IV contrast for diagnosis (are usually diagnosed on x-ray). Cancer or mass evaluations greatly benefit from the addition of IV contrast. When in doubt, phone your friendly neighborhood radiologist for a discussion. Typically, a standard 2 view chest x-ray (frontal and lateral) is a good place to start (yes, it still a good evaluation of the chest).

CT VS. MRI

CT is the gold standard for chest imaging secondary to its widespread availability, high resolution and rapid imaging protocols. MRI provides advantages over CT imaging particularly when evaluating mediastinal masses, typically in conjunction with CT. Traditionally, MRI has been limited due to poor image quality from susceptibility to respiratory and cardiac motion; however, new techniques have made vast improvements with new MRI techniques offering advanced evaluation of lung cancers, cardiac imaging, and vascular pathology.

IMAGE INTERPRETATION

Interpretation of CT chest studies via a systematic approach is very important. Every radiologist develops and utilizes a dedicated search pattern to evaluate each case. I would encourage you to design your own search pattern. A common search pattern for chest imaging is: lungs, heart, great vessels, thoracic inlet, bones, and superior abdomen. Always use the appropriate windows for each part. For example, interrogate the lungs on a lung window and the upper abdomen on a soft tissue window.

CASE 39

CASE AUTHOR: Gregory Puthoff

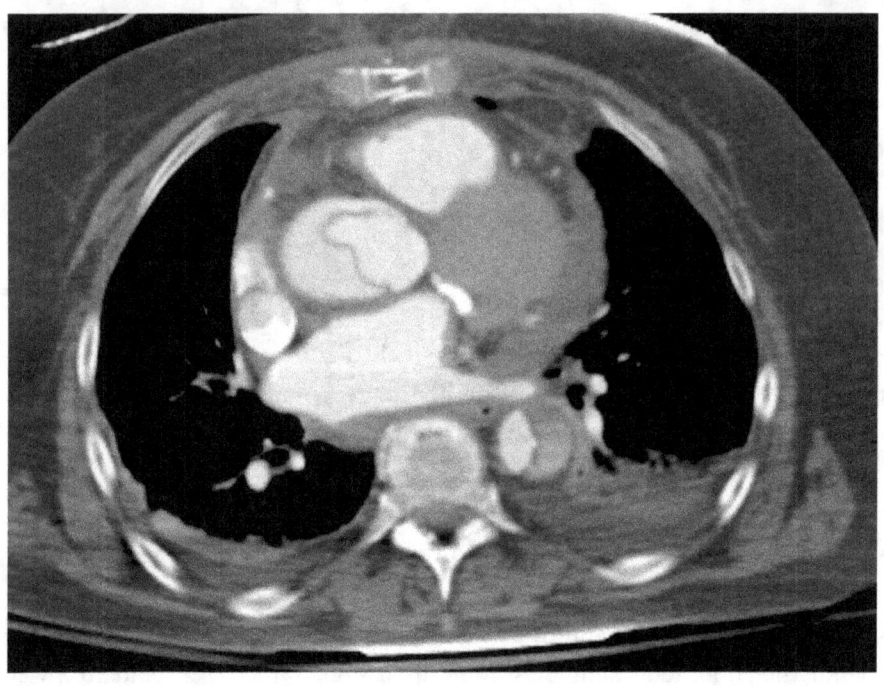

Best CT Study for Diagnosis:
CTA Chest with IV contrast

Key to DX
Linear band (intimal flap) of low attenuation bisecting the vascular lumen.

Facts
May be due to trauma, hypertension, connective tissue disorders, or vasculitis.
Patients classically present with tearing chest pain radiating to the back.
The most common association is with hypertension in elderly males.
Can involve either or both the ascending and descending aorta.

TX
Depends on which part of the thoracic aorta is involved. Stanford A (proximal involvement of the ascending aorta with or without the descending) is surgical and Stanford B (distal involvement of only the descending thoracic aorta) is medical therapy aimed at controlling hypertension.

THORACIC AORTIC DISSECTION

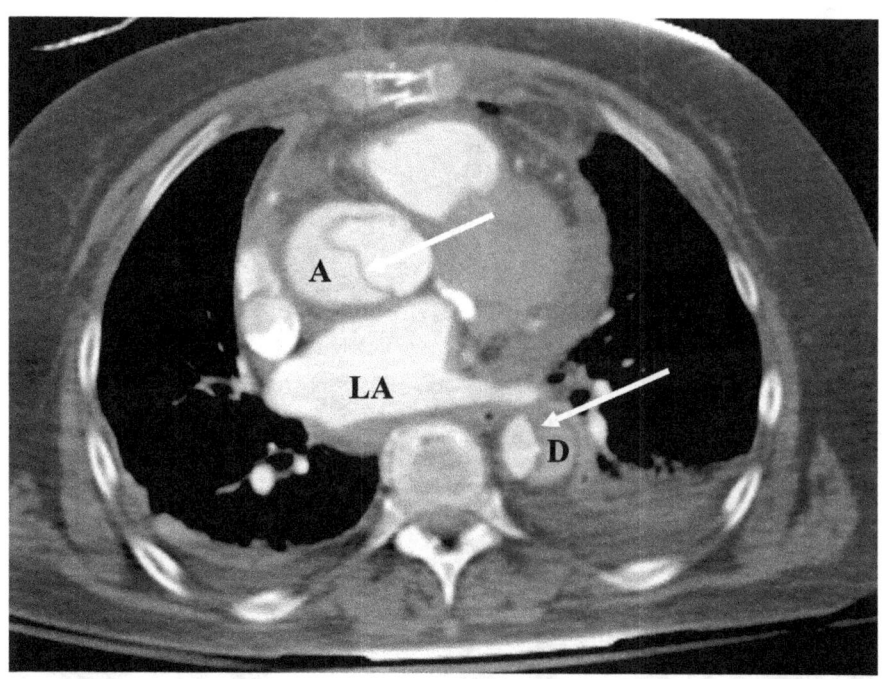

Study Above:
CT Chest with IV contrast at the level of the left pulmonary artery.

Radiographic findings:
Low attenuation band (intimal flap) is seen traversing the ascending and descending thoracic aorta representing an intimal flap (arrows).

Tips
Follow the dissection to the aortic root to exclude coronary artery involvement, which can cause myocardial infarction.
Follow dissection into the aortic arch to exclude great vessel or vertebral artery involvement.

Normal Anatomy
LA - Left atrium, A - Ascending thoracic aorta, D - Descending thoracic aorta

Further Reading
Murillo M, Molvin L, Chin AS. Aortic dissection and Other Acute Aortic Syndromes: Diagnostic Imaging Findings from Acute to Chronic Longitudinal Progression. *RadioGraphics* 2021 41:2, 425-446

CASE 40

CASE AUTHOR: Gregory Puthoff

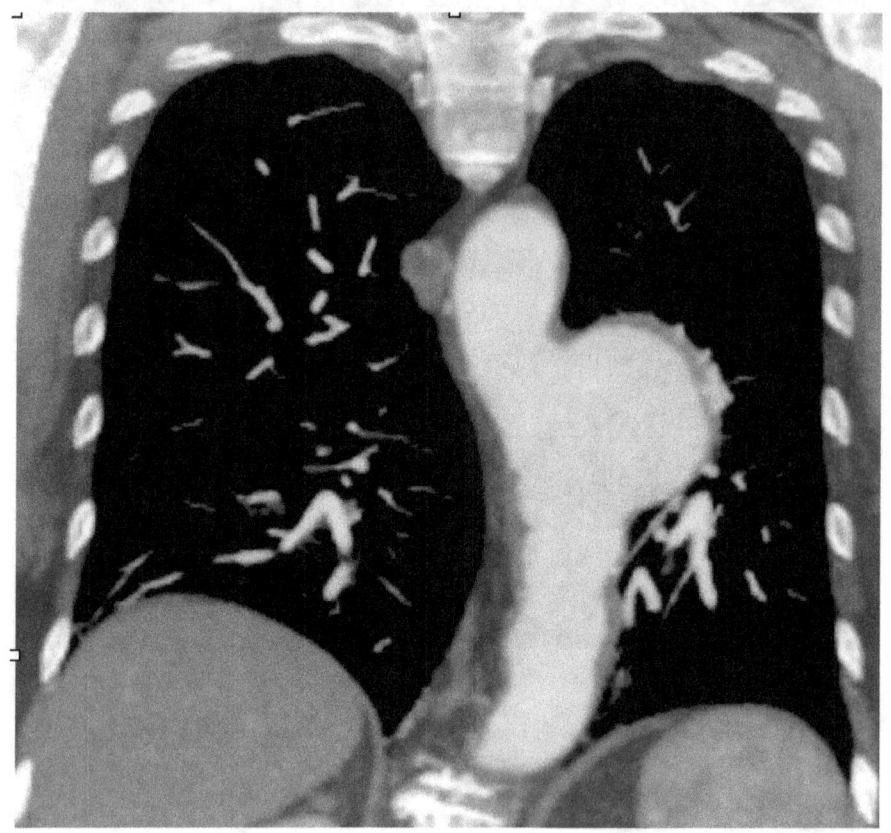

Best CT Study for Diagnosis:
CTA Chest with IV contrast

Key to DX
Enlarged thoracic aorta.

Facts
Usually asymptomatic until rupture or dissection occurs.
Commonly accepted size for thoracic aneurysm is greater than 5cm.
Risk factors include hypertension, dyslipidemia, and smoking.
The larger the aneurysm, the greater chance of rupture!

TX
Control of hypertension.
Endovascular stent grafting or open surgical repair.

THORACIC AORTIC ANEURYSM

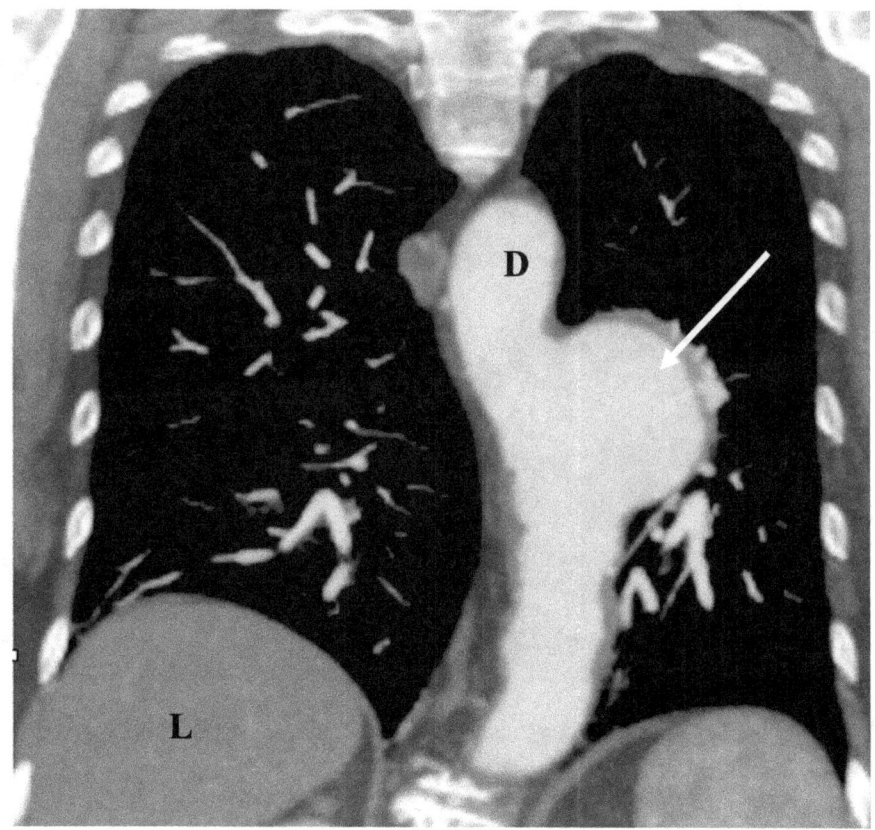

Study Above:
CTA Chest with IV contrast, coronal reformat.

Radiographic findings:
Focal enlargement of the descending thoracic aorta (arrow).

Tips
IV contrast is not needed to assess vessel size.
If dissection is a concern, IV contrast must be administered to diagnose (like the previous case).
Any portion of the thoracic aorta larger than 5.0 cm is considered aneurysmal.

Normal Anatomy
L – Liver, D - Descending thoracic aorta

Further Reading
Agarwal PP, Chughtai A, Matzinger FR, Kazerooni EA. Multidetector CT of thoracic aortic aneurysms.. *Radiographics*. 2010 Mar;29(2):537-52.

CASE 41

CASE AUTHOR: Gregory Puthoff

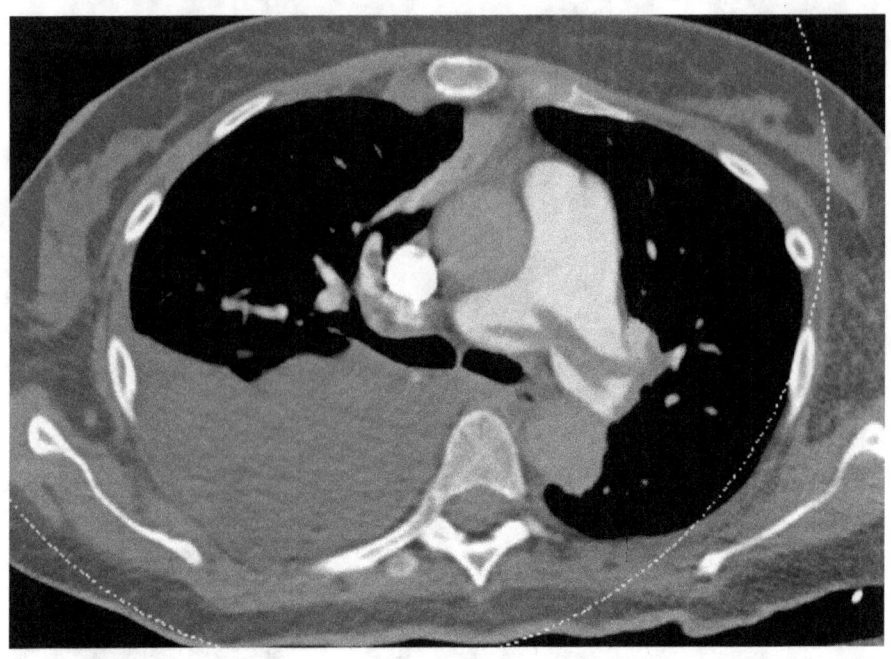

Best CT Study for Diagnosis:
CTA Chest with IV contrast

Key to DX
A low-density filling defect within the pulmonary artery.

Facts
Patients classically present with tachycardia, shortness of breath, and dyspnea.
ECG may show T wave depression in V1 to V4 or a new right bundle branch block.
D-dimer is elevated (usually above 400).
Risk factors include periods of inactivity, clotting disorders, and carcinoma.

TX
Intravenous anticoagulation therapy should be started.
Consider ultrasound doppler of the lower extremities to find a source.
IVC filter may be needed in patients who fail or have contraindications to anticoagulation therapy.

PULMONARY EMBOLI

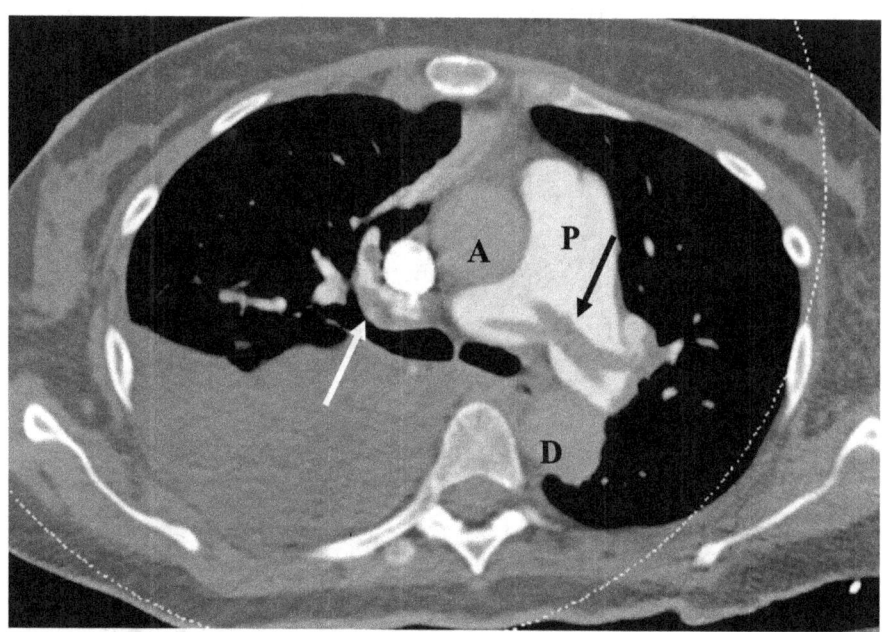

Study Above:
CTA Chest with IV contrast (PE protocol) at the level of the main pulmonary artery.

Radiographic findings:
A low density linear shaped filling defect is present at the bifurcation point of the pulmonary trunk consistent with a large saddle embolus (black arrow). Also noted is a filling defect in one of the branches of the right pulmonary artery (white arrow).

Tips
Intravenous contrast must be given to assess the vessel lumen.
Typically, emboli are multiple and more common in the lower lobes.
If a patient cannot receive IV contrast, consider Nuclear V/Q scan.
Coronal and sagittal reformats are very helpful.
Check for signs of right heart strain (right ventricle wider than left and bowing of the interventricular septum, RV/LV ratio > 1).

Normal Anatomy
P - Pulmonary trunk, A - Ascending thoracic aorta, D - Descending thoracic aorta

Further Reading
Sista AK, Kuo WT, et al. Stratification, Imaging, and Management of Acute Massive and Submassive Pulmonary Embolism. Radiology 2017 284:1, 5-24

CASE 42

CASE AUTHOR: Gregory Puthoff

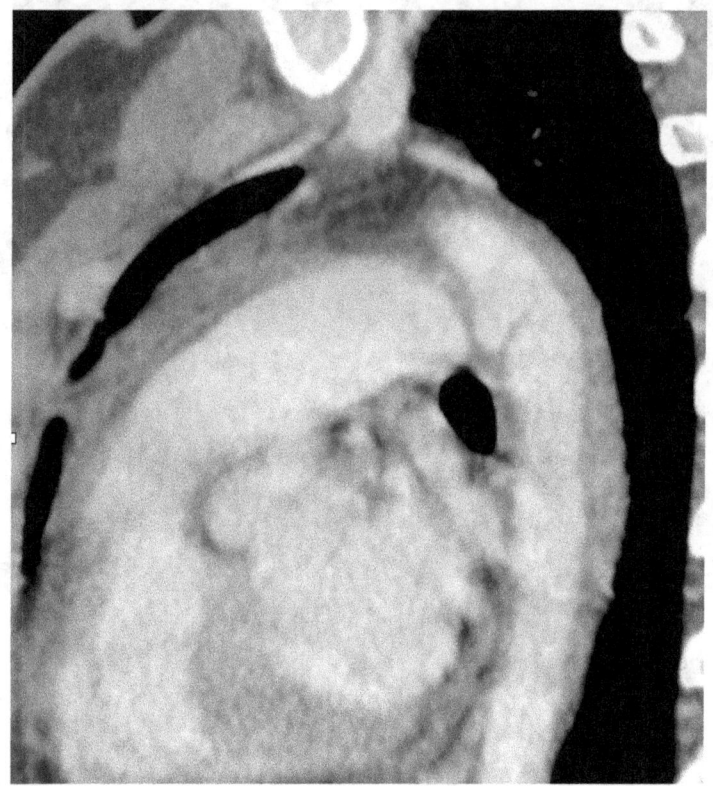

Best CT Study for Diagnosis:
CTA Chest with IV contrast

Key to DX
Focal "outpouching" of the aortic lumen with intimal injury.

Facts
Patients may have chest pain, cough, upper extremity hypertension, or lower extremity hypotension.
These injuries are most commonly secondary to high-speed motor vehicle accidents.
These injuries have a high mortality rate with most patients dying at the scene of the accident.
The aortic isthmus is the most common location for injury secondary to the attachment of the ligamentum arteriosum.

TX
This is a surgical emergency and is typically repaired using an endovascular approach or if severe a traditional open thoracotomy.

ACUTE TRAUMATIC AORTIC INJURY

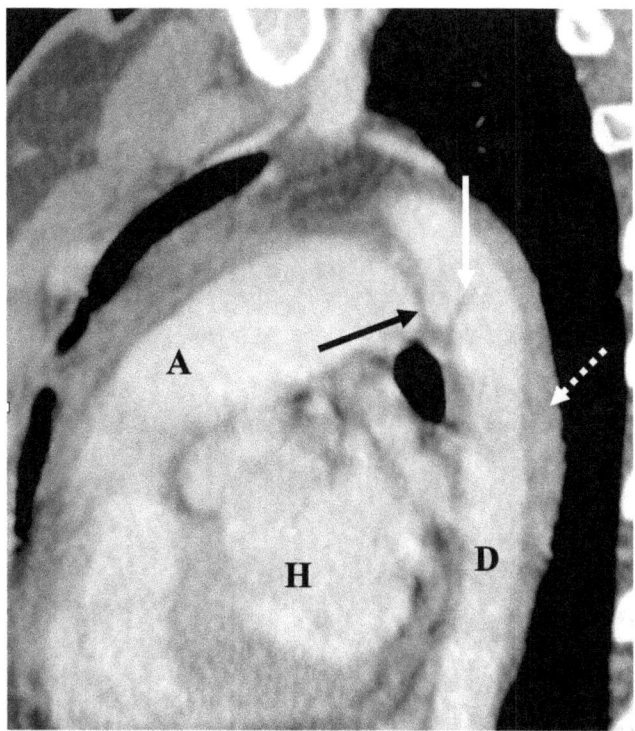

Study Above:
CTA Chest with IV contrast, sagittal reformat.

Radiographic findings:
A focal "outpouching" of the lumen along the anterior aspect of the descending thoracic aorta (black arrow). An associated intimal injury/flap is noted (white arrow). Periaortic hematoma is also noted (dashed arrow).

Tips
Look for a change in the morphology of the vessel.

Intravenous contrast must be given to assess the endoluminal or "inside" of the vessel.

Remember to interrogate the aorta just distal to the origin of the left subclavian artery (the region of the isthmus).

Coronal and sagittal reformats are very helpful.

Normal Anatomy
H- Heart, A - Ascending thoracic aorta, D - Descending thoracic aorta

Further Reading
Steenburg S, Ravenel J, et al. Acute Traumatic Aortic Injury: Imaging Evaluation and Management. Radiology 2008 248:3, 748-762

CASE 43

CASE AUTHOR: Gregory Puthoff

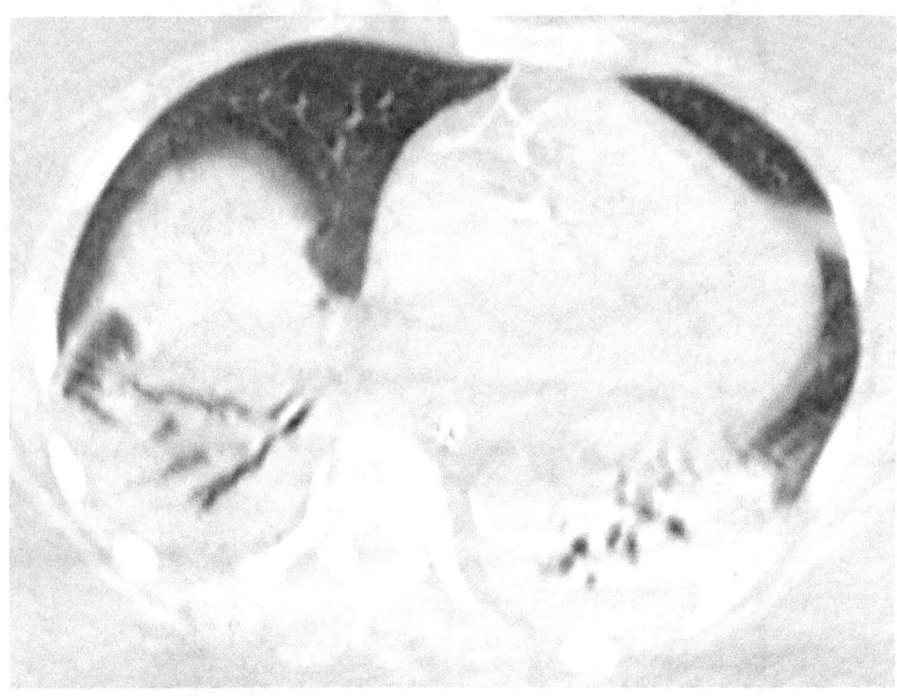

Best CT Study for Diagnosis:
CT Chest without IV contrast

Key to DX
Lobar shaped area of consolidation involving the lung parenchyma with associated "air bronchograms."

Facts
Patients may present with cough, fever, and chest pain.
The most common pathogens are *S. pneumoniae* (usually adults 40-60 years old), *H. influenzae* (usually children and COPD patients), *C. pneumoniae*, and *M. pneumoniae*.

TX
Antibiotic therapy is the mainstay.
Sputum samples may be necessary in complex cases to guide medical therapy.

PNEUMONIA

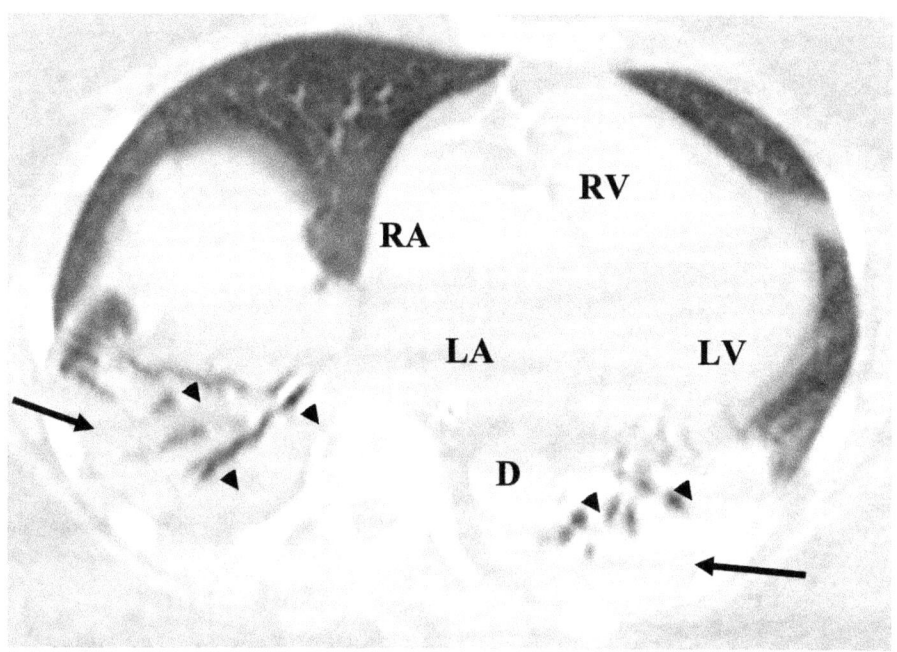

Study Above:
CT Chest without IV contrast at the level of the lower chest.

Radiographic findings:
Dense airspace consolidation (meaning non-aeration without visualization of the lung parenchyma) involving the lower lobes (arrows). Note all the branching air bronchograms traversing the lower lobes (arrowhead).

Tips
Air bronchograms are not always present.
A follow up CT or chest radiograph should be performed to demonstrate resolution of the pneumonia (4-6 weeks).
Lower lobe pneumonia can present with abdominal pain mimicking an abdominal process.

Normal Anatomy
LV - Left ventricle, RV - Right ventricle, LA - Left atrium, RA - Right atrium, D - Descending thoracic aorta

Further Reading
Walker CM, et al. Imaging pulmonary infection: classic signs and patterns. AJR Am J Roentgenol. 2014 Mar;202(3):479-92

CASE 44

CASE AUTHOR: Madison Kocher

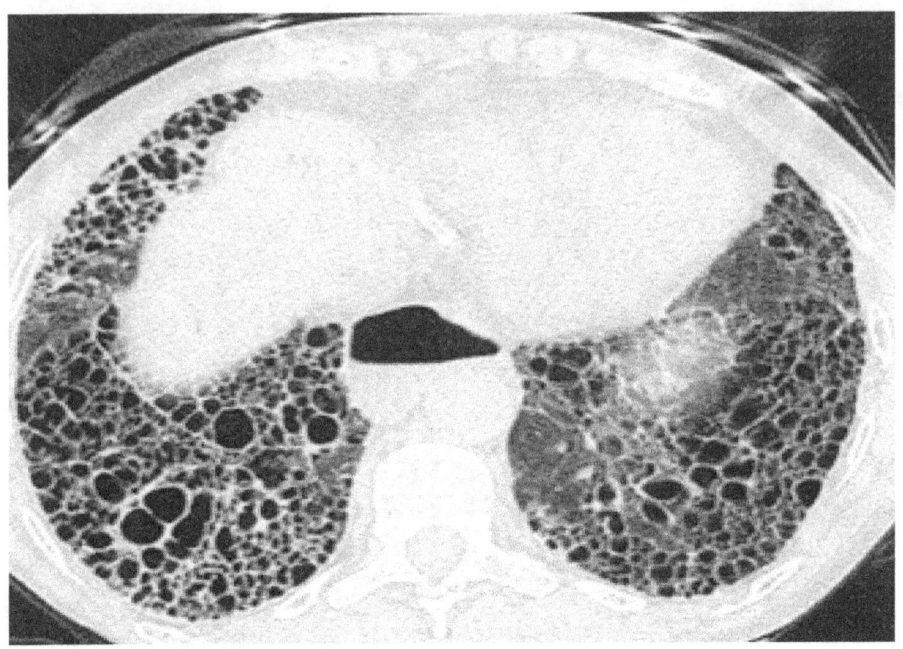

Best CT Study for Diagnosis:
CT Chest without IV contrast or High Resolution CT (HRCT) non-contrast

Key to DX:
Basilar, peripheral predominant reticular opacities and honeycombing with associated traction bronchiectasis.

Facts:
One of the most common types of interstitial lung disease (ILD).
Patients present with progressive shortness of breath and cough.
Etiology is predominantly idiopathic, but ILD can also be caused by connective tissue disease, drug toxicity, chronic hypersensitivity pneumonitis, and asbestosis.
Patients are typically over the age of 50 years with men affected slightly more than women.
Idiopathic pulmonary fibrosis is the name of the clinical syndrome associated with a UIP pattern.
Median survival is approximately 2.5-3.5 years.
CT has a high degree of accuracy in the diagnosis.

TX:
Does not respond to steroid treatments.
Lung transplantation.

USUAL INTERSTITIAL PNEUMONIA

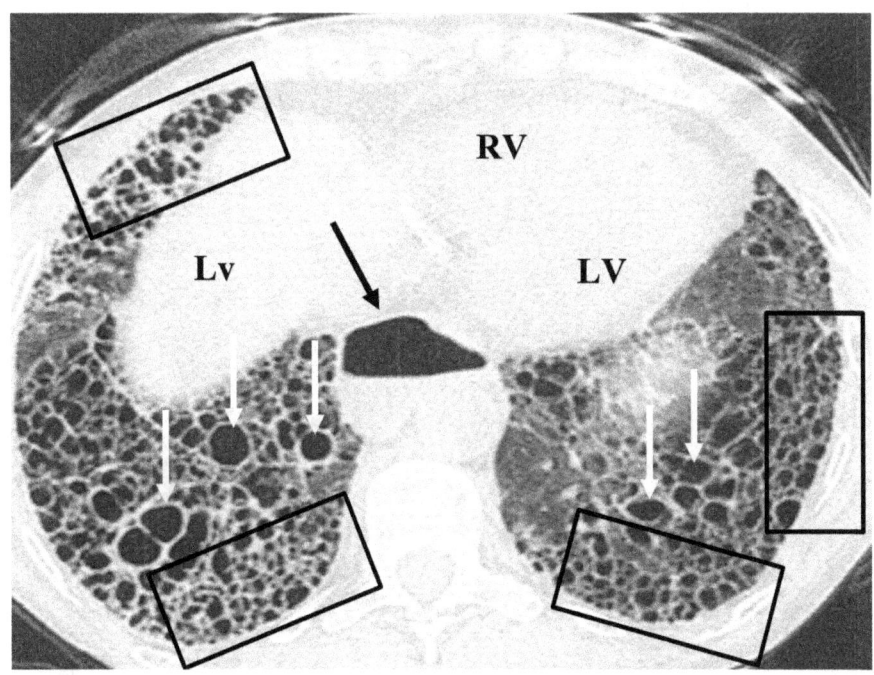

Study Above:
HRCT non-contrast at the level of the lower chest in lung window.

Radiographic Findings:
Peripheral and basilar predominant reticulations, traction bronchiectasis (white arrows), and multiple layers of cystic honeycombing (boxes). Incidentally noted is a dilated and fluid filled esophagus in a patient with known connective tissue disease (black arrow).

Tips:
Honeycombing is a very common finding in UIP.
Findings such as micronodules, extensive ground glass opacities, or consolidation suggest an alternative diagnosis.
Recognize the high degree of diagnostic accuracy with CT imaging and the important prognostic value.

Normal Anatomy:
LV – Left ventricle, RV – Right ventricle, Lv - Liver

Further Reading
Hansell DM. Classification of diffuse lung diseases: why and how. Radiology. 2013 Sep; 268(3):628-40

CASE 45

CASE AUTHOR: Gregory Puthoff

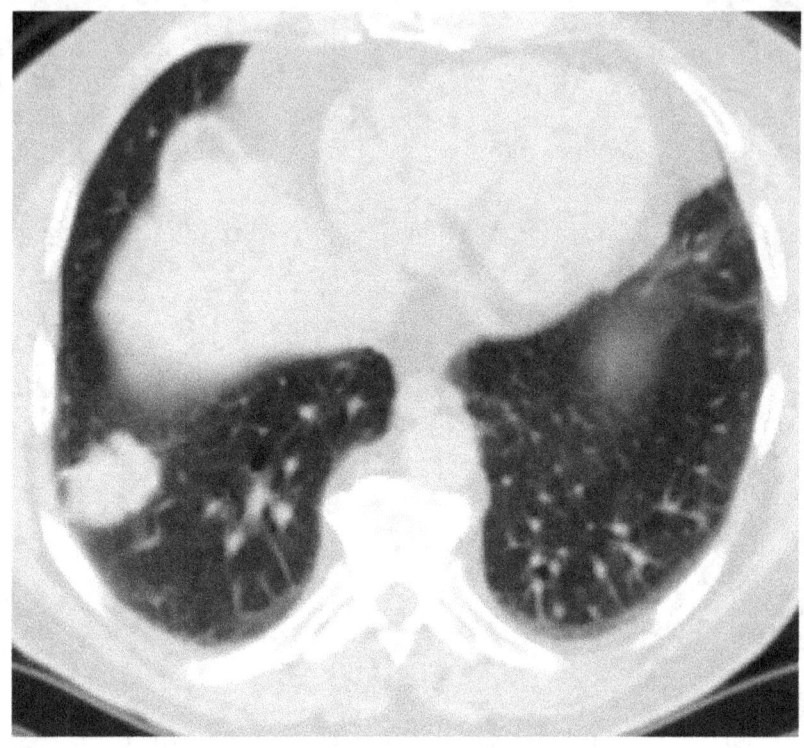

Best CT Study for Diagnosis:
CT Chest without IV contrast

Key to DX
Focal mass within the lung parenchyma.

Facts
Patients may present with dyspnea, weight loss, and hemoptysis.
The majority of cases are related to smoking.
Lung cancer has 2 basic types: small cell and non-small cell.
Small cell carcinoma is highly aggressive and has a high association with smokers.
Squamous cell carcinoma typically cavitates as it grows.

TX
Diagnosis is usually made with percutaneous CT guided sampling.
Treatment depends on the stage of disease and cell type. A combination of surgery, radiation, and chemotherapy are utilized.

LUNG MASS

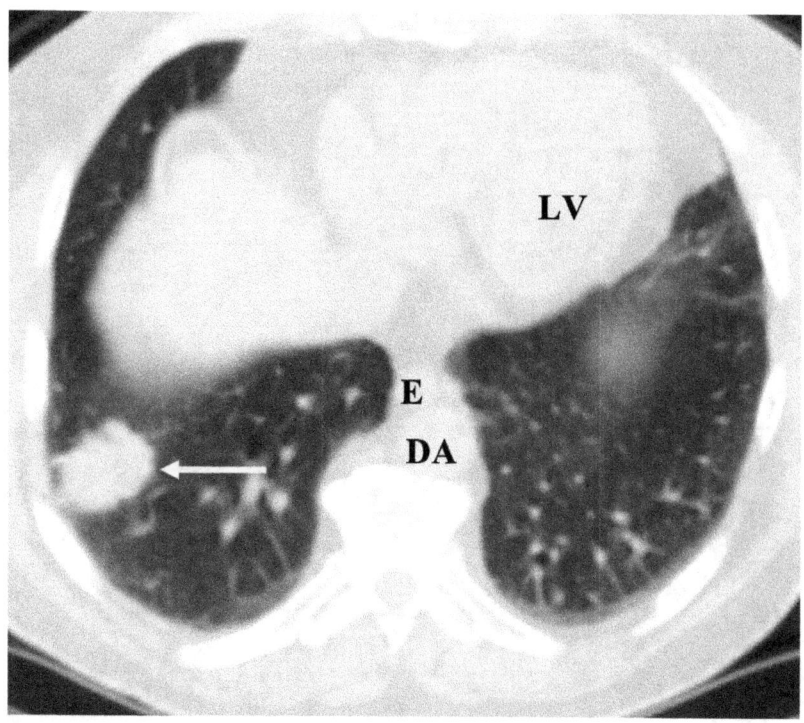

Study Above:
CT Chest without IV contrast at the level of the lung bases.

Radiographic findings:
A right lower lobe, lobulated mass (arrow).

Tips
Check for associated lung nodules and lymph nodes (larger than 1 cm is abnormal).
The term nodule is reserved for lesions less than 3 cm.
Realize that the larger a nodule is, the more likely it is to be malignant.
A spiculated nodule is typically malignant.
Interrogate adrenal glands and bones for metastatic involvement.
TMN classification, T1 lesions are less than 3 cm.

Normal Anatomy
LV - Left ventricle, DA - Descending aorta, E – Esophagus

Further Reading
Galvin J, Franks TJ. Lung Cancer Diagnosis: Radiologic Imaging, Histology, and Genetics. Radiology 2013 268:1, 9-11

CASE 46

CASE AUTHOR: Madison Kocher

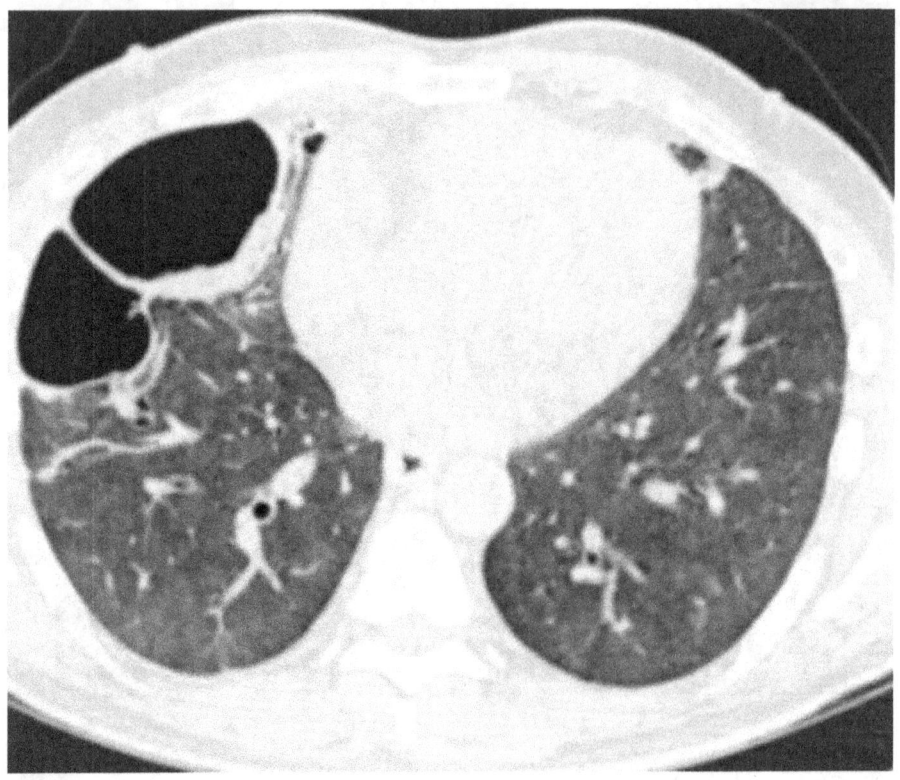

Best CT Study for Diagnosis:
CT Chest without IV contrast

Key to DX:
A transient, gas-filled lesion in the lung parenchyma that is usually thin-walled. They can have adjacent consolidation, ground glass opacities, or a thick wall if acute and caused by infection.

Facts:
Frequently caused by pneumonia, trauma, or inhalation of hydrocarbon fluid.
Patient will not have direct symptoms, only from the initial trauma or infection.
Appear during the healing phase of infection, particularly when caused by *Pneumococcus, Staphylococcus, E. coli,* or *Klebsiella.*
Mechanism is likely a combination of parenchymal necrosis and ball-valve effect.

TX:
Usually spontaneously resolves if caused by trauma.
Will also spontaneously resolve in the setting of treated pneumonia.

PNEUMATOCELE

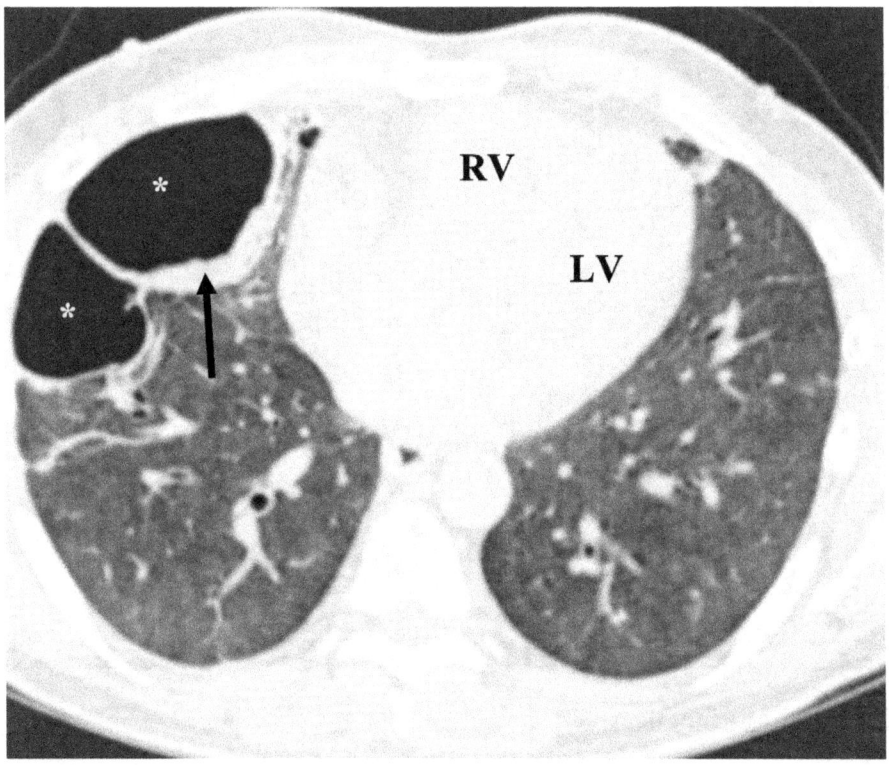

Study Above:
High Resolution CT (HRCT) non-contrast at the level of the lower chest in lung window.

Radiographic Findings:
Gas-filled lesion in the lung (asterisks) in a patient recovering from COVID-19 pneumonia. The cyst on the right has a thin wall and the cyst on the left has a thicker wall (arrow) with adjacent consolidation.

Tips:
May have thin or thick walls depending on acuity and initial etiology. Realize that pneumatoceles self-resolve and are likely a sign of healing.

Normal Anatomy:
LV – Left ventricle, RV- Right ventricle

Further Reading
Cantin L, Bankier AA, and Eisenberg RL. Multiple Cyst like Lung Lesions in the Adult. *American Journal of Radiology*. 2010; 194:W1-W11.

CASE 47

CASE AUTHOR: Gregory Puthoff

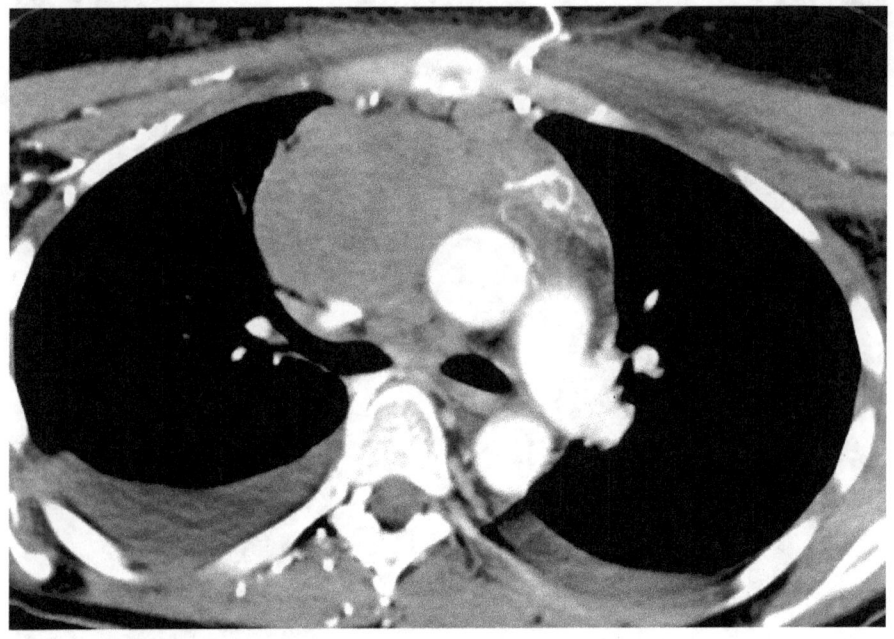

Best CT Study for Diagnosis:
CT chest with IV contrast

Key to DX
Marked enlargement of the mediastinal lymph nodes.

Facts
The differential diagnosis for enlarged lymph nodes includes lymphoma, infection, sarcoidosis, or metastatic lymph nodes.
The common types of lymphoma are Hodgkin lymphoma and non-Hodgkin lymphoma.
Non-Hodgkin lymphoma (NHL) is more common than Hodgkin.
"B" symptoms include fever, night sweats, and weight loss.
Hodgkin lymphoma results from the transformation of B-cells into pathognomonic binucleated Reed-Sternberg cells.
Most NHLs arise from B cells with the minority originating from T cells.
NHL is thought to be related to viral exposure.

TX
Includes combinations of chemotherapy, radiation therapy, and/or surgery.

LYMPHOMA

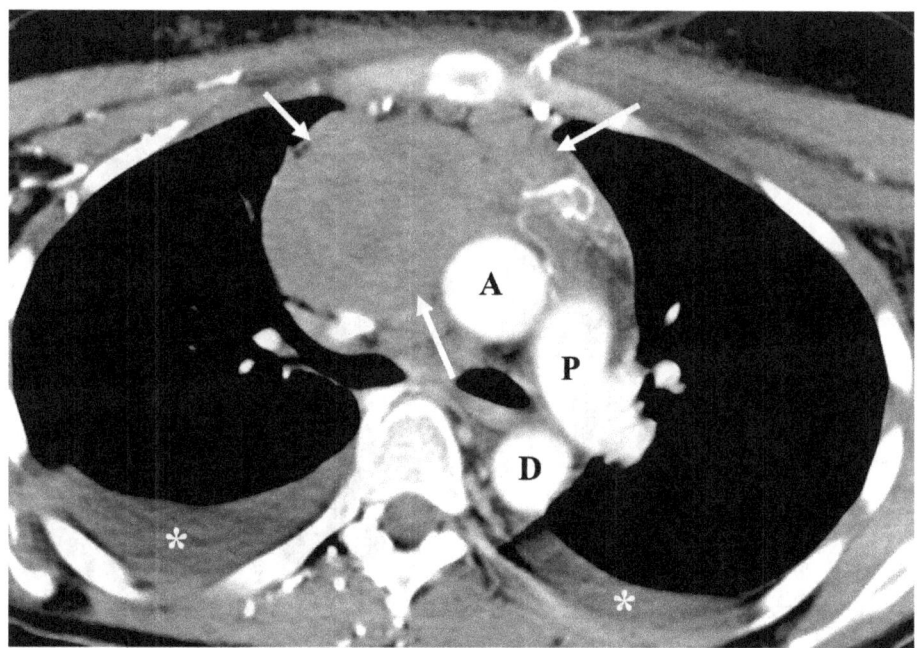

Study Above:
CT Chest with IV contrast at the level of the main pulmonary artery.

Radiographic findings:
There are two oval shaped soft tissue masses (arrows). These nodal masses are in the superior mediastinum and prevascular space. Notice that the aorta is being deviated to the left. Incidentally noted are bilateral small pleural effusions (*).

Tips
Check for associated supraclavicular and axillary lymph nodes.
With massive adenopathy, check the bronchi patency.
Vascular compression may also occur which may lead to thrombus formation or occlusion (SVC syndrome).

Normal Anatomy
A - Ascending thoracic aorta, D - Descending thoracic aorta, P - Pulmonary artery

Further Reading
Johnson S, et al. Imaging for Staging and Response Assessment in Lymphoma Radiology 2015 276:2, 323-338

CASE 48

CASE AUTHOR: Madison Kocher

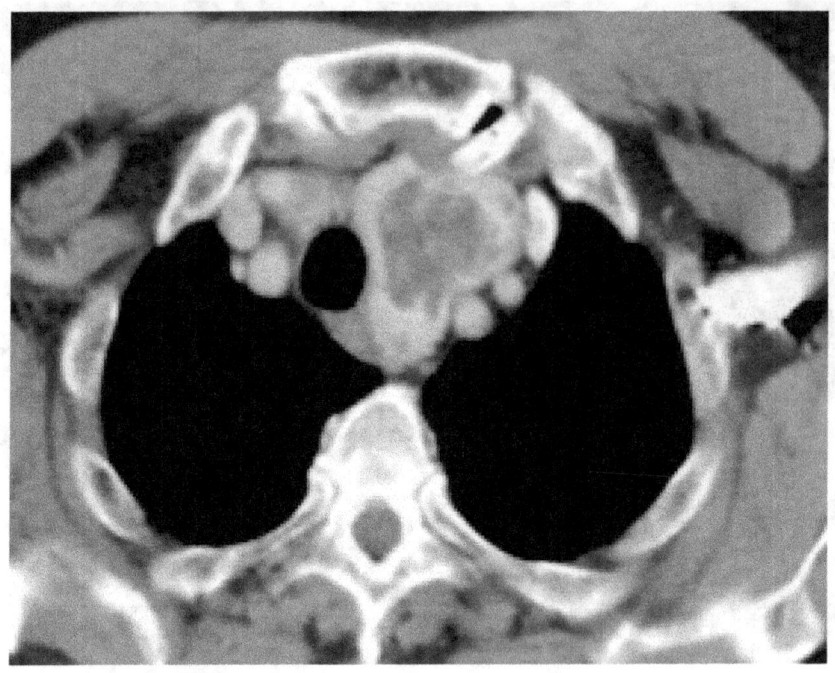

Best CT Study for Diagnosis:
CT Neck with IV contrast

Key to DX:
Thyroid extending below the plane of the thoracic inlet.

Facts:
There are multiple acceptable definitions of this entity. Most commonly it is defined as the thyroid extending below the plane of the thoracic inlet or having more than 50% of its mass lying inferior to the thoracic inlet.

If there is mass effect, the most frequent symptoms are palpable mass, dyspnea, dysphagia, or hoarseness.

CT is sometimes necessary to evaluate the full size and for operative planning. Extension to the aortic arch and beyond may necessitate the need for a thoracic surgical approach.

TX:
Conservative management if the patient is asymptomatic.

If causing mass-effect symptoms, surgical resection via cervical or thoracic approach can be curative.

RETROSTERNAL GOITER

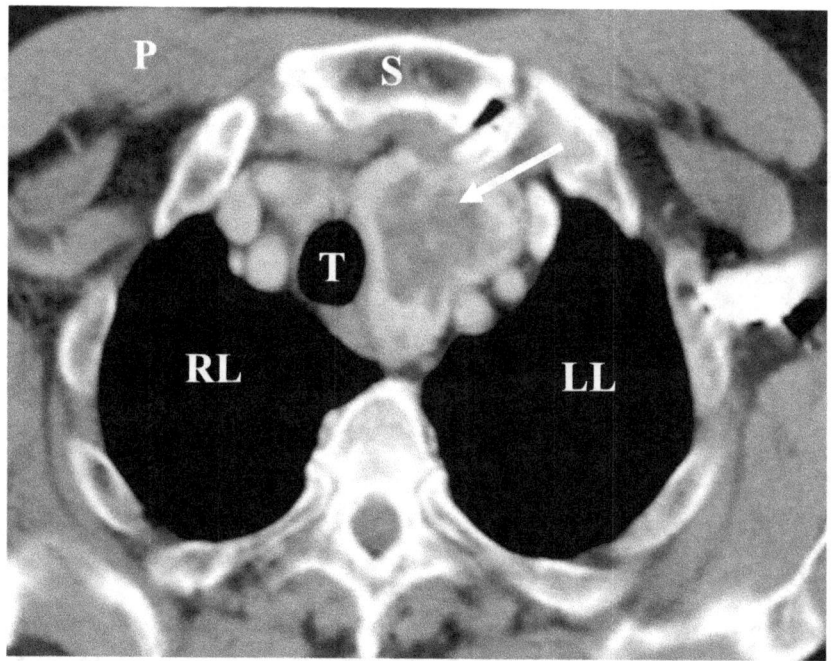

Study Above:
CT Chest with IV contrast; axial image on the left below the level of the thoracic inlet and coronal reformat on the right.

Radiographic Findings:
Heterogeneously enhancing thyroid goiter (arrow) extending into the thoracic inlet. There is mass effect on the trachea (T) with mild rightward displacement.

Tips:
Usually located in the anterior mediastinum and retains a connection with the thyroid gland.
1-16% risk of associated malignancy.
Dedicated thyroid ultrasound is helpful to evaluate and classify nodules.
Radiologic evaluation can be important in determining surgical approach.

Normal Anatomy:
T – Trachea, RL – Right lung, LL – Left lung, S – Sternum, P - Pectoralis

Further Reading
Buckley JA and Stark P. Intrathoracic mediastinal thyroid goiter: imaging manifestations. *AJR*. 1999; 173:471-475.

CASE 49

CASE AUTHOR: Rocky Saenz

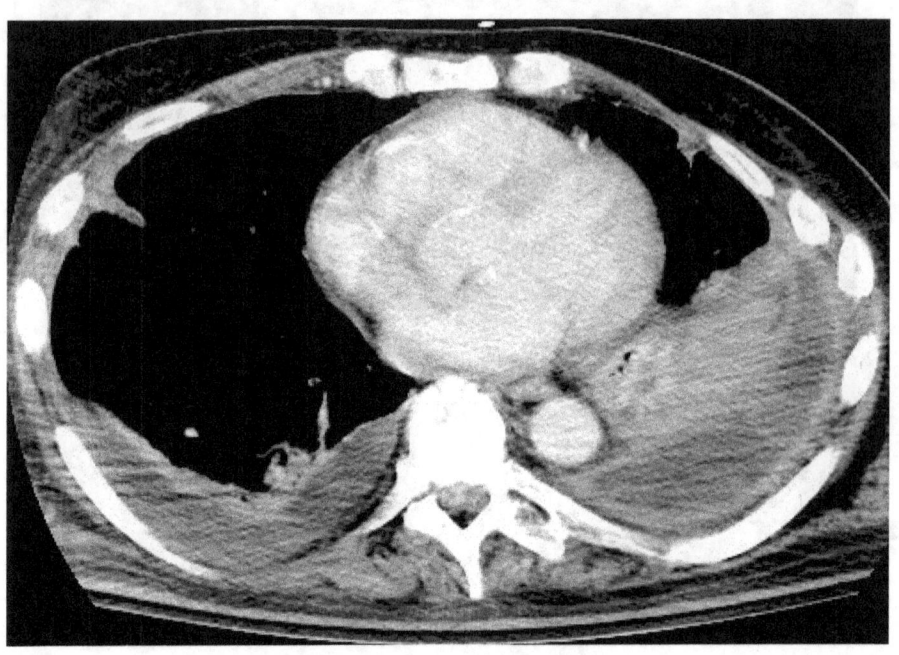

Best CT Study for Diagnosis:
CT Chest with IV contrast

Key to DX
Loculated pleural fluid collection with contrast enhancing borders.

Facts
Empyema refers to infection and pus in the pleural space.
Patients will usually present with fever and leukocytosis.
These are usually secondary to *Streptococci* and *Staphylococci*.
Intravenous contrast is necessary in order to visualize pleural enhancement.
The thickened, enhancing pleura is called the "split pleura" sign.
"Split pleura" sign may also be seen with malignant effusion, post-surgical changes, and hemothorax.

TX
CT guided drainage with pig-tail catheter placement. Radiology to the rescue!

EMPYEMA

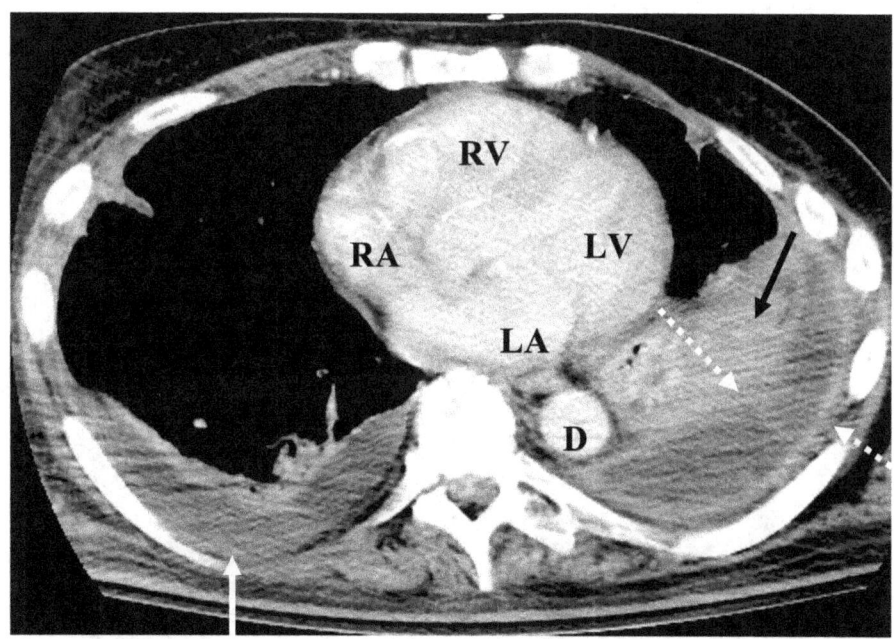

Study Above:
CT Chest with IV contrast at the level of the heart.

Radiographic findings:
Within the left chest, there is a loculated fluid collection with contrast enhancing borders representing the pleura (dashed arrows). Within the right lung base, there is a pleural effusion (solid white arrow). There is a component of left basilar consolidation (black arrow).

Tips
The key to diagnosis is noting the contrast enhancing periphery.
Do not confuse this with an abscess. An abscess is surrounded by lung parenchyma and typically round.
Empyema is crescentic in shape and outside the lung.

Normal Anatomy
LV - Left ventricle, RV - Right ventricle, LA - Left atrium, RA - Right atrium, D - Descending thoracic aorta

Further Reading
Walker CM, et al. Imaging pulmonary infection: classic signs and patterns.. AJR Am J Roentgenol. 2014 Mar;202(3):479-92

CASE 50

CASE AUTHOR: Gregory Puthoff

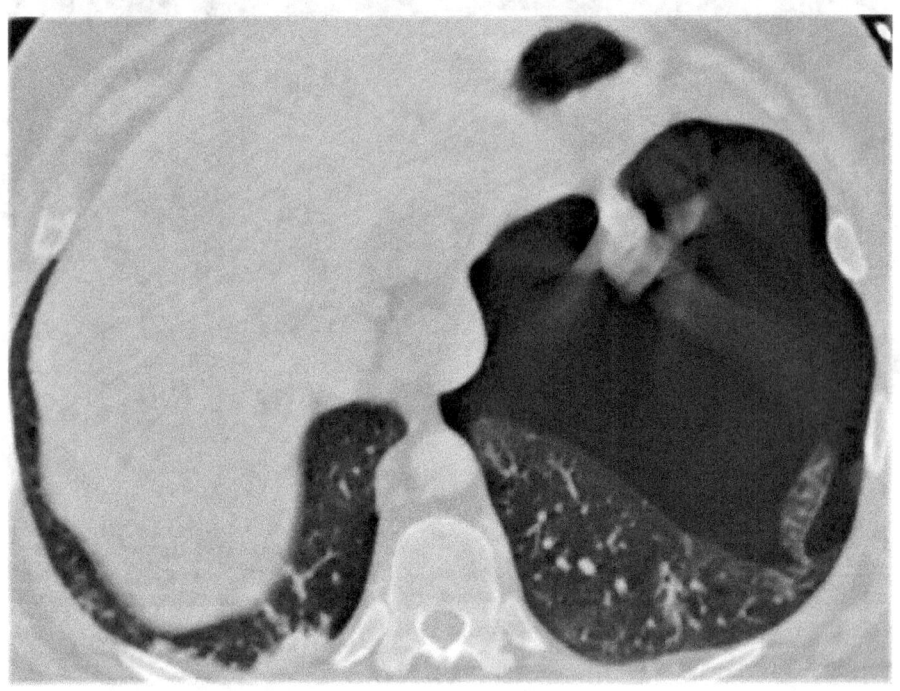

Best CT Study for Diagnosis:
CT Chest without contrast

Key to DX
Air filling the pleural space.

Facts
There are many etiologies of pneumothorax including trauma, iatrogenic, ruptured bleb, or metastasis.
When trauma is the cause, there may be associated pleural fluid/blood.
Chest radiographs performed in the supine position may miss 10%–50% of pneumothoraces due to the accumulation of air anteriorly and medially.
Tension physiology can occur when the air component of the pneumothorax becomes large and compresses the mediastinal vasculature or the heart.

TX
Chest tube placement with suction.
Tube placement depends on clinical symptoms because measuring the size of a pneumothorax may be inaccurate.

PNEUMOTHORAX

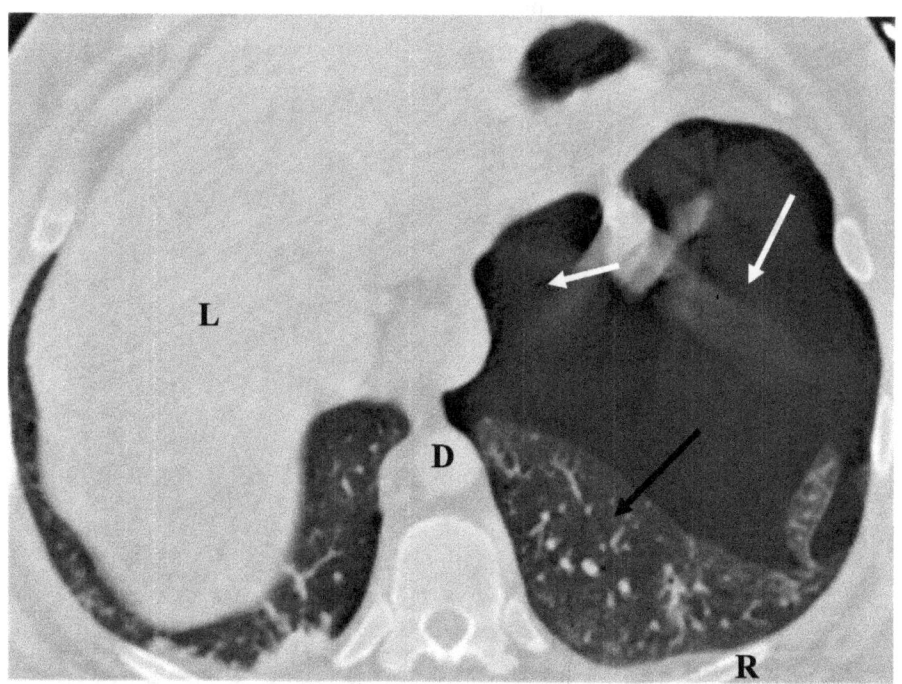

Study Above:
CT Chest with IV contrast at the level of the lung bases.

Radiographic findings:
Air in the pleural space (white arrows). Aerated lung parenchyma (black arrow).

Tips
Check for rib fractures as a source for injury.
Hemothorax should be suspected when Hounsfield units of any pleural fluid is 35-55.
Always evaluate for tension physiology.

Normal Anatomy
L - Liver, D - Descending thoracic aorta, R - Rib

Further Reading
Lewis BT, Hamlin SA, Henry T, Little BP, et al. Imaging Manifestations of Chest Trauma. *RadioGraphics* 2021 41:5, 1321-1334

CASE 51

CASE AUTHOR: Gregory Puthoff

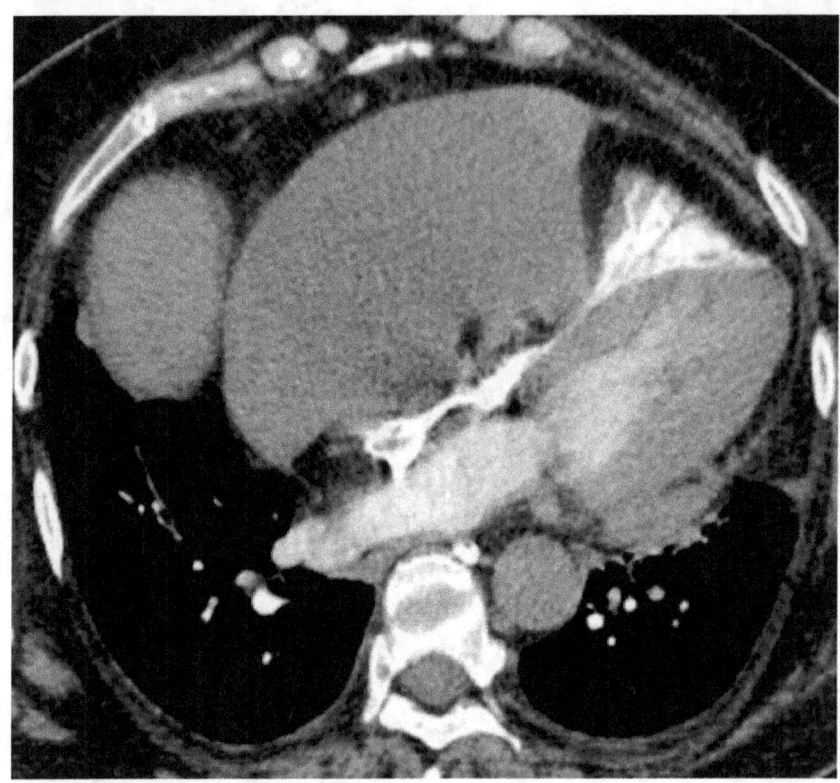

Best CT Study for Diagnosis:
CT Chest with IV contrast

Key to DX
Fluid accumulation within the pericardial sac.

Facts
Patients are usually asymptomatic but may present with chest pain.
Etiologies include infection, MI, trauma, metabolic disorders, or idiopathic.
May reduce the cardiac output either by constrictive or compressive physiology.
A pericardial rub may be heard on physical exam.
Echocardiography provides physiologic information a CT scan cannot.

TX
The underlying cause should be addressed.
Removal of the fluid (pericardiocentesis) may be necessary, particularly if the fluid results in altered cardiac output.

PERICARDIAL EFFUSION

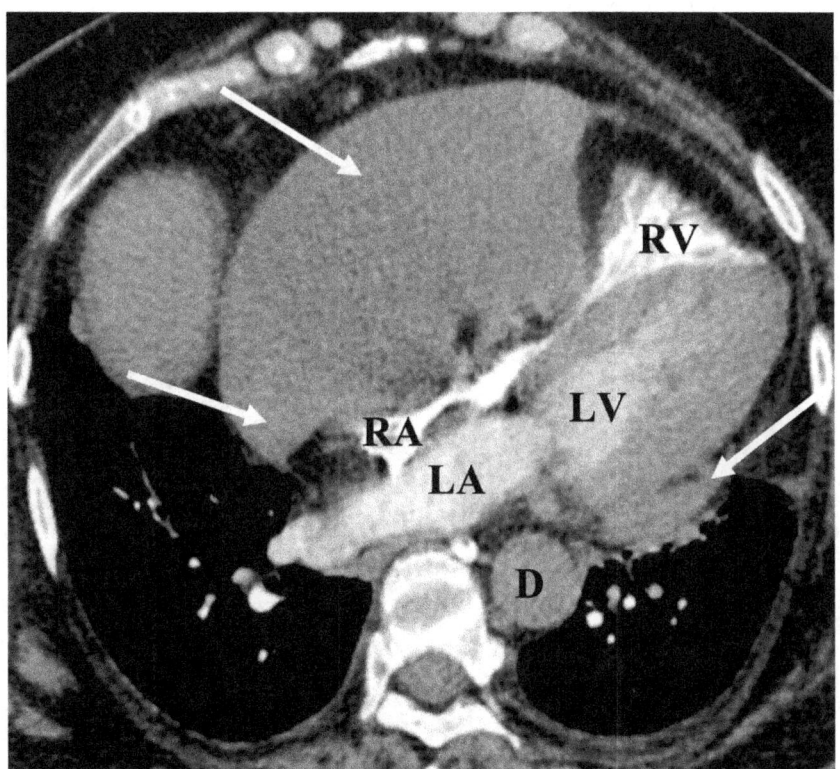

Study Above:
CT Chest with IV contrast at the level of the heart.

Radiographic findings:
Fluid attenuation is noted around the heart (arrows), maximally in the right pericardium. The large pericardial effusion is causing significant mass effect on the right ventricle, decreasing the chamber size.

Tips
Chronic pericarditis may have fine linear calcification of the pericardium.
Acute pericarditis may demonstrate peripheral enhancement of the pericardial sac.

Normal Anatomy
LV - Left ventricle, RV - Right ventricle, LA - Left atrium,
D - Descending thoracic aorta

Further Reading
Restrepo CS, et al. Imaging findings in cardiac tamponade with emphasis on CT. *Radiographics*. 2013 Oct;27(6):1595-610

CASE 52

CASE AUTHOR: Gregory Puthoff

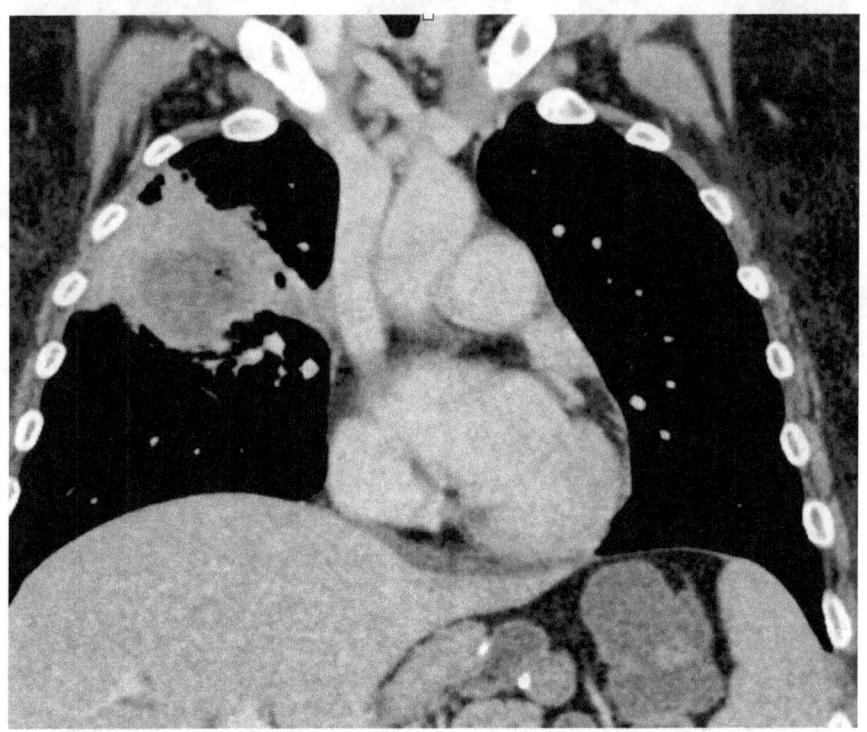

Best CT Study for Diagnosis:
CT Chest with IV contrast

Key to DX
Ovoid low attenuation lesion within the lung parenchyma with a fluid attenuated center and peripheral enhancement.

Facts
Symptoms may include ongoing cough, dyspnea, and fever.
Patients may present after failing outpatient antibiotic course.
Realize that this CT appearance may represent a necrotic tumor.
The most common aerobic pathogens are *streptococci* and *staphylococci*.
Consider *Nocardia, Mycobacteria,* or fungal origin in immunocompromised patients.

TX
IV antibiotics are needed. Surgical decompression may be necessary in advanced cases.
Percutaneous drainage catheter placement is controversial for management and may result in broncho-pleural fistula.

PULMONARY ABSCESS

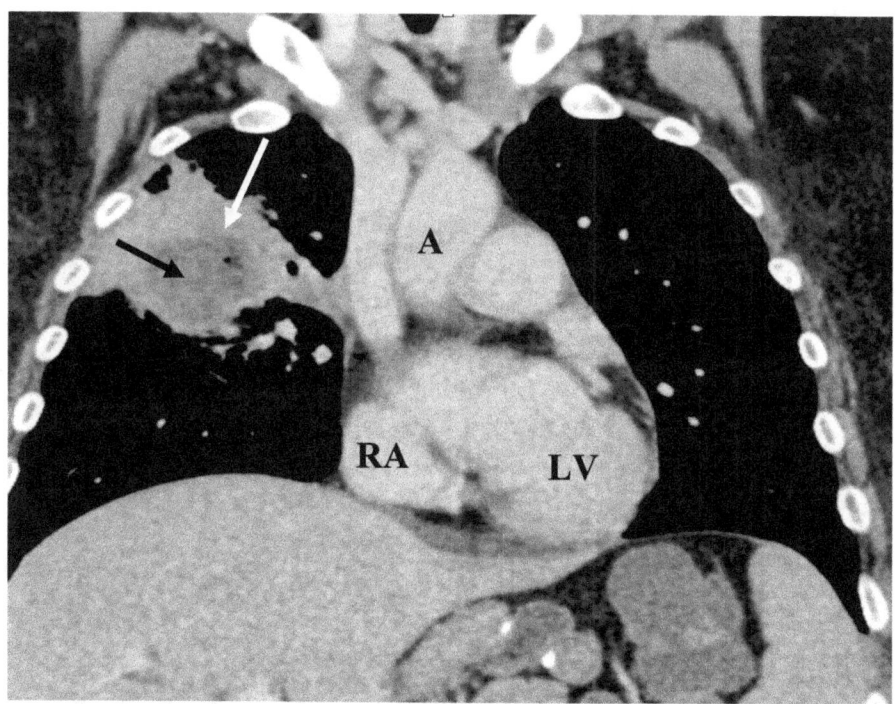

Study Above:
CT Chest with IV contrast at the level of the heart.

Radiographic findings:
A peripheral based lesion is seen involving the right upper lobe (white arrow). Note that the center of the lesion is fluid attenuation (black arrow).

Tips
Check the remaining lungs for other sites.
Interrogate mediastinum for adenopathy.
Consider empyema if the collection in question is crescentic in shape and not in the lung.
Always do a follow-up; typically 4-6 weeks after treatment to exclude an underlying tumor.

Normal Anatomy
LV - Left ventricle, RA - Right atrium, A - Ascending thoracic aorta

Further Reading
Walker CM, et al. Imaging pulmonary infection: classic signs and patterns. AJR Am J Roentgenol. 2014 Mar;202(3):479-92

CASE 53

CASE AUTHOR: Madison Kocher

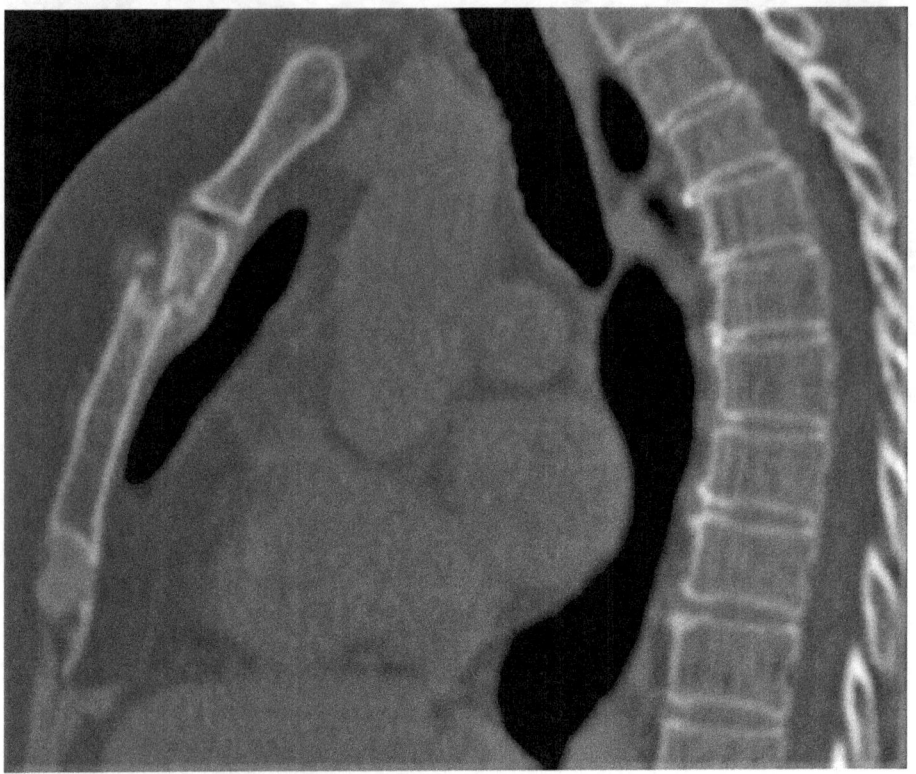

Best CT Study for Diagnosis:
CT Chest without IV contrast

Key to DX:
Cortical discontinuity of the sternum.

Facts:
Presence of a sternal fracture suggests high-energy blunt trauma and degree of displacement is proportional to the level of energy.
Can clinically present as acute coronary syndrome after trauma.
Although it can be diagnosed on a lateral chest radiograph, CT is necessary for further evaluation to exclude associated injuries.

TX:
Conservative management if non-displaced and no associated injuries.
Patients with suspected myocardial contusion should be monitored with ECG and cardiac enzymes. Operative fixation may be indicated for unstable or displaced fracture.

STERNAL FRACTURE

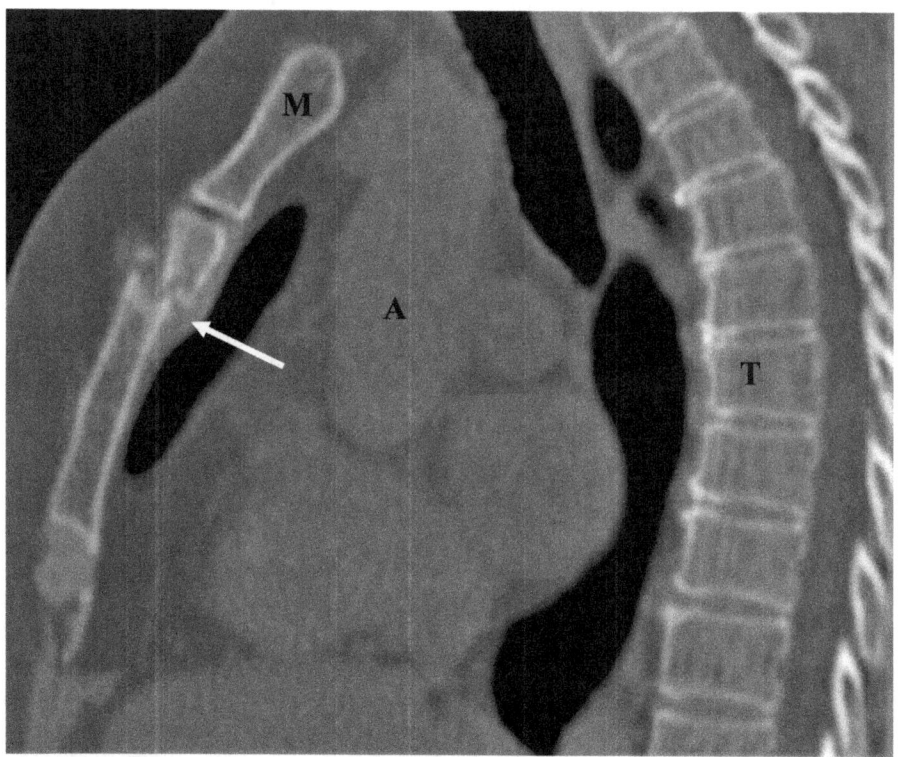

Study Above:
CT Chest without IV contrast; sagittal midline reformat in bone window.

Radiographic Findings:
Cortical irregularity at the mid aspect of the sternal body with displacement (arrow).

Tips:
Be sure to look for associated injuries including cardiac trauma, mediastinal hematoma, thoracic spine fracture, rib fracture, and lung contusions.

If there are no concomitant injuries, patients can be discharged after a normal ECG and normal cardiac enzymes. Hospitalization or observation is not required for an isolated sternal fracture.

Normal Anatomy:
A – Aorta, T – Thoracic spine, M - Manubrium

Further Reading
Restrepo CS, Martinez S, & Lemos DF, et. al. Imaging appearances of the sternum and sternoclavicular joints. *Radiographics*. 2009; 29:839-859.

CASE 54

CASE AUTHOR: Gregory Puthoff

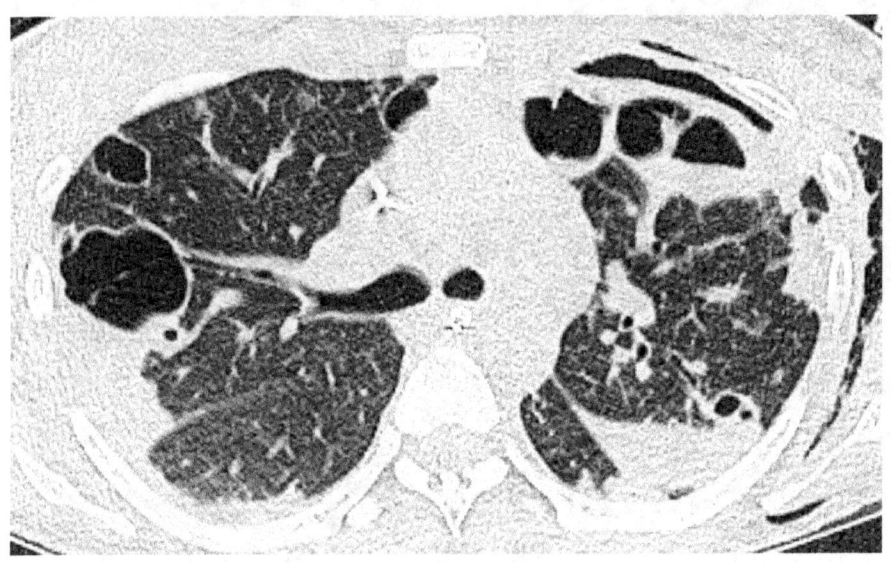

Best CT Study for Diagnosis:
CT Chest with IV contrast

Key to DX
Multiple bilateral cavitary pulmonary lesions.

Facts
Patients may present with low-grade fever, night sweats, or malaise.
IV drug abusers and immunocompromised patients are at highest risk.
Correlation with echocardiogram is helpful to exclude cardiac valve vegetations.

TX
Antibiotic therapy.
Consider cardiac consultation with echocardiogram.

SEPTIC EMBOLI

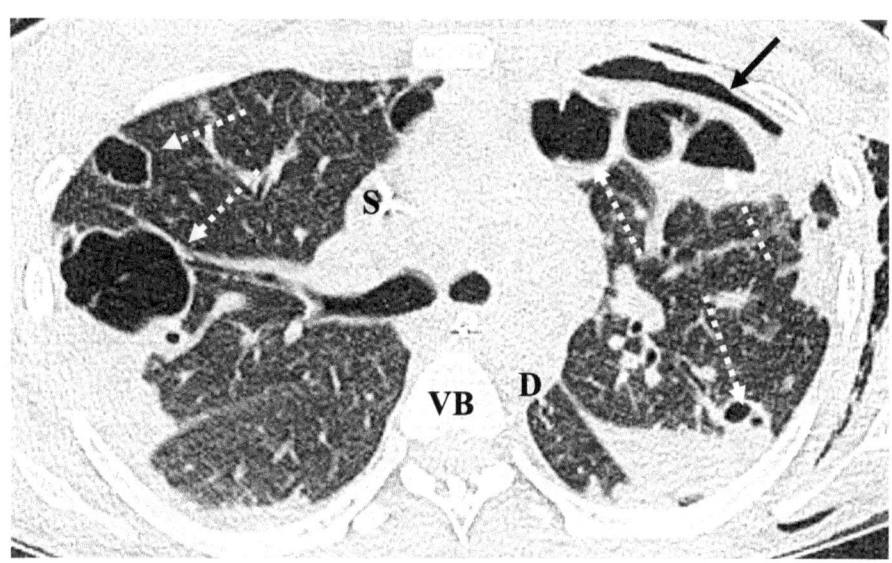

Study Above:
CT Chest without IV contrast at the level of the carina.

Radiographic findings:
Multiple cavitary nodules are present in the right and left lungs (dashed arrows). Note that the majority of the nodules are cavitary with air-fluid levels. Small left anterior pneumothorax (black arrow).

Tips
Check for cardiac valve vegetations.
Interrogate adrenal glands and bones for metastatic involvement.
Nodules in septic emboli may be cavitary or solid and are often a mixture of both.

Normal Anatomy
S - Superior vena cava, VB - Vertebral body, D - Descending thoracic aorta

Further Reading
Dodd JD, Souza CA, Müller NL. High-resolution MDCT of pulmonary septic embolism: evaluation of the feeding vessel sign.. AJR Am J Roentgenol. 2006 Sep;187(3):623-9.

CASE 55

CASE AUTHOR: Madison Kocher

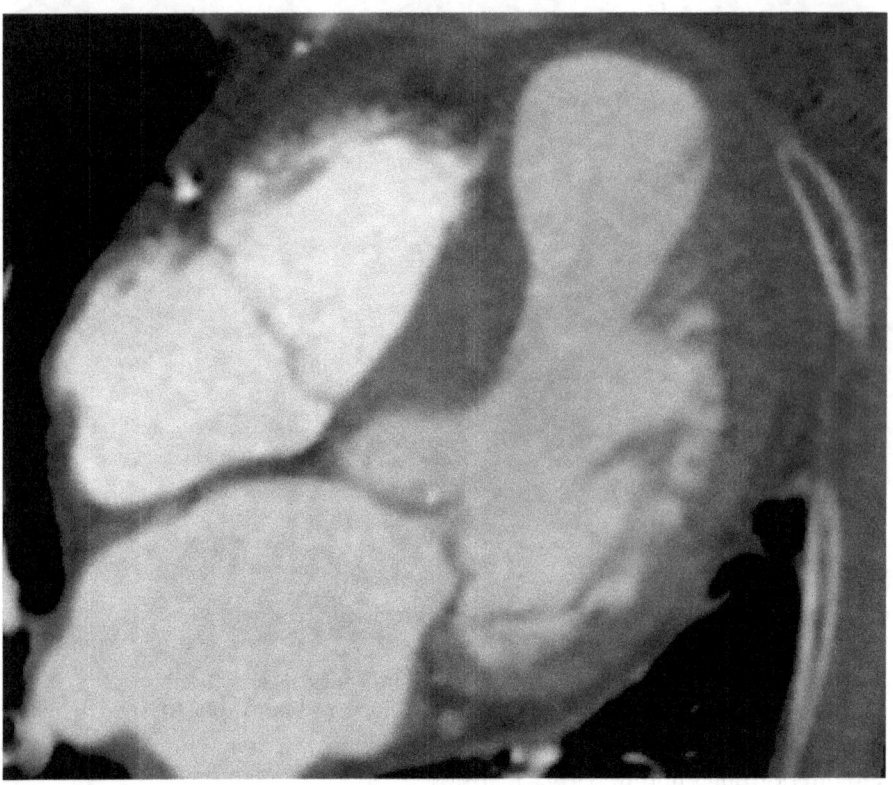

Best CT Study for Diagnosis:
CT Cardiac with IV Contrast

Key to DX:
Left ventricular myocardial wall thinning with ventricular outpouching.

Facts:
Differentiation should be made between aneurysms and pseudoaneurysms, as their prognoses vary widely.
This specific outpouching contains some elements of the myocardium.
Most common cause is transmural myocardial infarction.
Most commonly occur in the apical, anterior, or anterolateral wall secondary to a left anterior descending artery territory infarction.
These are likely to rupture only in the early postinfarction time period.

TX:
Low risk of rupture and is usually managed medically.
Surgical repair reserved for complicated cases and cases associated with heart failure or refractory arrhythmia.

LEFT VENTRICULAR ANEURYSM

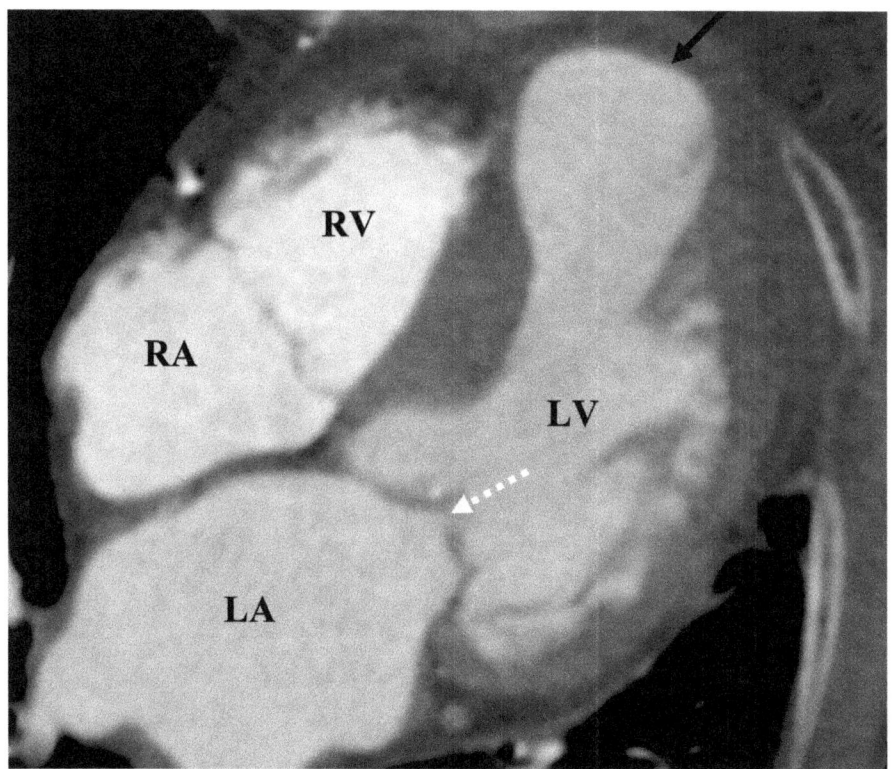

Study Above:
CT Cardiac with IV Contrast, four-chamber view.

Radiographic Findings:
Left ventricular myocardial wall thinning with wide-necked outpouching from the apical wall (black arrow).

Tips:
A true left ventricular aneurysm usually has a wide neck and left ventricular myocardial wall thinning.
Unlikely to rupture in the chronic phase and conservative management can be pursued.

Normal Anatomy:
RV – Right ventricle, LV – Left ventricle, LA – Left atrium, RA – Right atrium, Dashed Arrow – Mitral valve

Further Reading
Konen E, Merchant N, Gutierrez C, Provost Y, Mickleborough L, Paul NS, and Butany J. True versus false left ventricular aneurysm: differentiation with MR Imaging – Initial Experience. *Radiology* 2005; 236:65-70

CASE 56

CASE AUTHOR: Gregory Puthoff

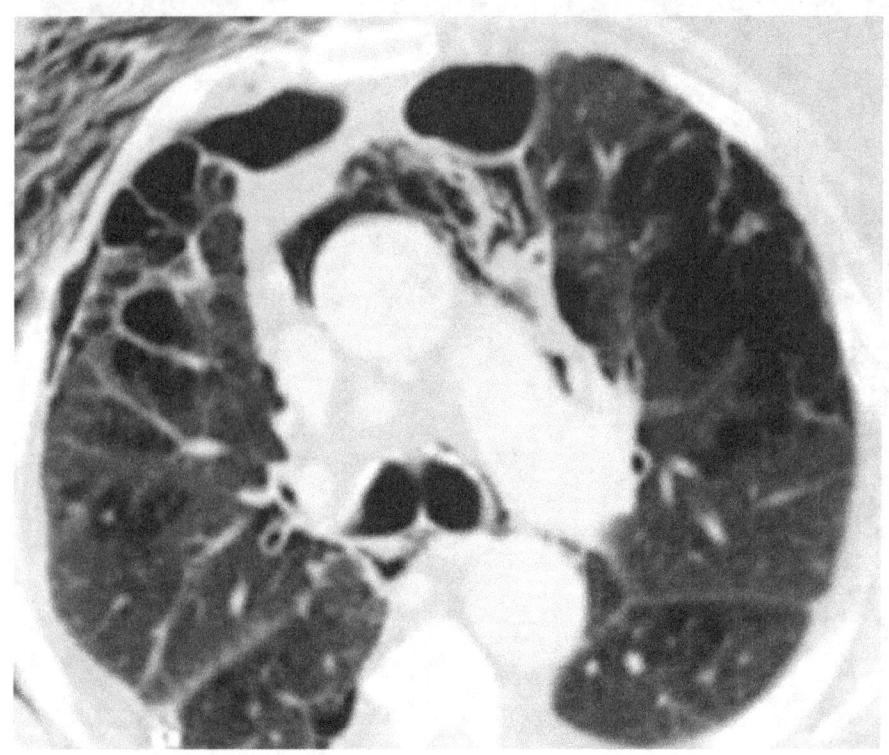

Best CT Study for Diagnosis:
CT Chest without IV contrast

Key to DX
Air outlining the heart and mediastinal structures.

Facts
Patients often present with severe chest/neck pain, cough, and dyspnea.
Physical exam may reveal palpable crepitus (when air extends into the neck or subcutaneous soft tissues) and "Hamman's crunch" upon auscultation (rasping sound synchronous with heartbeat).
May be spontaneous or traumatic in etiology.
Other causes include: alveolar rupture from increased intrathoracic pressure (asthmatics, valsalva, coughing), laceration of the tracheobronchial tree or esophagus, and extension of air from the neck or retroperitoneum.

TX
Typically self-limiting and usually resolves within a week. However, greater than 50% mortality rate with Boerhaave syndrome (esophageal rupture following vomiting).

PNEUMOMEDIASTINUM

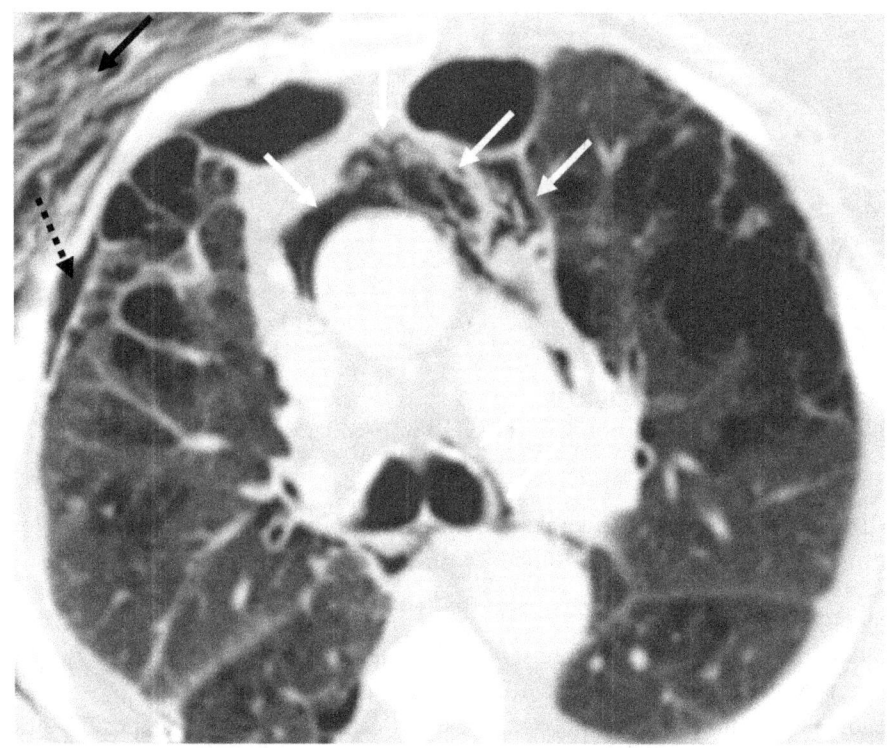

Study Above:
CT Chest with IV contrast at the level of the carina.

Radiographic findings:
Air is seen surrounding the mediastinal structures (white arrows) with extensive anterior chest wall subcutaneous emphysema (black arrow). Small right pneumothorax present (dashed black arrow).

Tips
Enlarging pneumomediastinum suggests injury to the trachea or esophagus. Bronchoscopy or esophagram may be necessary if visceral injury is a concern.
Pneumothorax does not cause pneumomediastinum, though pneumomediastinum may cause pneumothorax.
High mortality rate when secondary to Boerhaave syndrome, otherwise pneumomediastinum generally follows a benign course.

Further Reading
Zylak CM, Standen JR, Barnes GR, and Zylak CJ. Pneumomediastinum Revisited *RadioGraphics* 2000 20:4, 1043-1057

CASE 57

CASE AUTHOR: Madison Kocher

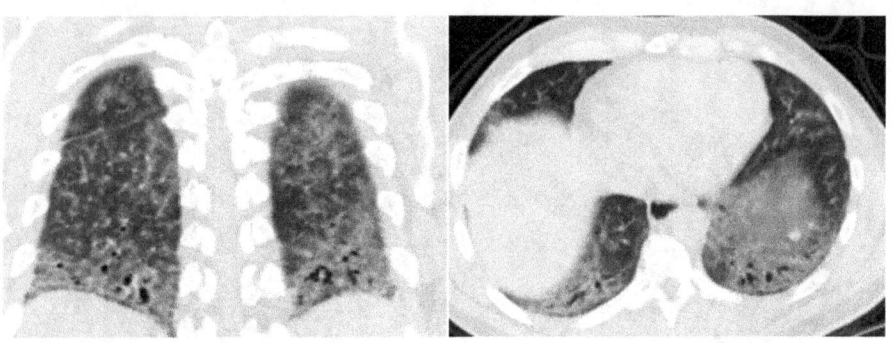

Best CT Study for Diagnosis:
CT Chest, High Resolution CT (HRCT) non-contrast.

Key to DX:
Bilateral lower lobe peripheral predominant ground-glass opacities, traction bronchiectasis, lower lobe volume loss, and fine reticulations.

Facts:
Patients present with gradual onset of shortness of breath, cough, and dyspnea. Affects men and women equally in the age range of 40-50 years.

Etiologies include idiopathic, toxic drug effects, occupational exposure, and hypersensitivity pneumonitis.

There is a high association with collagen vascular diseases including scleroderma, polymyositis, rheumatoid arthritis, and Sjogren syndrome.

Cellular subtype has a better survival rate (nearly 100%) as compared to the fibrotic lung type (5-year survival ranges from 45-90%), although both have a better survival rate than usual interstitial pneumonia (UIP).

TX:
Most respond to oral corticosteroids or immune-suppressing drugs.

Patients with the fibrotic subtype may benefit from anti-fibrotics or lung transplant for end-stage disease.

NONSPECIFIC INTERSTITIAL PNEUMONIA

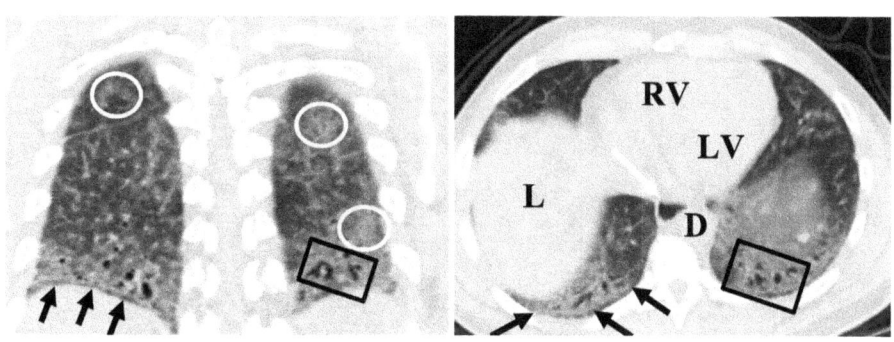

Study Above:
HRCT non-contrast. Image on the left is a coronal reformat posteriorly and the axial image on the right is at the level of the lower chest.

Radiographic Findings:
Peripheral and basilar predominant ground glass opacities (circles) with subpleural sparing (black arrows). Fibrotic changes are evident with architectural distortion, fine reticulations, and traction bronchiectasis (boxes). Also noted is a dilated and fluid filled esophagus in this scleroderma patient (white arrow).

Tips:
Must be bilateral and lower lobe predominant, as this is the characteristic pattern of lung involvement.
Realize that honeycombing may be present, as this can be found in the fibrotic NSIP subtype.
Subpleural sparing is a specific finding for NSIP.

Normal Anatomy:
RV – Right ventricle, LV – Left ventricle, L – Liver, D – Descending thoracic aorta

Further Reading
Kligerman SJ, Groshong S, Brown KK, and Lynch DA. Nonspecific interstitial pneumonia: radiologic, clinical, and pathologic considerations. *Radiographics*. 29:73-87; 2009.

CASE 58

CASE AUTHOR: Gregory Puthoff

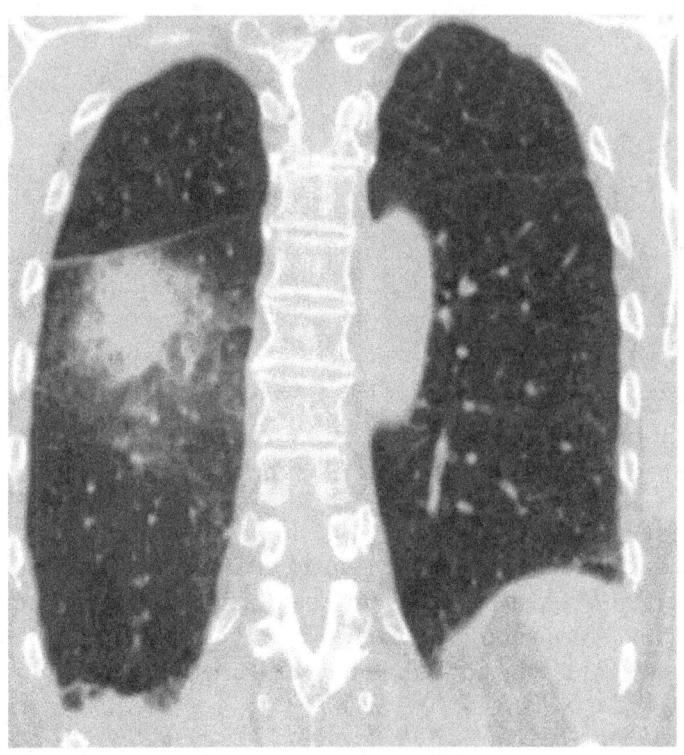

Best CT Study for Diagnosis:
CT Chest without IV contrast

Key to DX:
Mass-like attenuation with surrounding groundless halo.

Facts:
Patients present with shortness of breath, cough, and hemoptysis.
Requires profound neutropenia (CD4 count <50).
Commonly encountered in patients receiving chemotherapy.
High mortality for untreated infections.
Surrounding groundless halo is secondary to direct invasion of lung parenchyma by the fungi causing coagulative necrosis.

TX:
Most patients require hospitalization and aggressive IV anti-fungal treatment.

ANGIOINVASIVE ASPERGILLOSIS

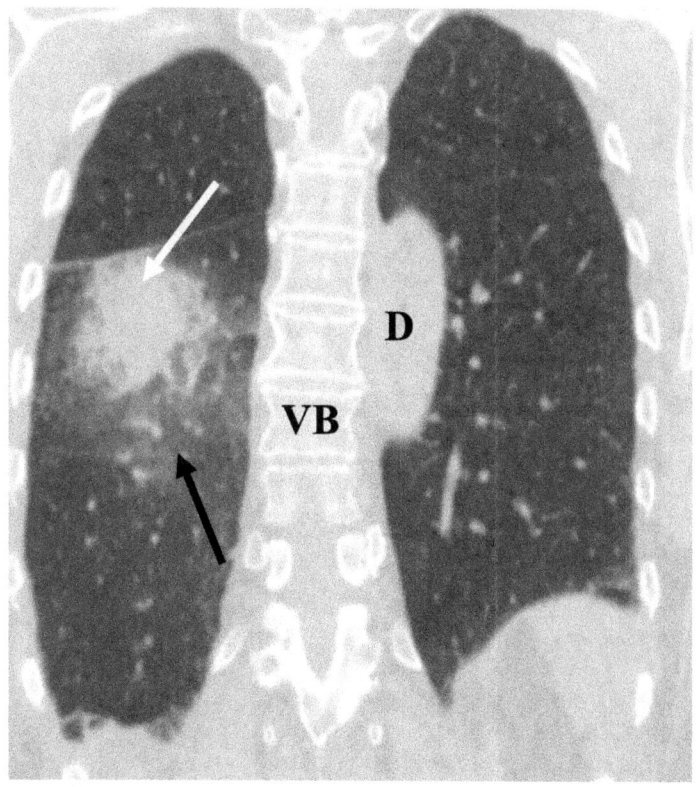

Study Above:
CT of chest without IV contrast, coronal reformat of the posterior lungs.

Radiographic Findings:
Mass-like airspace disease (white arrow) in the superior segment of the right lower lobe with surrounding ground glass halo (black arrow).

Tips:
Urgent identification and communication required to initiate lifesaving antifungals.
Can be singular or multiple.
Follow-up after treatment to monitor for scarring or cavity formation.

Normal Anatomy:
D– Descending thoracic aorta, VB – Vertebral body

Further Reading
Franquet T, Müller NL, Giménez A, Guembe P, and Bagué S. Spectrum of Pulmonary Aspergillosis: Histologic, Clinical, and Radiologic Findings. *Radiographics*. 2001; 21:4,825-837.

CASE 59, PEDIATRIC

CASE AUTHOR: Tammam Beydoun

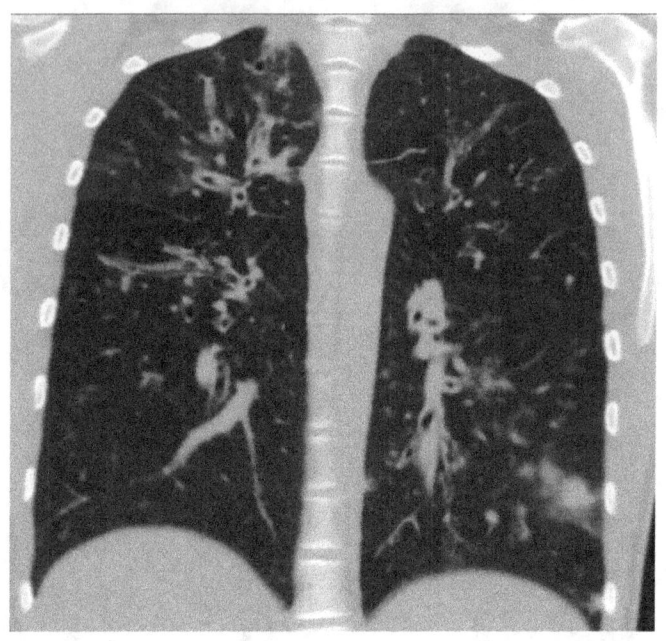

Best CT Study for Diagnosis:
CT Chest without IV contrast – High resolution protocol

Key to DX
Diffuse bronchiectasis, bronchial wall thickening, and mucus plugging.

Facts
Most diagnosed by 5 years of age.
Thick mucoid secretions secondary to abnormal cystic fibrosis transmembrane regulator (CFTR) protein.
Patients with recurrent respiratory infections (commonly *P. aeruginosa, S. aureus* and *H. influenza*).
Associated with pancreatic exocrine insufficiency, biliary cirrhosis, and pansinusitis.

TX
Bronchodilators and aggressive promotion of airway clearance (i.e. chest physiotherapy).
Antibiotic therapy for prophylaxis and during acute airspace disease.
End stage cases require bilateral lung transplant.

CYSTIC FIBROSIS EXACERBATION

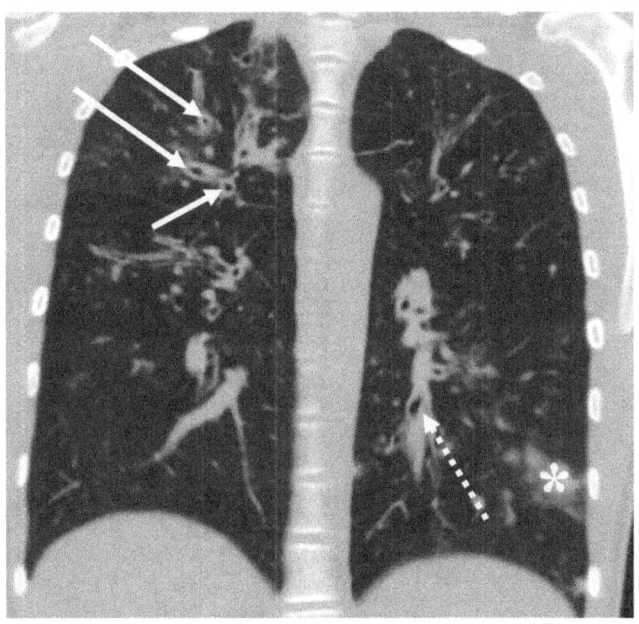

Study Above:
High resolution CT chest in multiple intensity projection (MIP) coronal reconstruction to better demonstrate pathology.

Radiographic findings:
Diffuse bronchiectasis (dilated bronchi) with wall thickening (white arrows), more dominant in the upper lobes. Air-fluid level consistent with mucus plugging (dashed arrow). Focal consolidation with adjacent ground-glass opacity suspicious for acute infection (asterisk).

Tips
Upper lobe predominance.
These patients receive a significant amount of radiation from repeat radiography.
CT is more sensitive than pulmonary function tests at detecting early disease.
Hyperinflation signifies air trapping due to 'ball valve' plugging of airway by mucus.
Radiographs in lateral decubitus with inspiration and expiration views may be helpful in non-cooperative patients (toddlers/infants) to evaluate for air trapping.
Disease may be masked under general anesthesia with controlled lung volumes.

Further Reading
Brody AS, Klein JS, Molina PL, Quan J, Bean JA, Wilmott RW. High-resolution computed tomography in young patients with cystic fibrosis: distribution of abnormalities and correlation with pulmonary function tests. J Pediatr. 145(1):32-8, 2004

CASE 60

CASE AUTHOR: Gregory Puthoff

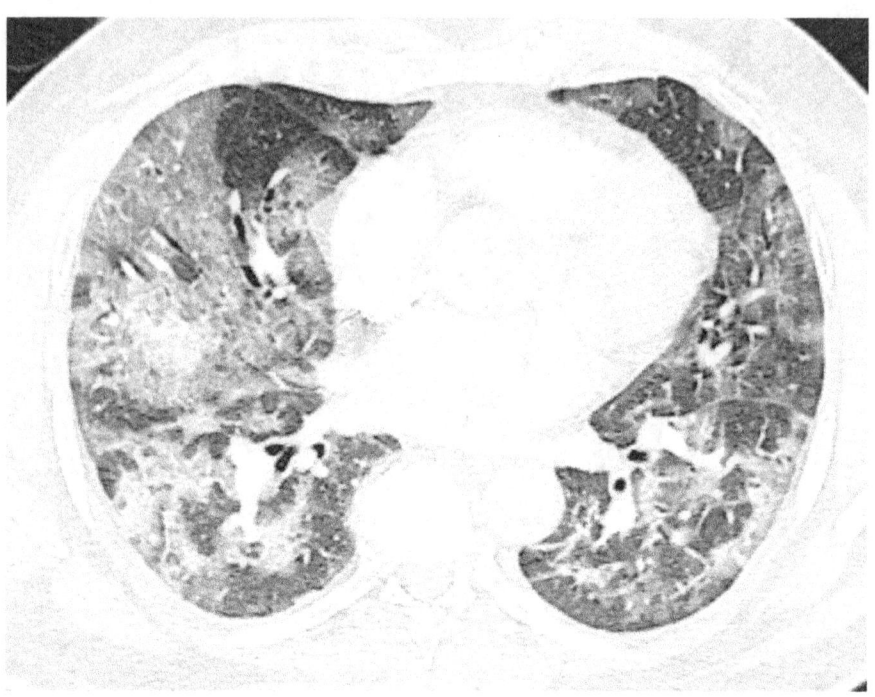

Best CT Study for Diagnosis:
CT Chest without contrast

Key to DX:
Multifocal peripherally oriented ground glass opacities and solid airspace disease.

Facts
Patients present with shortness of breath, cough, and fever.
Understanding of COVID pneumonia is ongoing.
Multiple stages of COVID pneumonia: early stages demonstrate predominantly ground glass airspace disease and later stages demonstrate signs of fibrosis.

TX
Predominantly supportive care with proposed pharmacologic treatments including steroids and immunotherapy.

COVID PNEUMONIA

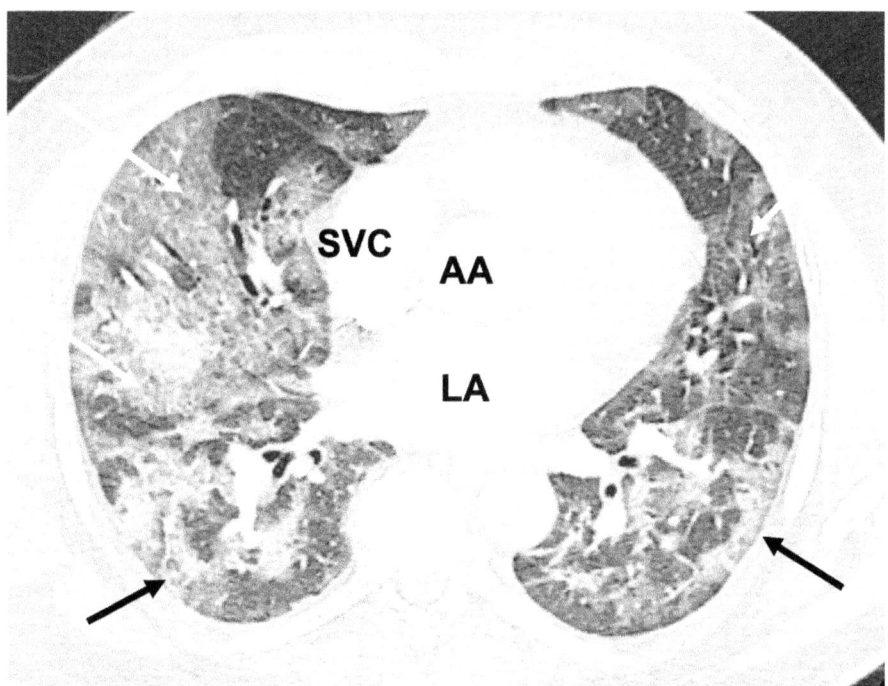

Study Above:
CT chest with contrast at the level of the heart.

Radiographic findings:
Multifocal ground glass opacities (white arrows) and solid airspace disease throughout the lung parenchyma which demonstrates predominantly peripheral distribution and involves the subpleural lung (black arrows).

Tips
False negatives have been reported. A symptomatic patient with CT findings of COVID should be retested.
CTA PE study should be considered as many patients are experiencing in-situ pulmonary artery thrombosis.
Do not neglect other differential diagnostic considerations of diffuse pulmonary pathology.

Normal Anatomy
AA - Ascending aorta, LA - Left atrium, SVC - Superior vena cava

Further Reading
Kwee, TC., and Kwee, RM. Chest CT in COVID-19: What the *Radiologist* Needs to Know. *RadioGraphics*, 40(7), 1848-1865. 2020.

CHAPTER 5
ABDOMINAL AND PELVIC CT

ABDOMEN

TO CONTRAST OR NOT TO CONTRAST
Most pathology in the acute setting requires administration of IV contrast. I always say if the pathology ends with "itis" order IV contrast. If bowel pathology is of concern, then oral contrast is also recommended. There are some abdominal diagnoses that do not require IV or oral contrast, including renal/ureteral stones, retroperitoneal hemorrhage, and pneumoperitoneum. For a visceral injury, IV contrast must be given as small visceral lacerations are not visible without IV contrast. In addition, trauma imaging requires delayed imaging (i.e., a second scan after portal venous standard imaging about 3 to 5 minutes after injection) in order to exclude active hemorrhage.

CT VS. MRI
CT is the gold standard for abdominal imaging. MRI is used on occasion for lesion characterization as an adjunct to CT. The classic example would be an indeterminate liver mass. The same concerns remain with MRI abdominal imaging (see "CT vs. MRI" in Chapter 1, brain imaging).

IMAGE INTERPRETATION
When attempting to interpret abdominal CT studies, it is best to take an organ by organ approach. This entails checking each organ one at a time by viewing each image of the organ continuously. The pathology is located when an irregular area is noted in or around an organ. Do not forget to check the osseous structures, lung bases, vessels, musculature, and abdominal walls. Remember that fat stranding in the abdomen or pelvis is typically indicative of pathology. Fat stranding is non-specific, and may represent an acute or chronic process related to infection, inflammation, neoplasm, or a traumatic process.

R Saenz DO, FAOCR

CASE 61

CASE AUTHOR: Maqsood Kahn

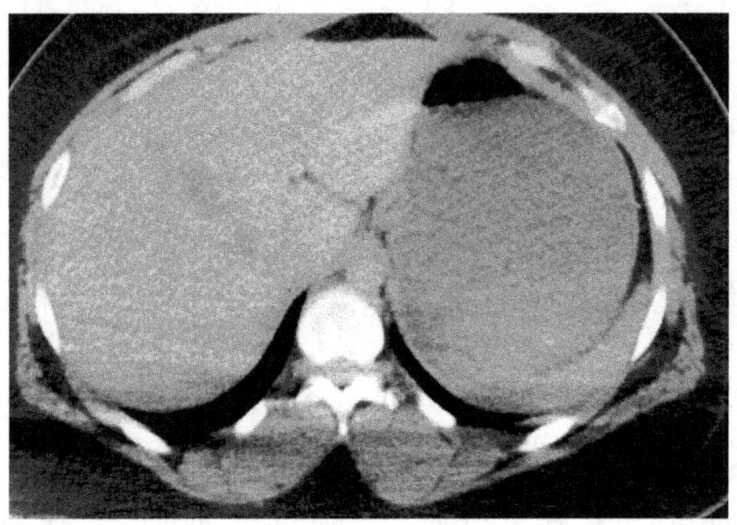

Best CT Study for Diagnosis:
CT Abdomen with IV contrast

Key to DX
Linear low attenuation traversing the liver parenchyma.

Facts
The liver is the most commonly injured organ.
Most liver injuries are treated non-surgically.

TX
Must be based on the patient's hemodynamic status not just CT AAST Grade (see below).

American Association for the Surgery of Trauma, Grades:
I Hematoma Subcapsular, <10% surface area or Laceration, <1 cm parenchymal depth
II Hematoma Subcapsular, 10-50% surface area or Laceration 1-3 cm parenchymal depth
III Hematoma Subcapsular, >50% surface area or Laceration >3 cm parenchymal depth
IV Laceration involving 25-75% of lobe or 1-3 Coinaud's segments in a single lobe
V Laceration involving >75% of lobe or >3 Coinaud's segments within a single lobe or Vascular Juxtahepatic venous injuries i.e. vena cava/central major hepatic veins
VI Vascular Hepatic Avulsion

LIVER LACERATION

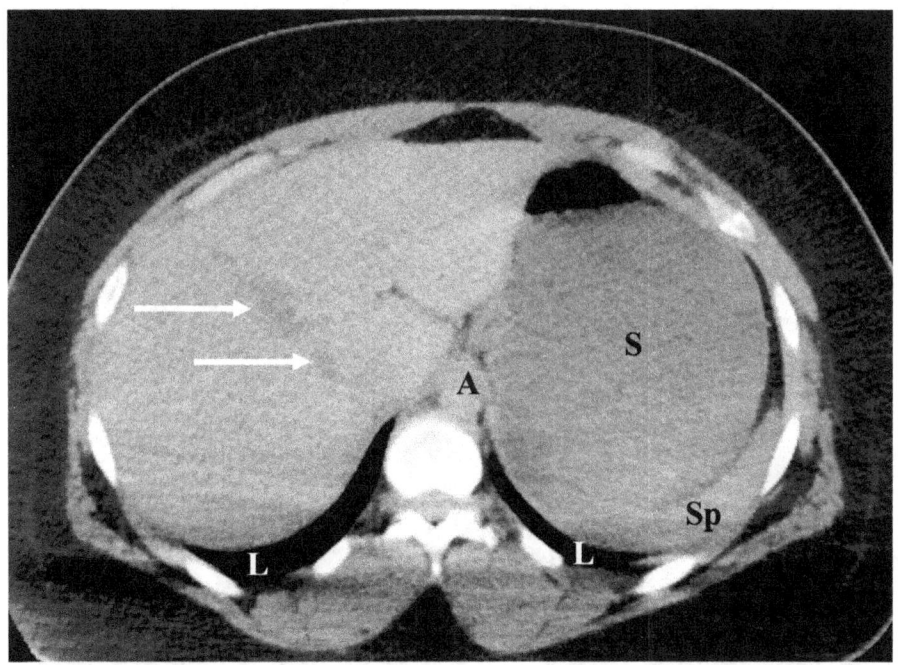

Study:
CT Abdomen with IV contrast at the level of the upper abdomen.

Radiographic Findings:
There is a linear area of hypoattenuation seen traversing the right hepatic lobe which is consistent with laceration (arrows), AAST Grade III.

Tips
Delayed imaging is necessary for all visceral trauma (AAST guidelines).
When an organ laceration is seen, evaluate for contrast pooling on delayed imaging which signifies sentinel clot (active extravasation).
Complications from biliary injury can result in biloma, abscess formation, arterio-biliary fistula, or stricture.
When grading, advance 1 grade for multiple injuries up to grade III.

Normal Anatomy
S – Stomach, Sp – Spleen, A – Aorta, L – Lung

Further Reading
Friedman J, Wilcyznski T, Maheshwar N, Bianco B. CT imaging and Interventional Radiology in Solid Organ Injury. JAOCR 2019; Vol. 8, Issue 3

CASE 62

CASE AUTHOR: Maqsood Kahn

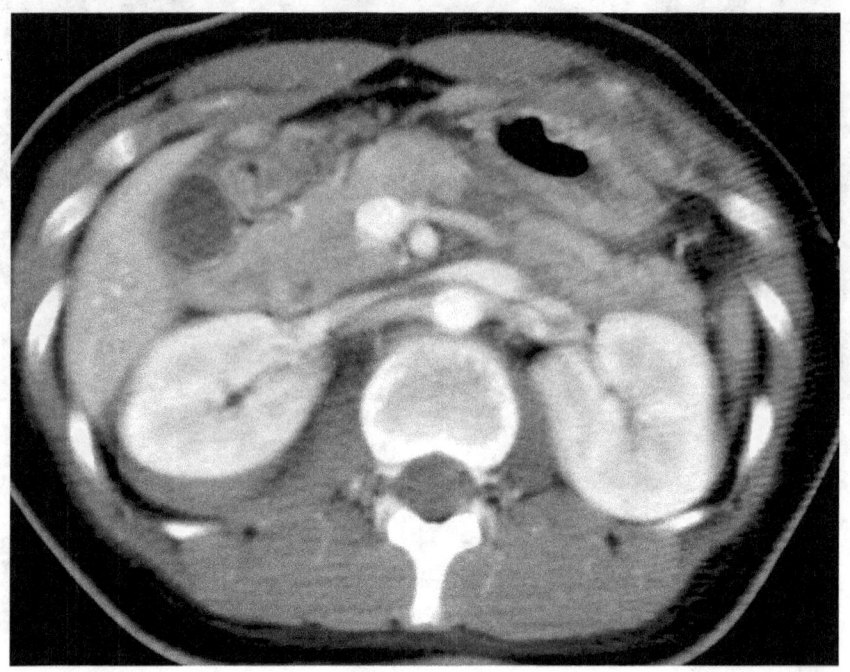

Best CT Study for Diagnosis:
CT Abdomen with IV contrast

Key to DX
Linear low attenuation traversing the pancreatic parenchyma.

Facts
Present with epigastric pain after injury such as handlebar or steering wheel impact.
Most commonly seen in young adults and children due to paucity of protective body fat. Associated clinical findings include seat belt sign and flank hematoma.

TX
Requires intervention with Grades III to V (surgical or endoscopic).

American Association for the Surgery of Trauma, Grades:
I Hematoma minor without duct injury or Laceration superficial without duct injury
II Hematoma major contusion without duct injury or Laceration major without duct injury or tissue loss
III Laceration distal transection or parenchymal injury with duct injury
IV Laceration proximal transection or parenchymal injury involving ampulla
V Laceration massive disruption of pancreatic head

PANCREATIC LACERATION

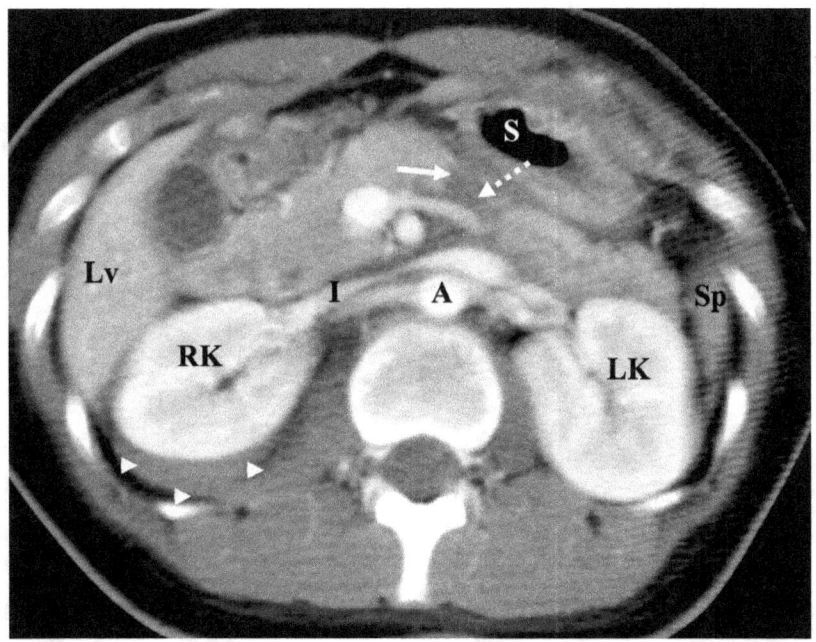

Study Above:
CT Abdomen with IV contrast at the level of the upper abdomen.

Radiographic Findings:
A linear area of hypoattenuation is seen traversing the distal pancreatic body consistent with a laceration (arrow), AAST Grade III. Low attenuation is present behind the pancreatic bed consistent with hemorrhage (dashed arrow). Right kidney crescent shaped low attenuation represents a subcapsular hematoma (arrowheads).

Tips
Delineate the laceration with respect to the pancreatic duct because duct injury necessitates intervention.
Pancreatic injuries are associated with other visceral injuries; so, double check!
Pancreatic injury is delineated into direct (as in this case) and indirect findings. Indirect signs can include parenchymal contusions (subtle small areas of hypoattenuation) and peripancreatic edema.

Normal Anatomy
S – Stomach, Sp – Spleen, A – Aorta, I - Inferior vena cava, Lv – Liver, RK - Right kidney, LK - Left kidney

Further Reading
Ayoob A, Lee J, Herr K, Lebedis C, et al. Pancreatic trauma: Imaging Review and Management Update. *Radiographics* 2020.

CASE 63

CASE AUTHOR: Elias Antypas

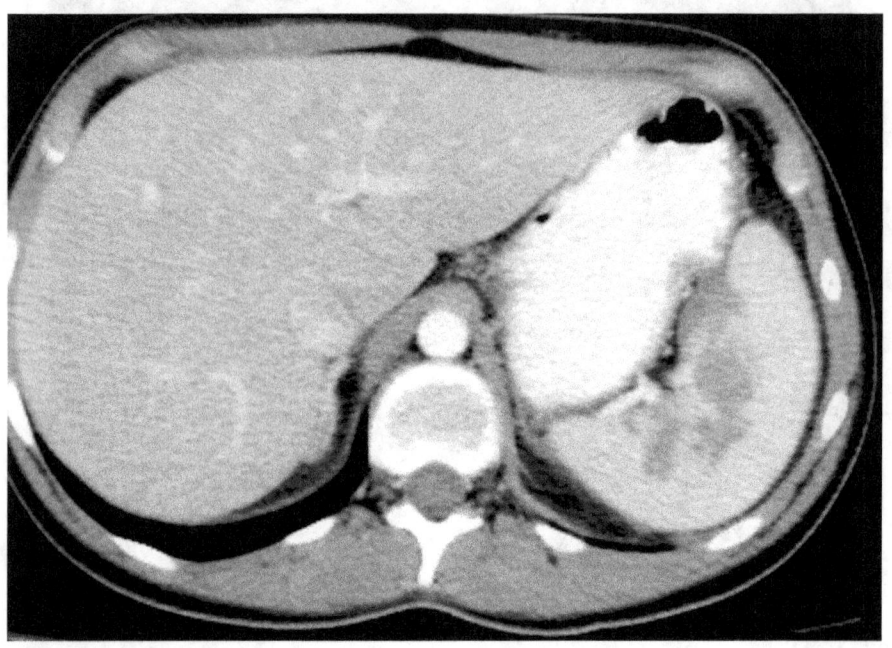

Best CT Study for Diagnosis:
CT Abdomen with IV contrast

Key to DX
Irregular, linear, or branching non-enhancing low attenuation in the splenic parenchyma.

TX
Conservative treatment with grades I-III. Patient's hemodynamic stability is paramount.

American Association for the Surgery of Trauma, Grades:
I Hematoma Subcapsular, <10% surface area or Laceration <1 cm parenchymal depth
II Hematoma Subcapsular, 10-50% surface or Laceration 1-3 cm parenchymal depth not involving a parenchymal vessel
III Hematoma Subcapsular, >50% surface area or Laceration >3 cm parenchymal depth IV Laceration of segmental or hilar vessels producing devascularization/infarct (>25%) V Shattered spleen or Vascular hilar injury with devascularized spleen

SPLENIC LACERATION

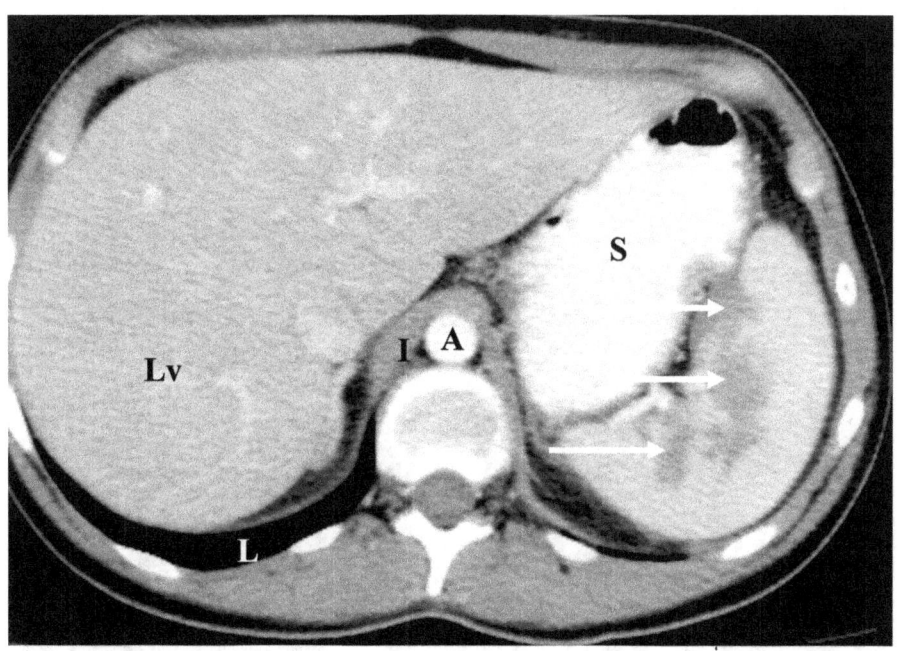

Study Above:
CT Abdomen with IV contrast at the level of the upper abdomen.

Radiographic Findings:
Linear, irregular branching areas of hypoattenuation seen traversing the spleen consistent with lacerations (arrows), AAST Grade III.

Tips
Don't forget to check delayed imaging for "sentinel clot" (highest density blood) which indicates active hemorrhage. This can occur without a discrete laceration.
When grading, advance 1 grade for multiple injuries up to grade III.

Normal Anatomy
S - Stomach, Lv - Liver, A - Aorta, I - Inferior vena cava, L - Lung

Further Reading
Uyeda JW et al; Active hemorrhage and vascular injuries in splenic trauma: utility of the arterial phase in MDCT. Radiology. 2014. 270(1):99-106.

CASE 64

CASE AUTHOR: Reehan Ali

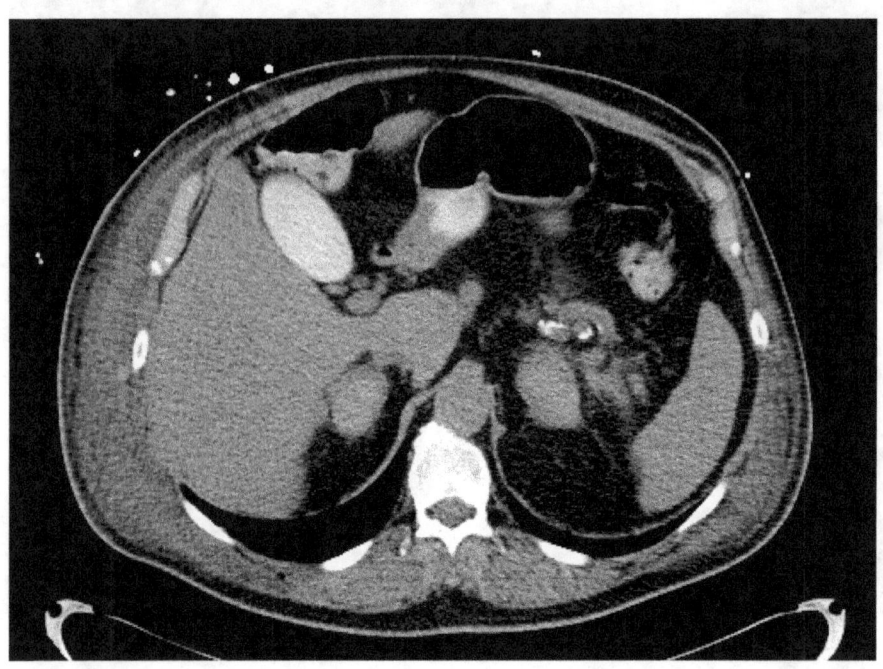

Best CT Study for Diagnosis:
CT Abdomen with IV contrast

Key to DX
Enlarged adrenal glands with increased attenuation.

Facts
May be associated with liver injury and IVC thrombosis.
Bilateral adrenal hemorrhage may result in adrenal insufficiency.

TX
Most of these injuries resolve spontaneously.

American Association for the Surgery of Trauma, Grades:
I Contusion
II Laceration involving only cortex (<2 cm)
III Laceration extending into medulla (> 2 cm)
IV >50% parenchymal destruction
V Total parenchymal destruction (massive hemorrhage) or avulsion from blood supply

ADRENAL HEMATOMA

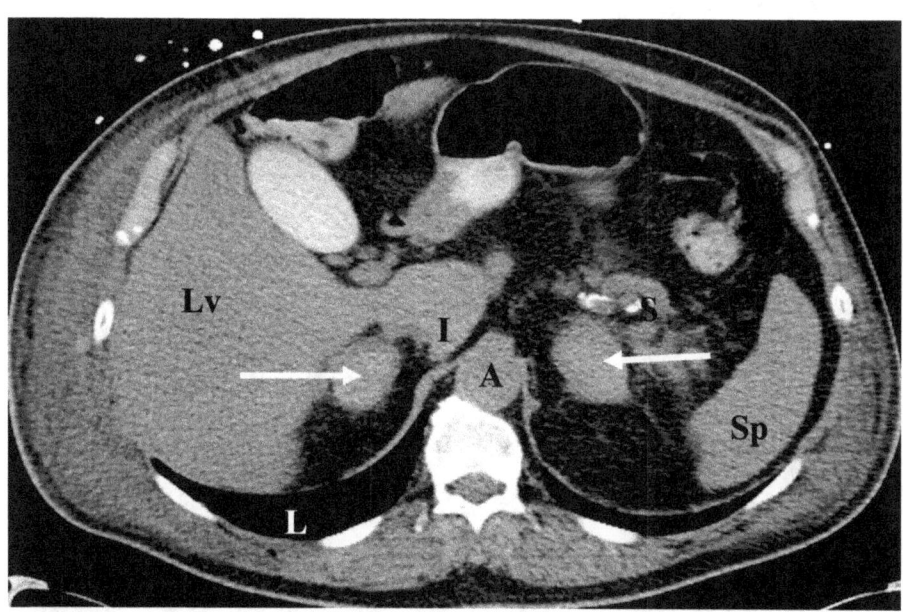

Study Above:
CT Abdomen without IV contrast at the level of the adrenal glands.

Radiographic Findings:
Large, round area of hyperattenuation replacing the adrenal glands consistent with hematomas (arrows). These hematomas are AAST Grade IV.

Tips
The right adrenal gland is most commonly injured.
Periadrenal fat stranding is a good clue for an adrenal injury.
When grading, advance 1 grade for bilateral injuries up to grade IV.
Adrenal hematoma may be mimicked by an adenoma (use CT washout study or MR imaging with in and out of phase sequences if in doubt).

Normal Anatomy
S - Stomach, Sp - Spleen, Lv - Liver, A - Aorta, I - Inferior vena cava, L - Lung

Further Reading
Udare, A., Agarwal, M., Siegelman, E. et al. CT and MR imaging of acute adrenal disorders. Abdominal Radiology 46, 290–302, 2021.

CASE 65

CASE AUTHOR: Reehan Ali

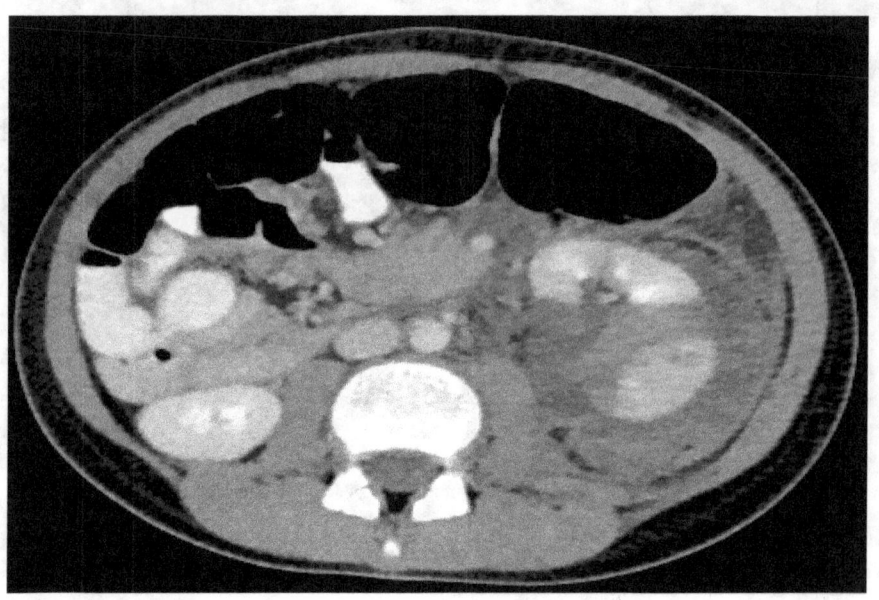

Best CT Study for Diagnosis:
CT Abdomen with IV contrast

Key to DX
Linear low attenuation traversing the renal parenchyma.

Facts
The most common cause is blunt trauma associated with motor vehicle accidents.
Urine extravasation is indicative of a Grade IV injury.

TX
AAST Grades I to III are typically treated non-surgically. Grades IV and V depend on the patient's hemodynamic stability.

American Association for the Surgery of Trauma, Grades:
I Subcapsular hematoma or contusion, without laceration
II Laceration ≤1 cm depth not involving the collecting system
III Laceration >1 cm not involving the collecting system
IV Laceration involving the collecting system with urinary extravasation OR laceration of the renal pelvis and/or complete ureteropelvic disruption OR vascular injury to segmental renal artery or vein OR segmental infarctions without associated active bleeding (i.e. due to vessel thrombosis) OR active bleeding extending beyond the perirenal fascia (i.e. into the retroperitoneum or peritoneum)
V Shattered kidney or Avulsion of renal hilum resulting in devascularized kidney

RENAL LACERATION

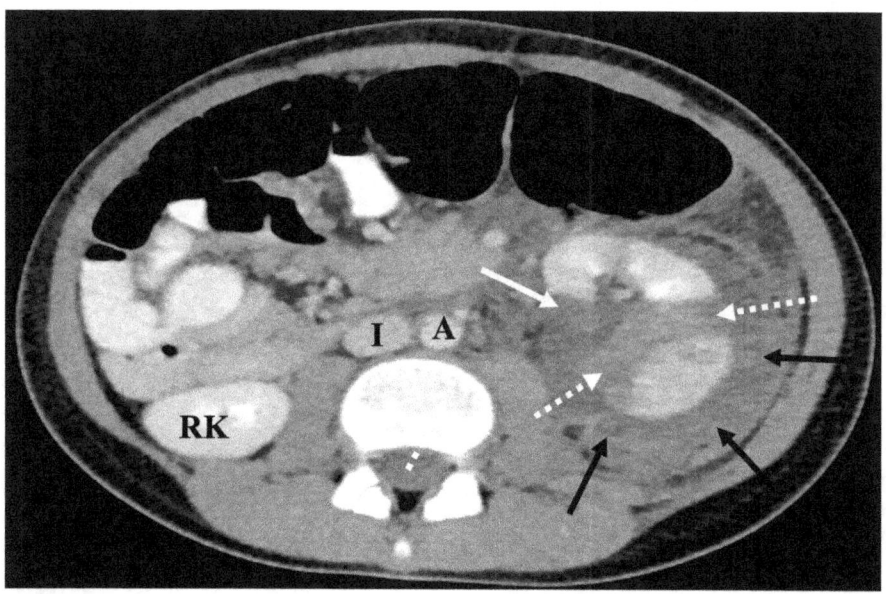

Study Above:
CT Abdomen with IV and oral contrast at the level of the kidneys.

Radiographic Findings:
A band of hypodense attenuation traverses the left renal cortex extending into the renal sinus consistent with a laceration (white dashed arrows). There is high density fluid in the left perinephric space consistent with perinephric hematoma (black arrows). Fluid density is seen in the hilum consistent with an urinoma (white arrow) from injury to the renal collecting system, AAST grade IV.

Normal Anatomy
RK - Right kidney, A - Aorta, I - Inferior vena cava

Further Reading
Kozar R, Crandall M, Shanmuganathan K et al. Organ Injury Scaling 2018 Update: Spleen, Liver, and Kidney. J Trauma Acute Care Surg. 85(6):1119-22, 2018.

CASE 66

CASE AUTHOR: Elias Antypas

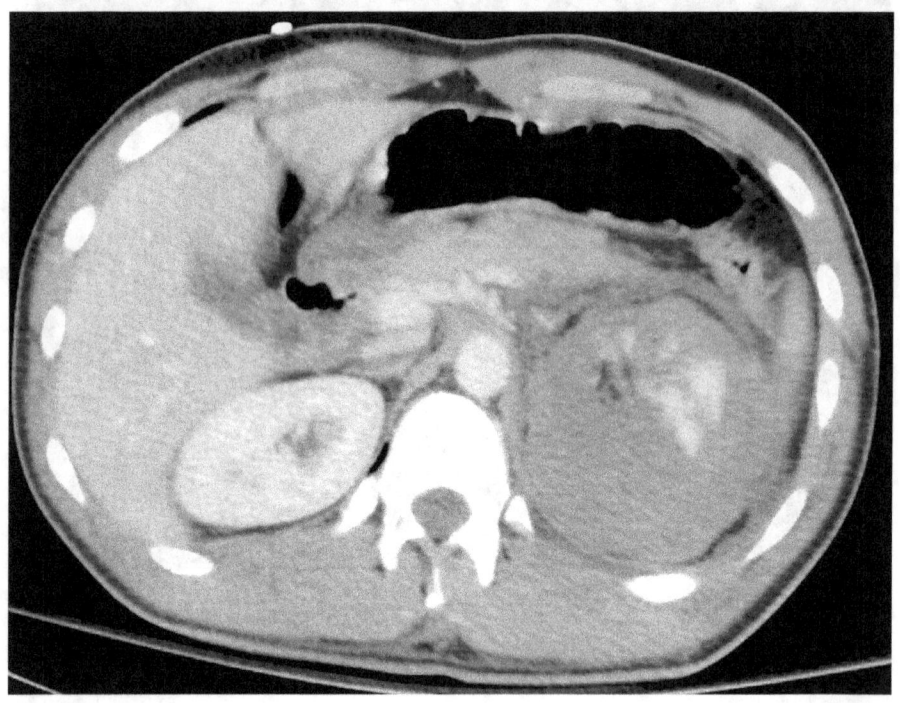

Best CT Study for Diagnosis:
CT Abdomen with IV contrast

Key to DX
Separated islands of vascularized or devascularized renal parenchyma.

TX
Most renal injuries are low grade and managed conservatively (98%). However, an advanced injury like this case requires intervention.
This patient presented after an ATV accident.
This patient had to undergo emergent nephrectomy (surgical removal) as he was hemodynamically unstable.

SHATTERED KIDNEY

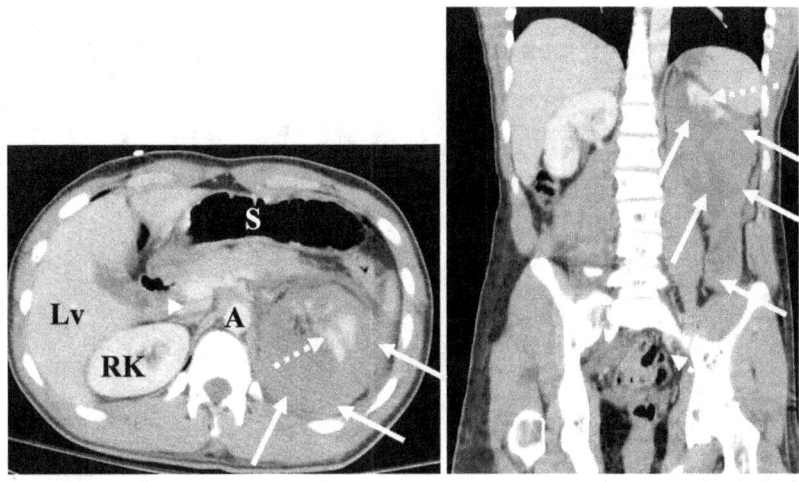

Study Above:
CT Abdomen and Pelvis with IV contrast, axial and coronal reformat (right).

Radiographic Findings:
Near complete low attenuation fills the left renal fossa extending into the pelvis (arrows), consistent with hematoma. Minimal areas of parenchymal contrast enhancement remain only in the left upper pole which indicates a significant vascular injury (dashed arrows). In addition, the inferior vena cava has a "flat" appearance instead of a round appearance (arrowhead).

Tips:
Multiphasic CT is the preferred modality. If laceration is evident on CT, delayed imaging at 10-12 minutes is helpful to evaluate for urine extravasation. Avulsion of ureteropelvic junction can be confirmed by extravasation of contrast enhanced urine during delayed imaging.

Normal Anatomy
S - Stomach, RK - Right kidney, Lv - Liver, A - Aorta, Arrowhead - Inferior vena cava

Further Reading
Berko NS et al. CT imaging of renal and ureteral emergencies. Curr Probl Diagn Radiol. 44(22):207-220, 2015.

CASE 67

CASE AUTHOR: Reehan Ali

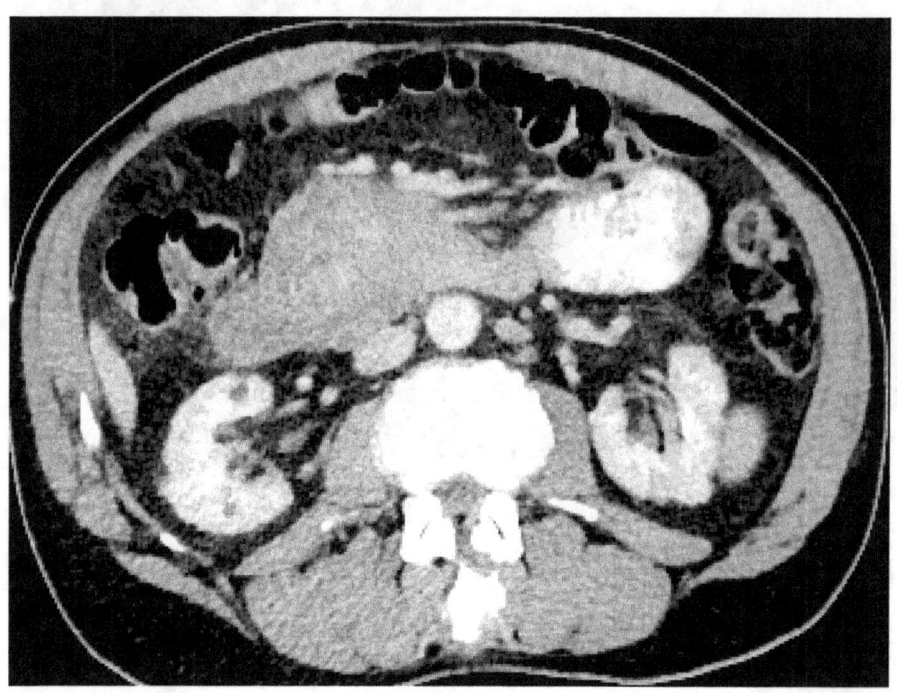

Best CT Study for Diagnosis:
CT Abdomen with IV contrast

Key to DX
Focal fluid attenuation adjacent to a bowel loop.

Facts
Common sites of injury are the proximal jejunum and near the ileocecal valve. Associated with anterior abdominal wall injury (look for seat belt sign).

TX
AAST Grades I to III are typically treated non-surgically. Must consider the patient's hemodynamic stability.

American Association for the Surgery of Trauma, Grades:
I Hematoma without devascularization OR partial thickness laceration, no perforation
II Laceration <50% of circumference
III Laceration > 50% of circumference without transection
IV Transection of the small bowel
V Transection of the small bowel with segmental tissue loss OR devascularized segment

BOWEL HEMATOMA

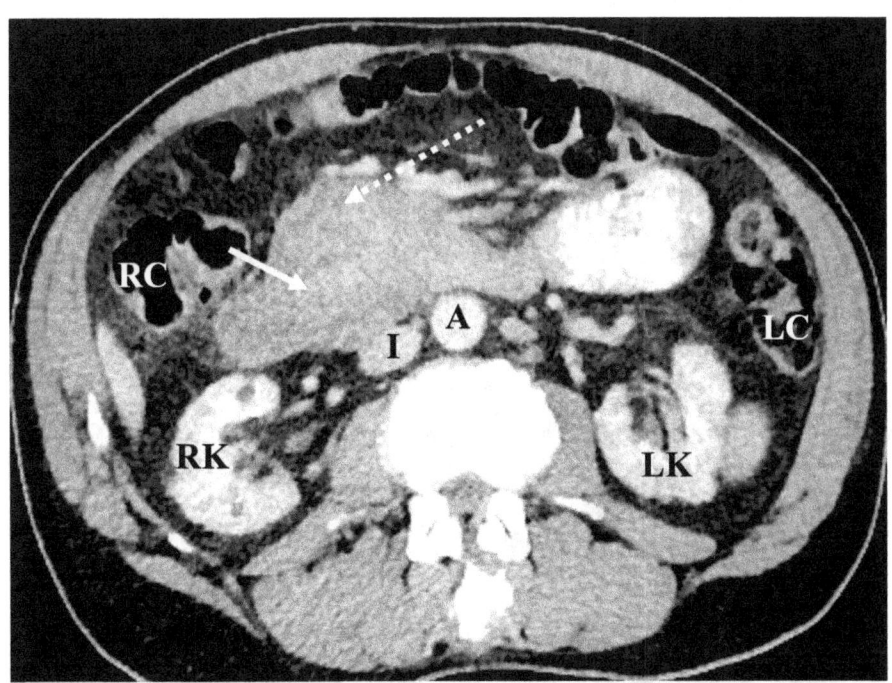

Study Above:
CT Abdomen with IV and oral contrast at the level of the duodenum.

Radiographic Findings
Presumed acute to subacute hematoma in the region of the second/third portion of the duodenum is seen. There is thickening of the duodenal wall (arrow) and heterogeneous fluid (hematoma) seen adjacent to the bowel wall (dashed arrow).

Tips
Assess the hematoma on delayed imaging for changes (enlargement indicates active bleeding).
All trauma cases should be done with multiple phases.
When grading, advance 1 grade for multiple injuries up to grade III.

Normal Anatomy
RK - Right kidney, LK - Left kidney, A - Aorta, I - Inferior vena cava, RC - Right colon,
LC - Left colon

Further Reading
Sugi MD, Menias CO, Lubner MG et al. CT Findings of Acute Small-Bowel Entities. *RadioGraphics*; 38(5):1352–1369, 2018.

CASE 68

CASE AUTHOR: Elias Antypas

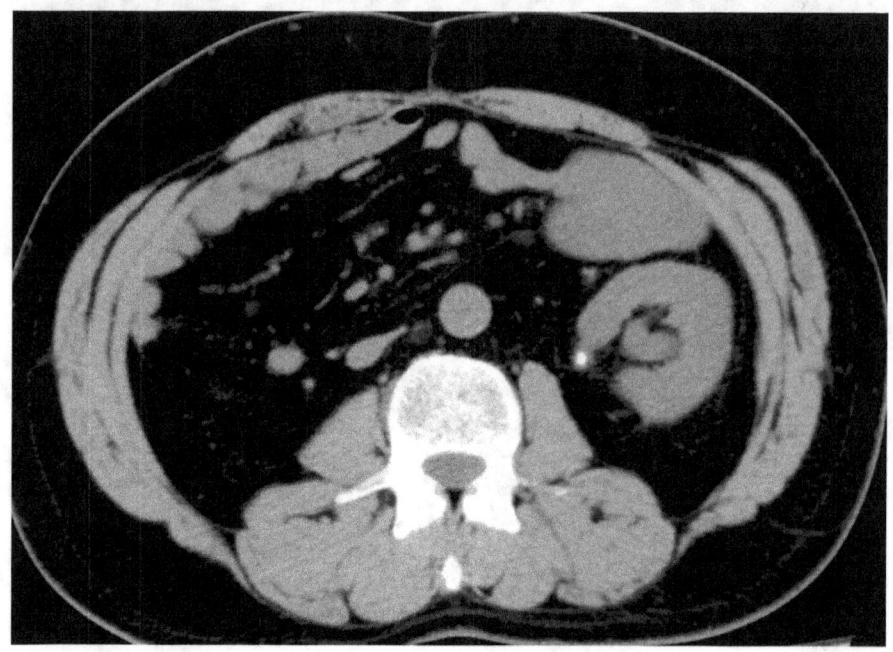

Best CT Study for Diagnosis:
CT Abdomen and Pelvis without contrast

Key to DX
Calcified density within the collecting system.

Facts
Patients will typically present with colicky flank pain. Nonspecific symptoms include abdominal pain, nausea, or vomiting. There is microscopic hematuria in 90% of patients.
If the stone becomes lodged in the distal ureter, it is usually associated with pain radiating into the ipsilateral groin.
Most commonly stones are calcium oxalate composition.
Up to 60% of stones less than 5 mm will pass spontaneously.
An obstructed kidney may spontaneously decompress creating an urinoma.

TX
Medical treatments depend on stone size. ESWL is used for proximal ureteral calculi < 1 cm and mid/upper pole < 2 cm. Nephrolithotomy is used for larger stone burden/treatment failure. If hypercalciuria is present, increasing fluid intake and decreasing dietary sodium and calcium to recommended levels is recommended.

NEPHROLITHIASIS

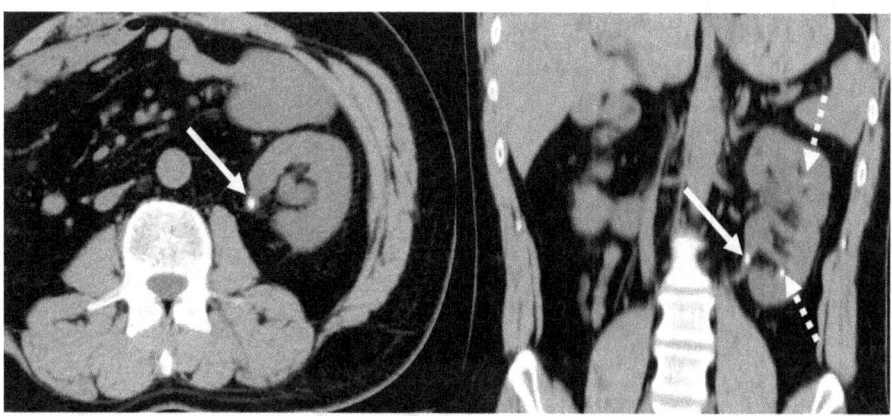

Study Above:
CT Abdomen without contrast, axial and coronal reformat (right).

Radiographic Findings:
Oval calcified structure in the proximal ureter is consistent with an ureterolith (arrows). Additionally, two other stones are seen (dashed arrows) in the left renal calyces and are non-obstructive.

Tips:
Non-contrast CT is the most sensitive to detect stones as intravenous contrast would hide stones (both stones and IV contrast are white).

Prone positioning may be helpful to distinguish UVJ obstructed stone vs bladder stone.

In patients with a history of nephrolithiasis, the presence or absence of obstruction may be the only imaging question and ultrasound can be used instead of CT (avoiding radiation and decreasing cost).

Further Reading
Berko NS et al. CT imaging of renal and ureteral emergencies. Curr Probl Diagn Radiol. 44(22):207-220, 2015.

CASE 69

CASE AUTHOR: Andrew Mizzi

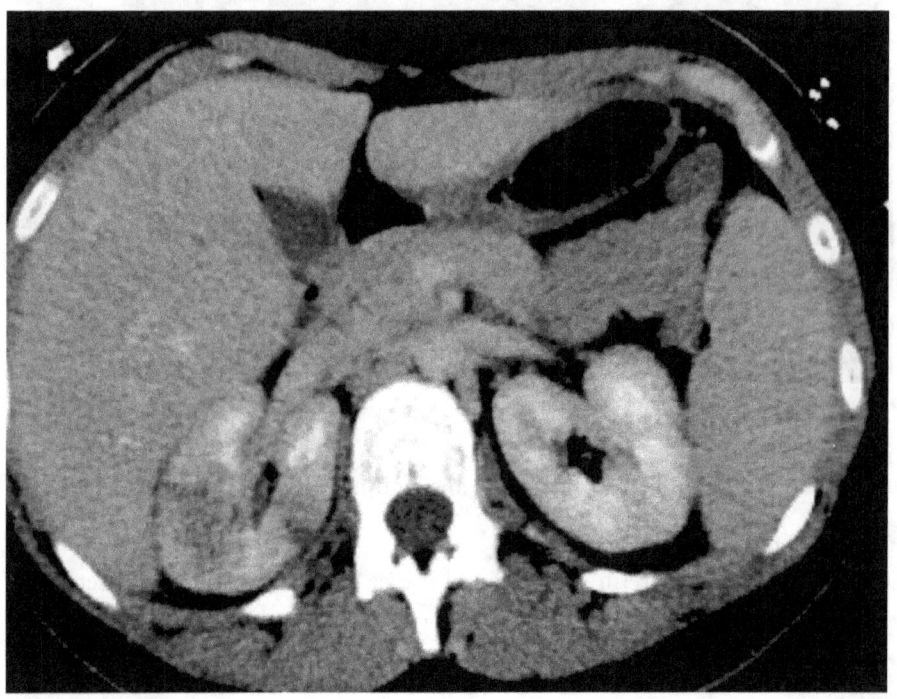

Best CT Study for Diagnosis:
CT Abdomen with IV contrast

Key to DX
Patchy low attenuation involving the renal parenchyma.

Facts
Patients usually present with dysuria, fever, and flank pain.
Starts as lower urinary tract infection. More common in females (shorter urethra).
Most common bug is Escherichia *coli*.
Complicating factors include emphysematous pyelonephritis, hydronephrosis, and abscess.

TX
Antibiotics to treat infection.

PYELONEPHRITIS

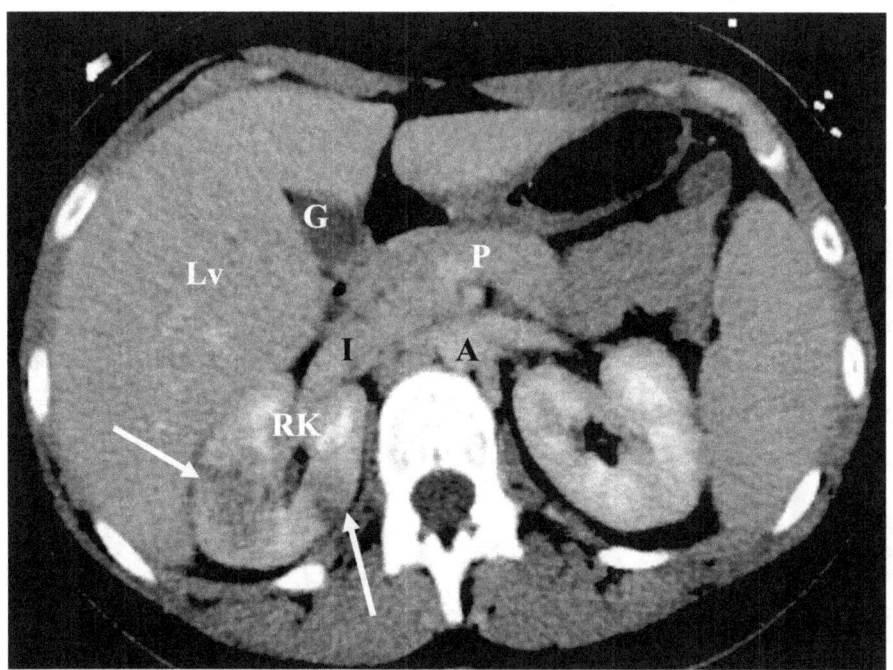

Study Above:
CT Abdomen with IV and oral contrast at the level of the mid kidneys.

Radiographic Findings:
Heterogeneous enhancement of the right renal cortex with focal patchy areas of low attenuation seen (arrows).

Tips
Check for a partially obstructing ureterolith which may be the cause.
Interrogate the kidney and collecting system for air which would signify a more serious infection. Emphysematous pyelonephritis (gas in parenchyma) is worse than emphysematous pyelitis (gas in the collecting system).

Normal Anatomy
A - Aorta, I - Inferior vena cava, G - Gallbladder, Lv - Liver, P – Pancreas, RK – Right kidney

Further Reading
Lacy,M.E., M.D., et al. When does acute pyelonephritis require imaging? Cleveland Clinic Journal of Medicine Aug, 86 (8) 515-517, 2019.

CASE 70

CASE AUTHOR: Juliann Giese

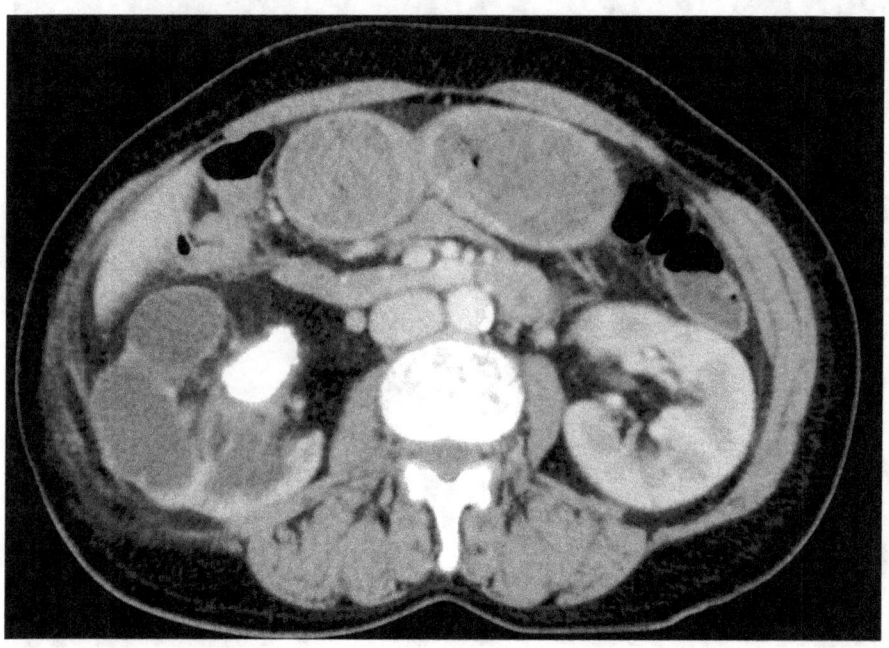

Best CT Study for Diagnosis:
CT Abdomen and Pelvis with IV Contrast

Key to DX
Enlarged kidney with dilated calyces and a staghorn calculus.

Facts
Most common in women with a history of chronic UTI and/or obstructive renal calculi.
May present with fever, flank pain, and palpable mass.
Rare disease entity (1% of renal infections).
Most common bugs are *E.coli* and *Proteus*.
Damaged renal parenchyma replaced by lipid-laden macrophages (xanthoma cells).

TX
Antibiotics prior to surgical intervention; open nephrectomy is often required.

XANTHOGRANULOMATOUS PYELONEPHRITIS (XGP)

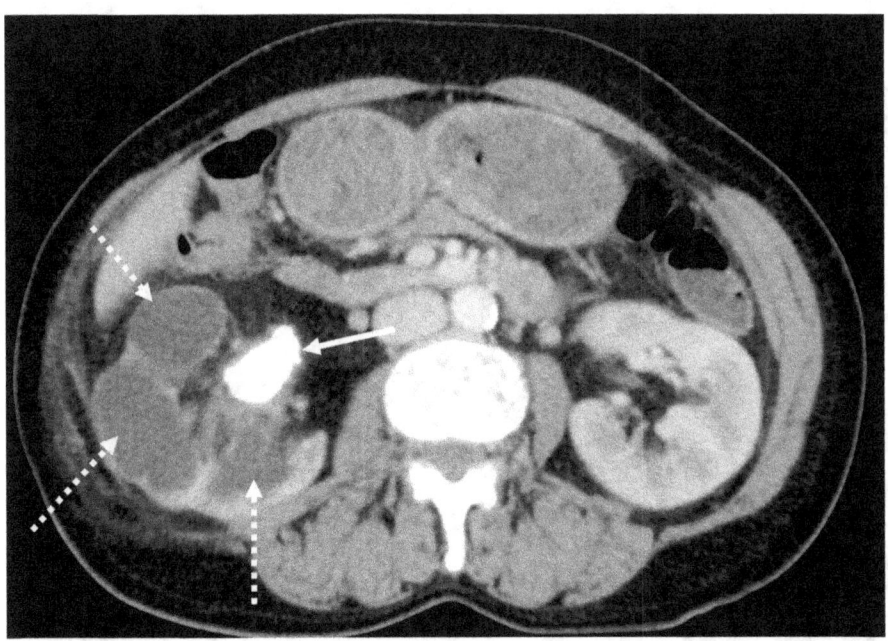

Study Above:
CT Abdomen and Pelvis with IV contrast at the level of the mid kidneys.

Radiographic findings:
The right kidney is enlarged and edematous with perinephric fat stranding and enlarged fluid-filled calyces mimicking a "bear paw" (dashed arrows). A large obstructive staghorn calculus is present within the renal pelvis (arrow).

Tips
Look for an enlarged non-functioning kidney with preserved reniform morphology, centrally obstructive staghorn calculus, dilated calyces (bear paw sign), and cortical thinning.
Histologic diagnosis is required to solidify diagnosis, which is often made at time of nephrectomy.
Top differential diagnoses include renal abscess, pyonephrosis, and malignancy. Evaluate for possible complications such as adjacent psoas muscle abscess and GI fistula formation.

Further Reading
Naeem, Muhammad, et al. "Imaging Spectrum of Granulomatous Diseases of the Abdomen and Pelvis." *RadioGraphics* 200172, 2021.

CASE 71

CASE AUTHOR: Andrew Mizzi

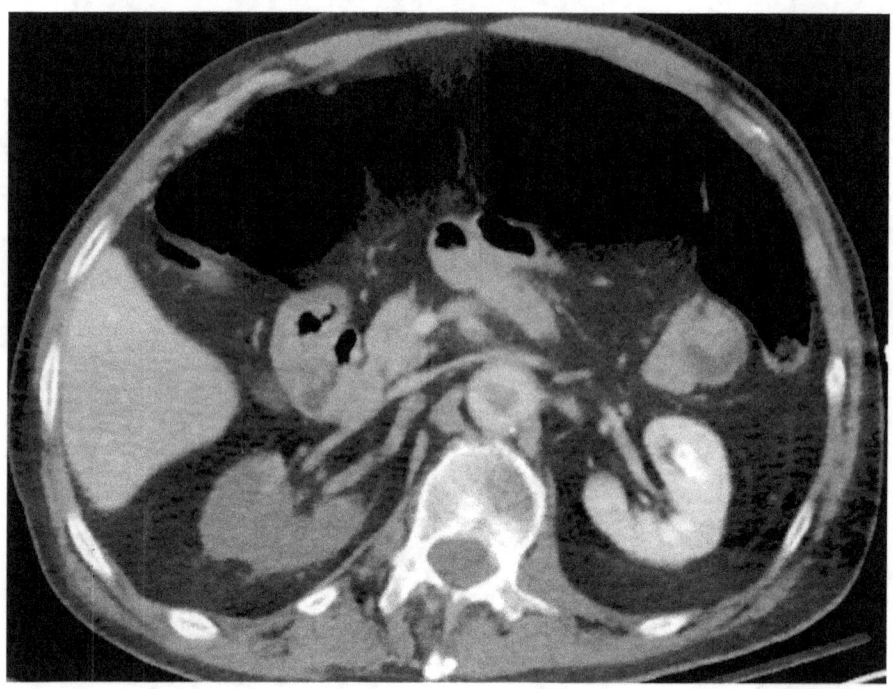

Best CT Study for Diagnosis:
CT Abdomen with IV contrast

Key to DX
Global or wedge shaped area of low attenuation involving the renal parenchyma.

Facts
Patients may present with flank pain, fever, and elevated white count.
This CT appearance is non-specific and could represent tumor, infection, or infarct.
Etiologies include thrombus/embolism, trauma, and renal artery stenosis.

TX
Underlying etiology must be addressed.
If etiology is renal artery stenosis, stenting or angioplasty may be of benefit.
Anticoagulants and thrombolytics may be useful.

RENAL INFARCT

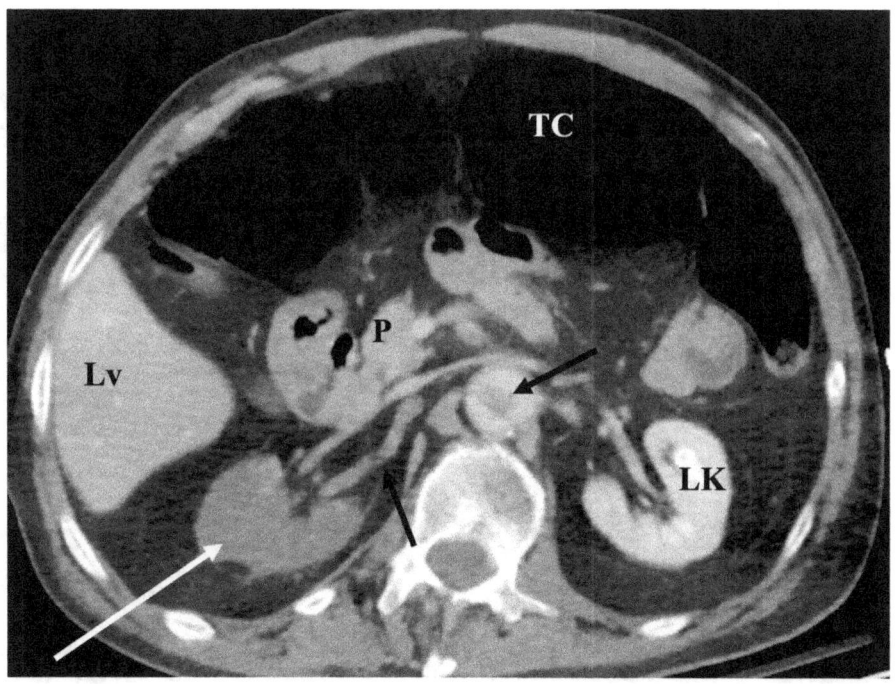

Study Above:
CT Abdomen with IV and oral contrast at the level of the mid kidneys.

Radiographic Findings:
Global low attenuation of the right kidney (white arrow). Note thrombi in the aorta and the right renal artery (black arrows).

Tips
Check the aorta and renal artery for thrombus.
Interrogate other organs for infarcts.

Normal Anatomy
LK - Left kidney, P - Pancreas, TC - Transverse colon, Lv - Liver

Further Reading
D. Radcliffe, M.D., H. Kotecha, D.O. JAOCR at the Viewbox: Spontaneous Renal Artery Dissection: J Am Osteopath Coll Radiol; Vol. 9, Issue 2, 2020.

CASE 72

CASE AUTHOR: Rocky Saenz

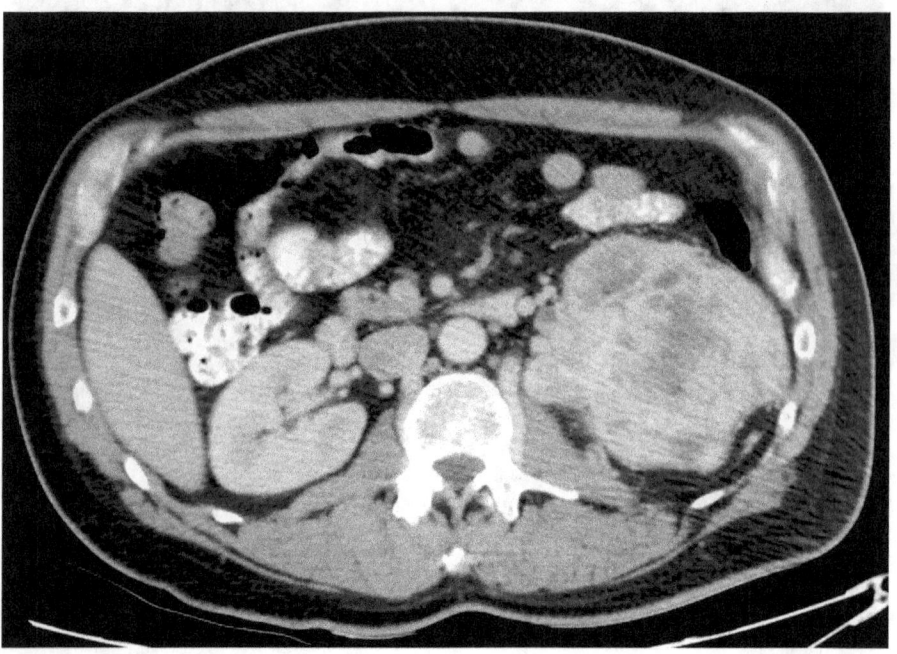

Best CT Study for Diagnosis:
CT Abdomen with IV contrast

Key to DX
Focal soft tissue lesion involving the left kidney.

Facts
Most common primary malignancy of the kidney is renal cell carcinoma.
Less likely renal malignancies include lymphoma and transitional cell carcinoma.
Classic clinical triad for renal cell carcinoma: flank mass, hematuria, and pain.
Any solid renal mass should be considered malignant until proven otherwise.

TX
CT guided biopsy for diagnosis.
Surgical removal for malignancy

RENAL CELL CARCINOMA

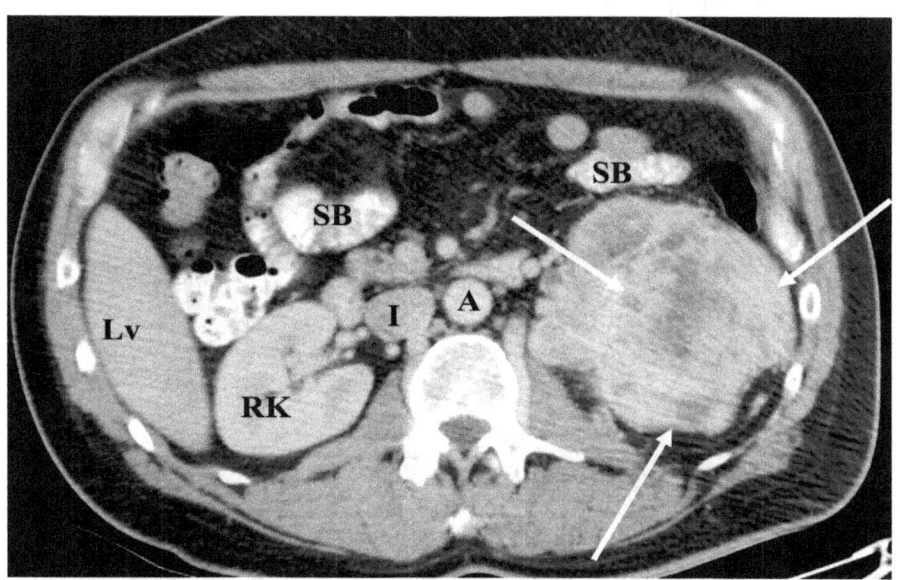

Study Above:
CT Abdomen with IV and oral contrast at the level of the mid kidneys.

Radiographic Findings:
An irregular, contrast enhancing soft tissue mass is seen projecting from the left renal parenchyma (arrows).

Tips
Dynamic CT with IV contrast (renal mass protocol) may be of benefit to confirm mass.
Coronal reformats may be very helpful in detection of a mass.
Interrogate the ipsilateral collecting system and bladder for "drop" metastases.

Normal Anatomy
RK - Right kidney, A - Aorta, I - Inferior vena cava, Lv - Liver, SB – Small bowel

Further Reading
Hötker AM, Karlo CA, Zheng J, Moskowitz CS, Russo P, Hricak H, Akin O. Clear Cell Renal Cell Carcinoma: Associations Between CT Features and Patient Survival.. AJR. 2016 Mar;1-8(1-8):1-8.

CASE 73

CASE AUTHOR: Juliann Giese

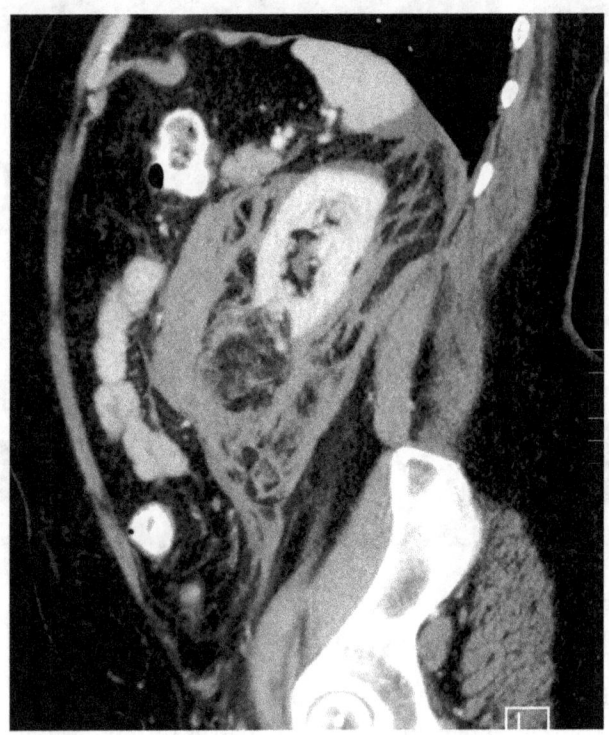

Best CT Study for Diagnosis:
CT Abdomen and Pelvis with IV contrast (dynamic-phase renal mass protocol)

Key to DX
Hemorrhaging fat-containing renal mass with hematoma.

Facts
Spontaneous, non-traumatic renal hemorrhage into the subcapsular and peri-renal spaces.
Most common cause is renal angiomyolipoma (AML), a benign, fat-containing mass.
AMLs have an increased risk of rupture when larger than 4 cm.
AMLs are most commonly seen in middle-aged females, however, 20% of lesions are associated with tuberous sclerosis and are often bilateral.
Associated with Lenk's triad of acute flank pain, palpable flank mass, and hypovolemic shock (Lenk's triad is present in 25% of cases, but flank pain is seen in 75%).

TX
If stable, conservative management and follow-up interventional radiology embolization.
If unstable, aggressive hydration, blood transfusion, and nephrectomy.

WUNDERLICH SYNDROME

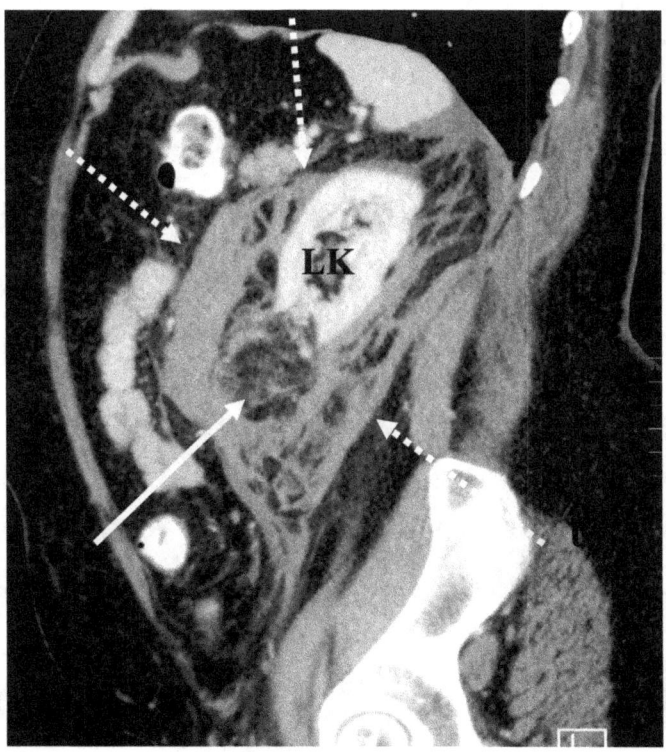

Study Above:
CT Abdomen and pelvis with IV and oral contrast, sagittal reformat of the left kidney.

Radiographic findings:
Sagittal view demonstrates complex fluid surrounding the left kidney (LK) compatible with perirenal hemorrhage (dashed arrows). Hypoattenuating fat-containing lower pole renal mass is noted consistent with AML (arrows).

Tips
CT diagnosis of AML is made by finding a focus of fat measuring less than -40 HU.
Size of lesion directly correlates with risk of spontaneous rupture.
Don't forget AMLs do enhance, so don't consider RCC as a diagnosis.
Wunderlich syndrome is most commonly caused by a hemorrhagic mass (such as AML or RCC) followed by a vascular abnormality, such as polyarteritis nodosa.

Further Reading
Helley, Neal H., Matthew P. Borloz, and William J. Frohna. "Female with Flank Pain and Hypotension. Journal of Emergency Medicine (2013): e19-e20.

CASE 74

CASE AUTHOR: Juliann Giese

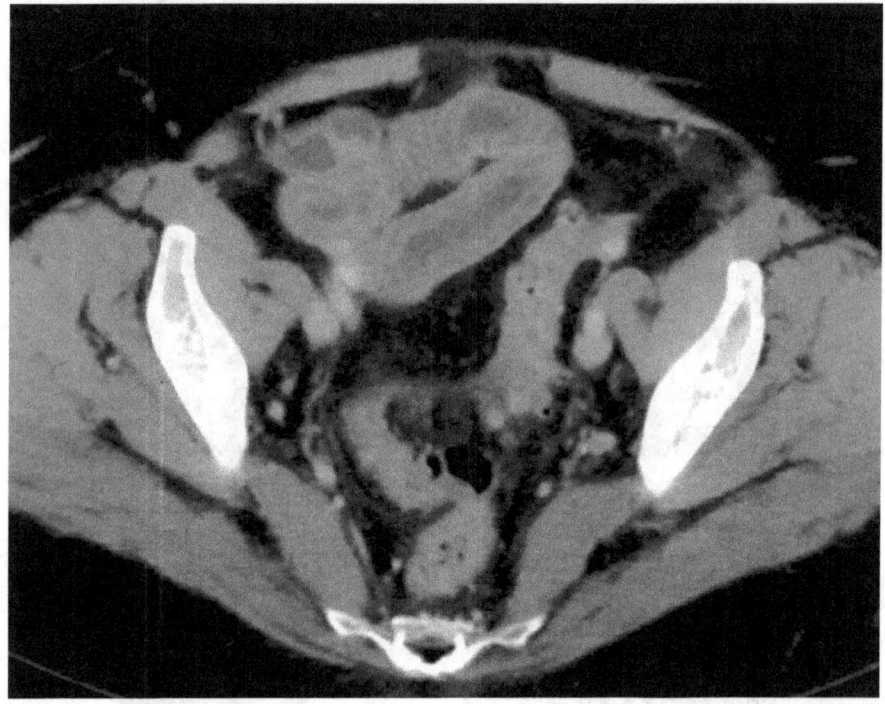

Best CT Study for Diagnosis:
CT Abdomen and Pelvis with IV contrast

Key to DX
Long-segment, circumferential small bowel wall thickening greater than 3 mm with wall hyperemia.

Facts
Patients may present with abdominal cramping, fever, and diarrhea.

CT appearance of bowel wall thickening is non-specific. Primary differential includes infectious, inflammatory, ischemic and carcinoma (3 I's and don't forget C, thanks R. Saenz). So pertinent patient history is essential!

TX
Typically supportive.
Endoscopic biopsy results and stool cultures are often needed for correct diagnosis.

ENTERITIS

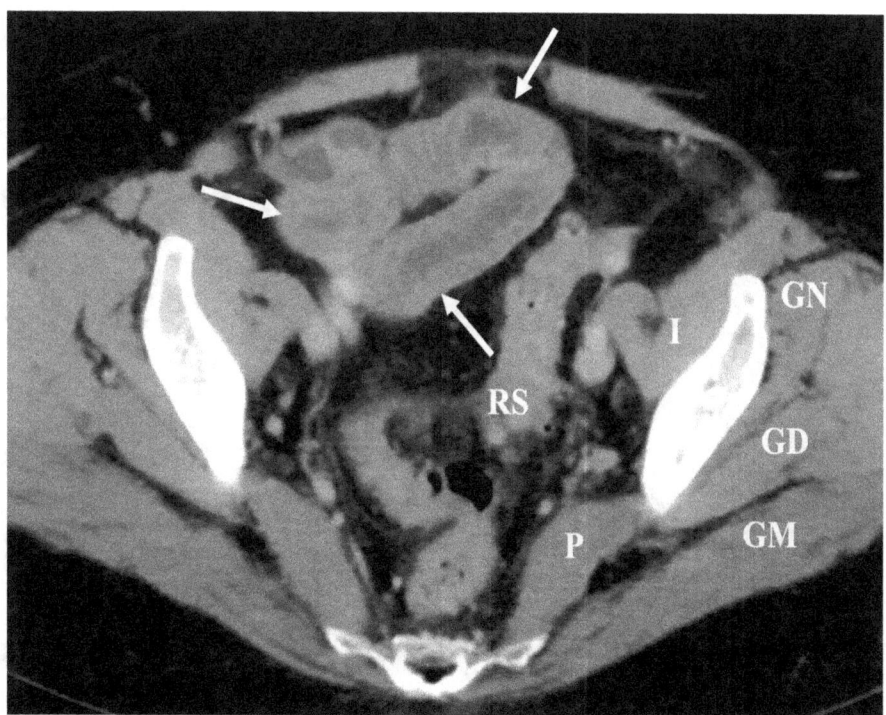

Study Above:
CT Pelvis with IV contrast at the level of the pelvis.

Radiographic Findings:
Long segment, circumferential bowel wall thickening with wall hyperemia of the ileum (arrows). Incidental note is made of rectosigmoid colon (RSC) diverticulosis without evidence of diverticulitis.

Tips
Remember small bowel wall thickness must measure greater than 3 mm to be abnormal.
Peripheral fat stranding may be present, which indicates an acute or subacute process.

Normal Anatomy
RS – Rectosigmoid colon, GN - Gluteus minimus, GD – Gluteus medius, GM - Gluteus maximus, P - Piriformis, I - Iliopsoas

Further Reading
Boyd, SK., Hobson, JJ., Cameron, JD., Saenz, RC. "CT Imaging of Large Bowel Wall Thickening". JAOCR, 2016; Vol. 5, Issue 2

CASE 75

CASE AUTHOR: Rocky Saenz

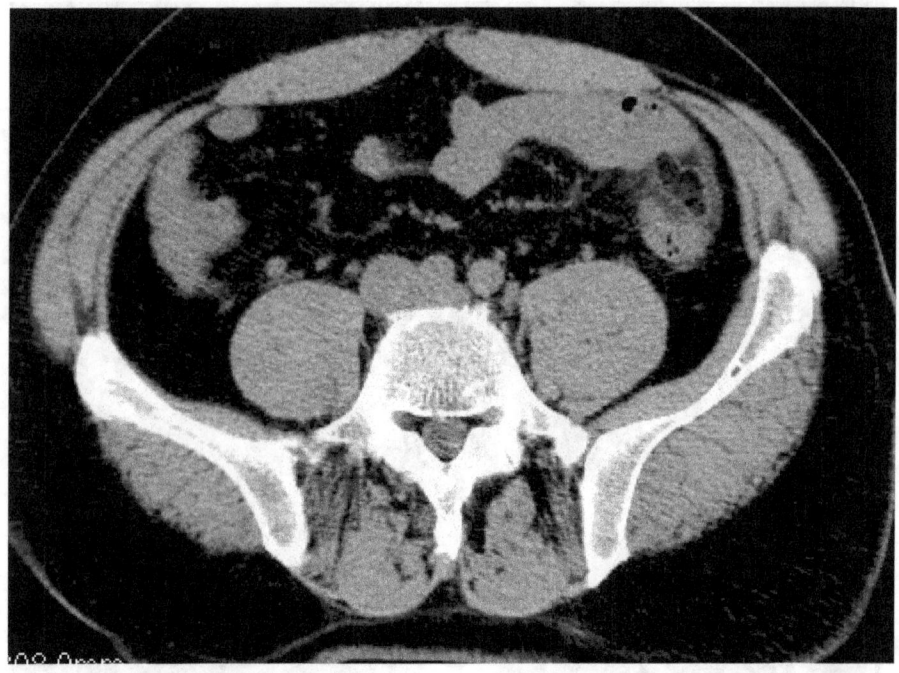

Best CT Study for Diagnosis:
CT Abdomen and Pelvis with IV contrast

Key to DX
Focal fat stranding surrounding a fatty mass adjacent to the colon.

Facts
Patients present with focal pain and a mildly elevated white count.
Epiploic appendages are normal fat structures associated with the colon.
This occurs due to strangulation of the epiploic appendage.
Epiploic appendagitis is not a surgical case!

TX
Usually supportive treatment with pain management, as it is usually self-limited.
Antibiotic therapy is debatable.

EPIPLOIC APPENDAGITIS

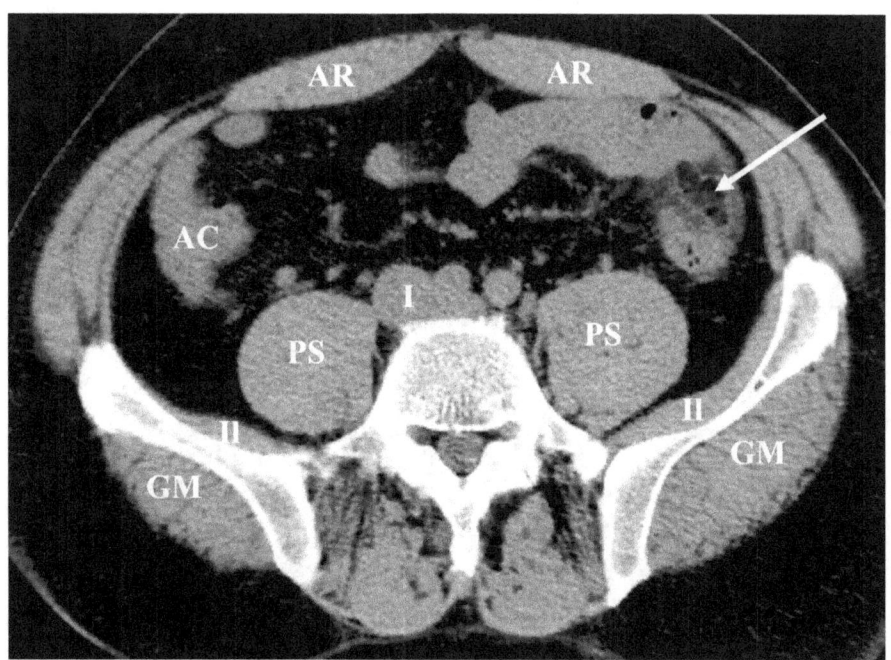

Study Above:
CT Pelvis without contrast at the level of the mid pelvis.

Radiographic Findings:
A globular focus of fat attenuation is noted anterior to the descending colon with associated peripheral fat-stranding. The fat globule represents the infarcted epiploic appendage (arrow) with surrounding inflammation.

Tips
Remember there is differential for pericolonic fat stranding: diverticulitis (most common), epiploic appendagitis, colitis, inflammatory bowel disease and adenocarcinoma (most common location sigmoid colon).
Diagnosis is diverticulitis when fat stranding surrounds a diverticulum.
Always check around bowel for microperforation (tiny adjacent air bubbles).

Normal Anatomy
PS - Psoas muscle, AC - Ascending colon, I - Inferior vena cava
GM - Gluteus maximus muscle, Il - Iliacus muscle
AR - Abdominus rectus muscles

Further Reading
Saenz RC. Top 3 Differentials in Gastrointestinal Imaging, A case Review. Chapter 3. Thieme. 2019.

CASE 76

CASE AUTHOR: Rocky Saenz

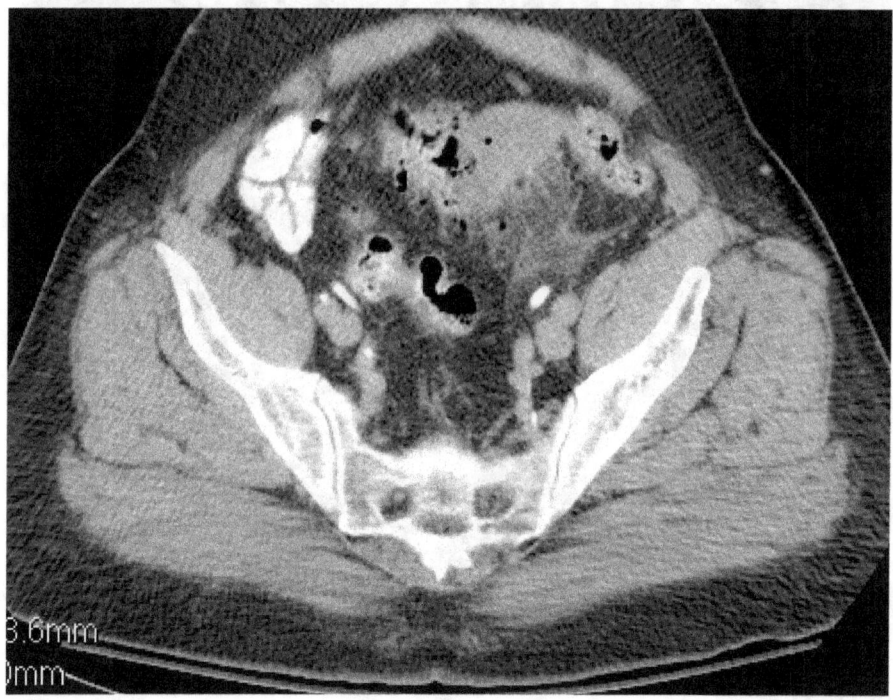

Best CT Study for Diagnosis:
CT Abdomen and Pelvis with IV and oral contrast

Key to DX
Focal fat-stranding surrounding a diverticulum.

Facts
Patients usually present with focal abdominal pain, cramping, and fever.
50% of adults over 50 have diverticulosis.
May be an elusive clinical diagnosis as any part of the colon can be involved.
Sigmoid colon is the most common location.

TX
Antibiotic treatment in non-complicated cases.
Complex cases with abscess formation may require CT drainage with catheter placement (Radiology to the rescue!).
Cases exacerbated by perforation may need surgical intervention.

DIVERTICULITIS

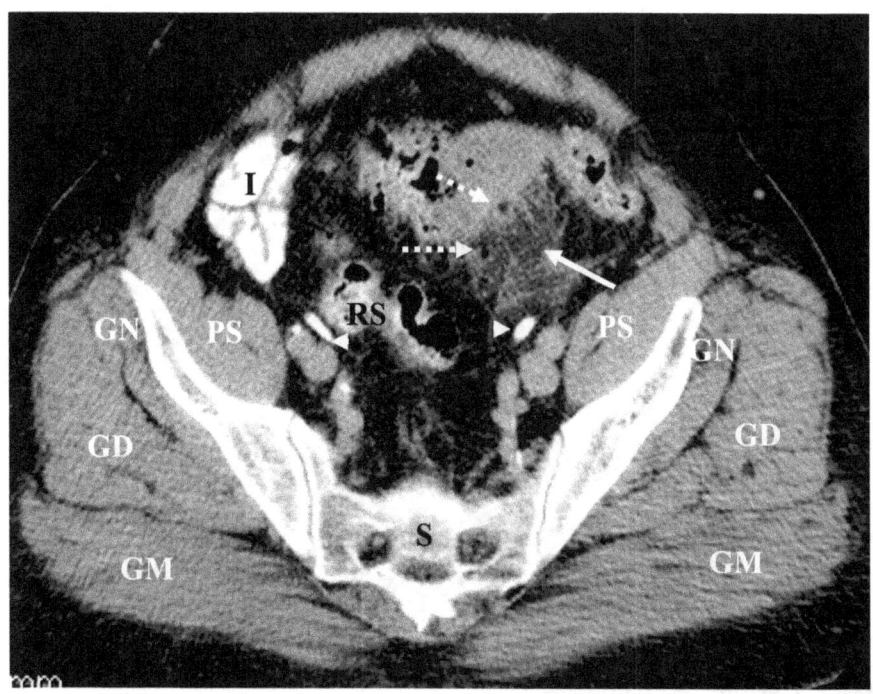

Study Above:
CT Pelvis with IV and oral contrast at the level of the mid pelvis.

Radiographic Findings:
Focal fat-stranding surrounding the sigmoid colon (arrow) centered around a couple of diverticula (dashed arrows).

Tips
Evaluate images closely for microperforation and abscess.
Recommend follow-up colonoscopy after 4-6 weeks in order to exclude an underlying mass.

Normal Anatomy
RS - Rectosigmoid junction, I - Ileum, GN - Gluteus minimus, GD – Gluteus medius,
GM - Gluteus maximus, S - Sacrum, Arrowheads – Ureters, PS – Psoas muscle

Further Reading
Saenz RC. Top 3 Differentials in Gastrointestinal Imaging, A case Review. Chapter 3. Thieme. 2019.

CASE 77

CASE AUTHOR: Gregory D. Puthoff

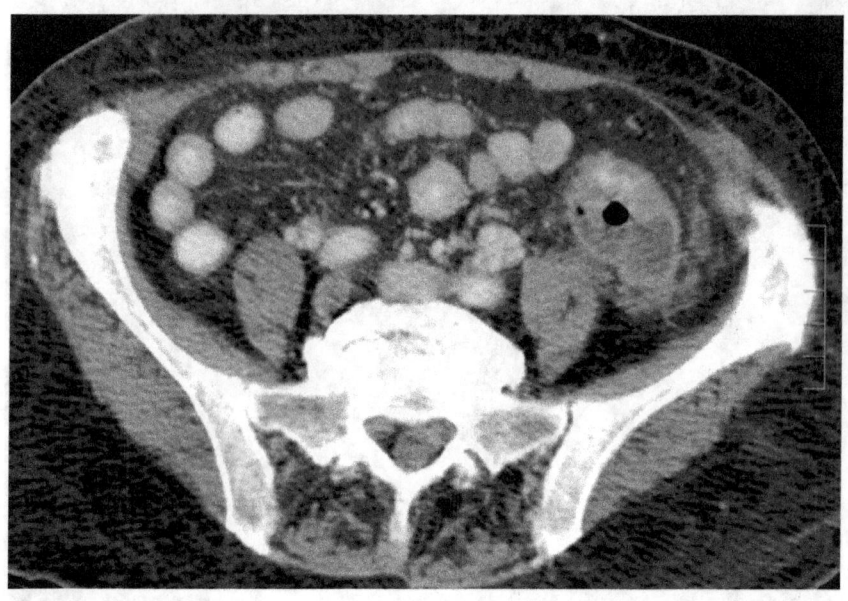

Best CT Study for Diagnosis:
CT Abdomen and Pelvis with IV and oral contrast

Key to DX
Irregular thick-walled peripherally enhancing pericolonic fluid collection +/- air.

Facts
Diverticulitis is inflammation of a preexisting colonic diverticulum secondary to obstruction and microperforation of the diverticulum.
Pericolonic abscesses occur after rupture (perforation) of a diverticulum secondary to inflammatory weakening of diverticular wall.
Air or necrotic debris within the fluid collection are not required for definitive diagnosis.

TX
CT guided percutaneous drainage with catheter placement and/or surgery.

DIVERTICULITIS WITH PERICOLONIC ABSCESS

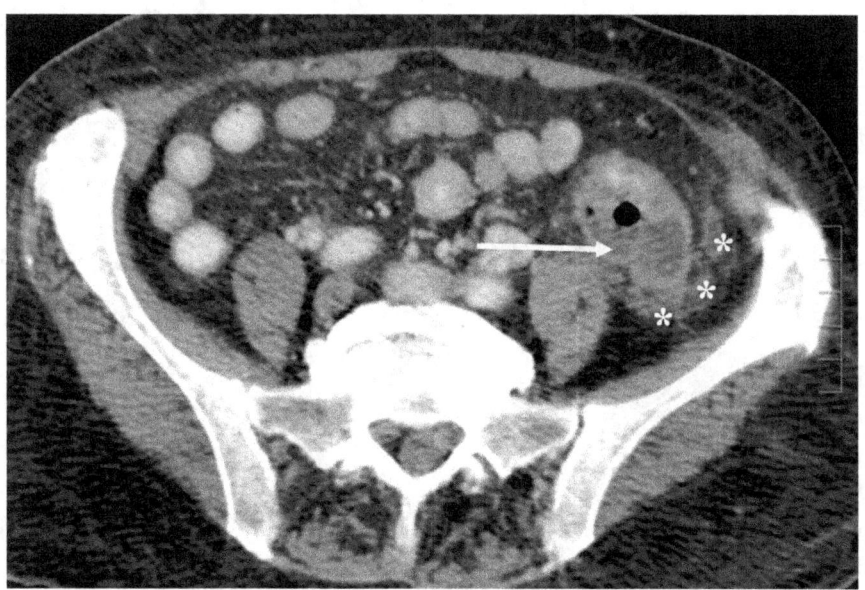

Study Above:
CT Abdomen and Pelvis with IV and oral contrast at the level of the mid pelvis.

Radiographic Findings:
An irregular, peripherally enhancing fluid collection with intraluminal air is identified within the left lower quadrant adjacent to the sigmoid colon (arrow). There is associated peripheral fat stranding (asterisks).

Tips
Microperforations, as seen in diverticulitis, do not typically produce pneumoperitoneum.
Microperforation will be easier to see with wide windows (so look at a lung window).
Interventional radiology CT guided drainage with catheter placement may eliminate need for surgery.
CT also helps delineate other complications of diverticulitis such as colovesicular fistula or contained perforations.

Further Reading
Boyd, SK., Hobson, JJ., Cameron, JD., Saenz, RC. "CT Imaging of Large Bowel Wall Thickening". JAOCR, 2016; Vol. 5, Issue 2

CASE 78

CASE AUTHOR: Zophia Martinez

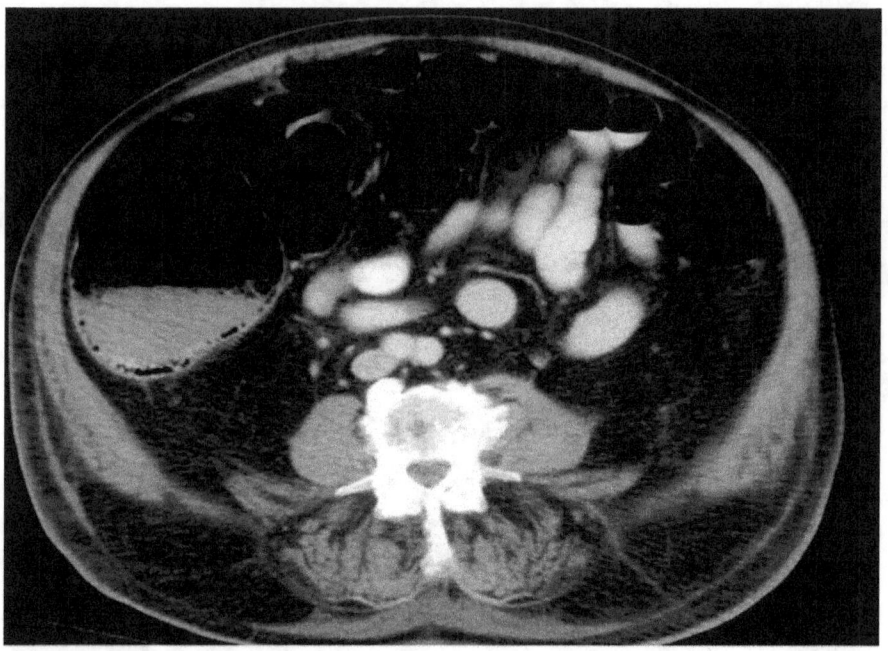

Best CT Study for Diagnosis:
CT Abdomen and Pelvis with IV and oral contrast

Key to DX
Air within the colon wall.

Facts
Clinical presentation varies and can range from mild abdominal pain and rectal bleeding to severe abdominal pain and hemodynamic instability.
Elevated serum lactic acid level may be seen, but serum lactate measurement lacks sensitivity (especially in early bowel ischemia).
Possible causes include arterial occlusion (including atherosclerosis, embolic disease, or procedural complications), venous occlusion, and low-flow states.
Right ischemic colitis has a poorer prognosis than left ischemic colitis (left colon ischemia tends to result from microvascular disease rather than acute arterial occlusion).

TX
Colonoscopy is needed for confirmation.
Conservative treatment for uncomplicated cases. Surgical intervention for severe cases.

ISCHEMIC COLITIS

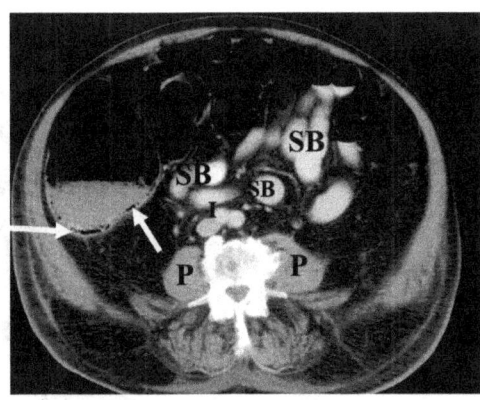
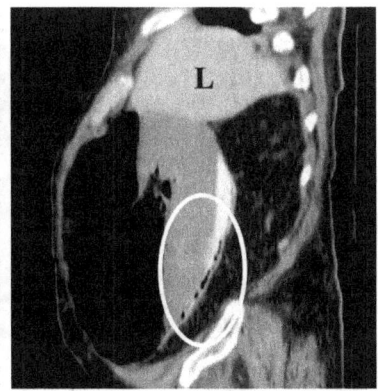

Study Above:
CT Abdomen with IV and oral contrast, axial image through the lower abdomen and sagittal reformat (right image).

Radiographic Findings:
Punctate pockets of air within the dependent wall of the ascending colon consistent with pneumatosis (white arrows on axial image, white oval on sagittal image).

Tips
Examine the dependent portions of the bowel for pneumatosis.
Look for air in the mesenteric vessels, including the intrahepatic portal veins.
Be aware of the watershed areas, including the splenic flexure and rectosigmoid colon, which are more susceptible to ischemia and low flow states.

Normal Anatomy
I - Iliac arteries, L - Liver, P - Psoas muscle, SB - Small bowel

Further Reading
Boyd, SK., Hobson, JJ., Cameron, JD., Saenz, RC. "CT Imaging of Large Bowel Wall Thickening". JAOCR, 2016; Vol. 5, Issue 2.

CASE 79

CASE AUTHOR: Zophia Martinez

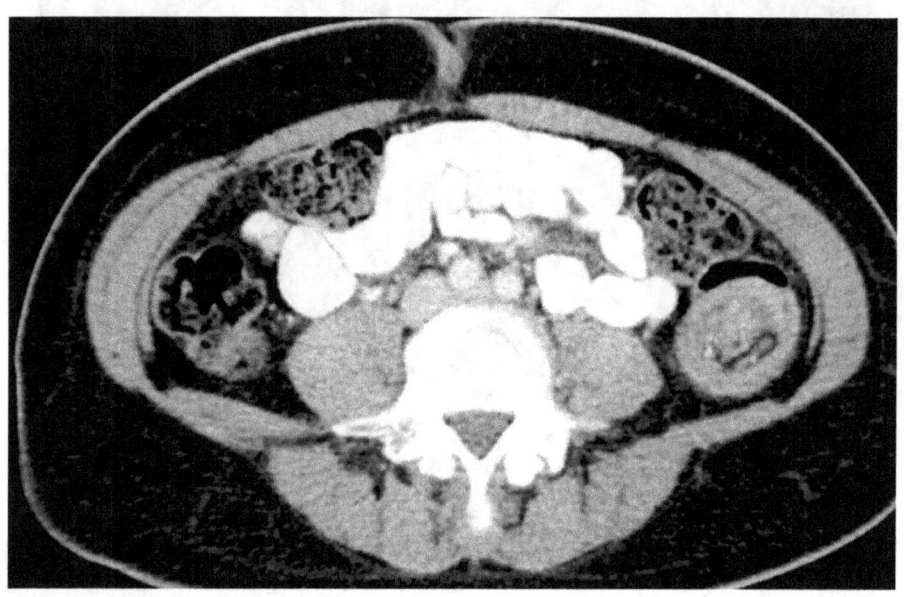

Best CT Study for Diagnosis:
CT Abdomen and Pelvis with IV and oral contrast

Key to DX
A loop of bowel protruding into itself.

Facts
Patients may present with colicky intermittent pain, diarrhea, bloody stools, and/or vomiting.
Intussusception is more common in children and is idiopathic in 90% of cases. In adults, the majority of cases are associated with a "lead point."
Adult colonic intussusception has a high association with the presence of a malignant tumor, while lead points in the small bowel are more often benign.
Transient asymptomatic small bowel intussusception is often encountered incidentally on CT and may be more common in adults than previously thought.

TX
Short segment small bowel intussusception is typically self-limited.
Adult colonic intussusception is typically treated with surgical resection.
Pediatric colonic intussusception is usually treated with pneumatic or hydrostatic reduction.

INTUSSUSCEPTION

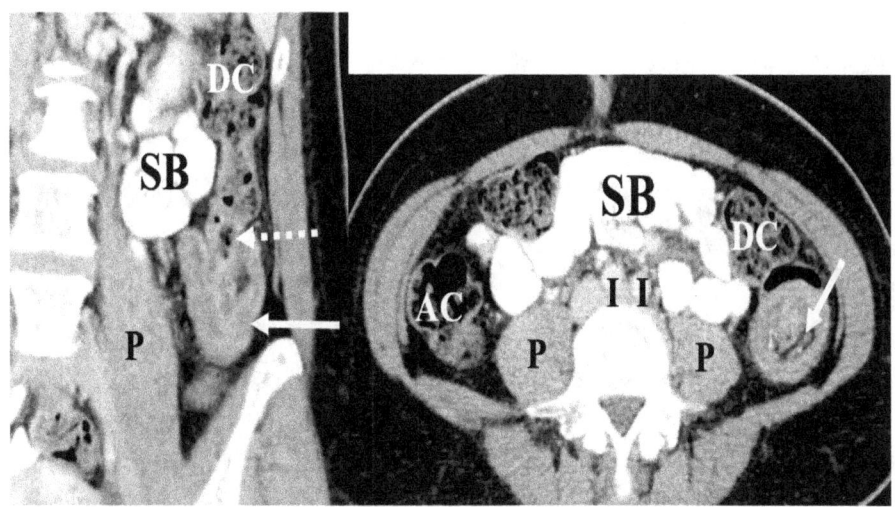

Study Above:
CT Pelvis with IV and oral contrast, axial image at the level of the upper pelvis and coronal reformat (left).

Radiographic Findings:
The colon is seen protruding into itself in the left lower quadrant consistent with a colo-colonic intussusception. The loop that is telescoping inward is the intussusceptum (dashed arrow). The receiving loop is the intussuscipiens (arrow). Axial image demonstrates a "target" shaped appearance of the colon in the left lower quadrant with central fat (arrow).

Tips
Mesenteric fat within a bowel loop is diagnostic.
Look for a loop within a loop (telescoping bowel).

Normal Anatomy
SB - Small bowel, P - Psoas, DC - Descending colon, AS- Ascending colon, I - Iliac arteries

Further Reading
Saenz RC. Top 3 Differentials in Gastrointestinal Imaging, A case Review. Chapter 3. Thieme. 2019.

CASE 80

CASE AUTHOR: Juliann Giese

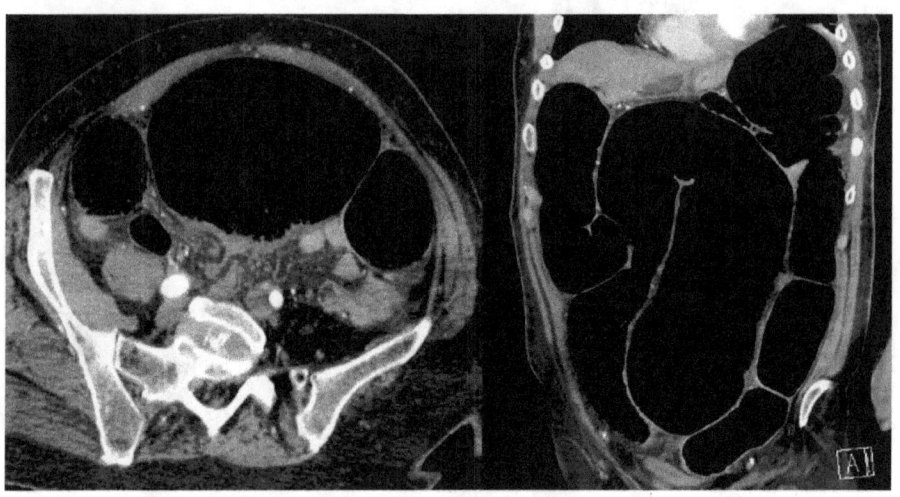

Best CT Study for Diagnosis:
CT Abdomen and Pelvis with IV and oral contrast

Key to DX
Ahaustral dilated colonic loop (> 6 cm) with an inverted "U" shape and abrupt luminal tapering at its base forming a closed-loop large bowel obstruction.

Facts
Abdominal emergency with a high mortality rate (25%) due to bowel ischemia.
Abnormal twisting of colon along its mesenteric axis resulting in closed loop large bowel obstruction.
Third leading cause of large bowel obstruction (after colon cancer and diverticulitis).
Most common locations: sigmoid (70%), cecum (25%), and transverse colon (5%).
Most common among elderly and debilitated neuropsychiatric patients.
Often related to chronic constipation, laxative abuse, and high-fiber diet.

TX
Colonoscopic decompression +/- rectal tube; usually followed by bowel resection.

COLONIC (SIGMOID) VOLVULUS

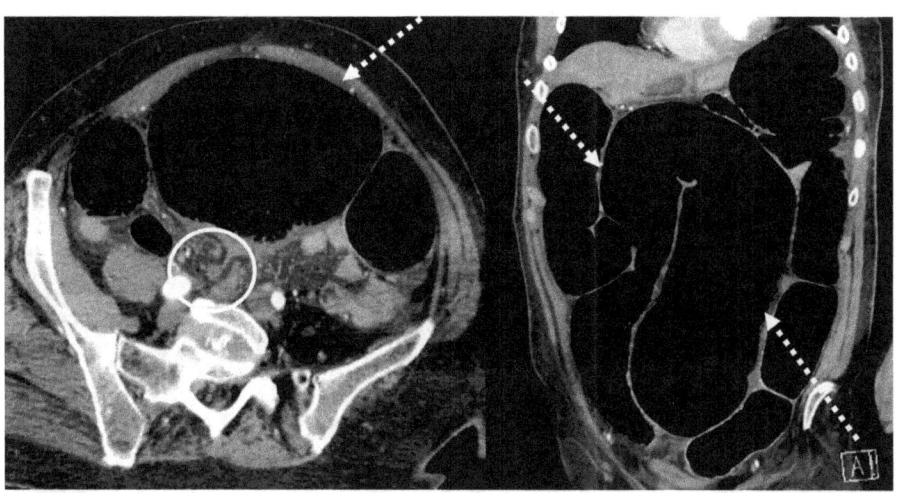

Study Above:
CT Abdomen and Pelvis with IV contrast, axial at the level of the mid pelvis and a coronal reformat (right).

Radiographic findings:
Dilated sigmoid lumen (dashed arrow) with tightly twisted mesentery centrally, also known as the "whirl sign" (circle). Coronal image demonstrates a large ahaustral gas-filled loop of sigmoid colon with an inverted U-shaped appearance, also known as the "coffee bean sign" (dashed arrows).

Tips
"Bird beak" sign is an additional finding that may be seen on CT and water-soluble enema with abrupt luminal tapering at the site of obstruction.

Evaluate for findings of closed loop obstruction, which may lead to ischemia and perforation.

Absence of rectal gas is a common finding in sigmoid volvulus.

Cecal volvulus presents as air-filled, dilated cecum with apex often pointing toward the left upper quadrant.

Further Reading
Levsky, Jeffrey M., et al. CT findings of sigmoid volvulus. AJR. 194.1 (2010): 136-143.

CASE 81

CASE AUTHOR: Juliann Giese

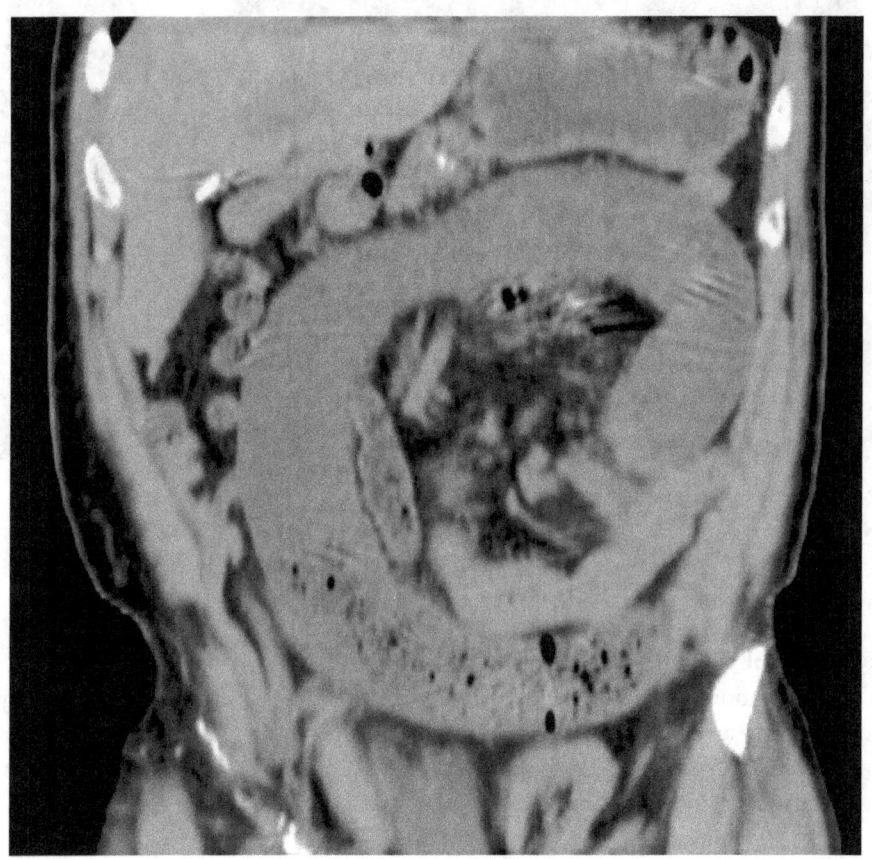

Best CT Study for Diagnosis:
CT Abdomen and Pelvis with IV contrast

Key to DX
A "C" or "U-shaped" loop of dilated small bowel (> 3 cm).

Facts
Most commonly caused by a single adhesive band, though can be seen in association with internal or external hernias.
Occurs when a segment of bowel is obstructed at two points.
As fluid and air accumulate within the obstructed loop, there is increasing risk for volvulus, strangulation, ischemia, and perforation.
Radially oriented "C" or "U-shaped" dilated bowel points to the site of obstruction.

TX
Prompt surgical intervention.

CLOSED-LOOP SMALL BOWEL OBSTRUCTION

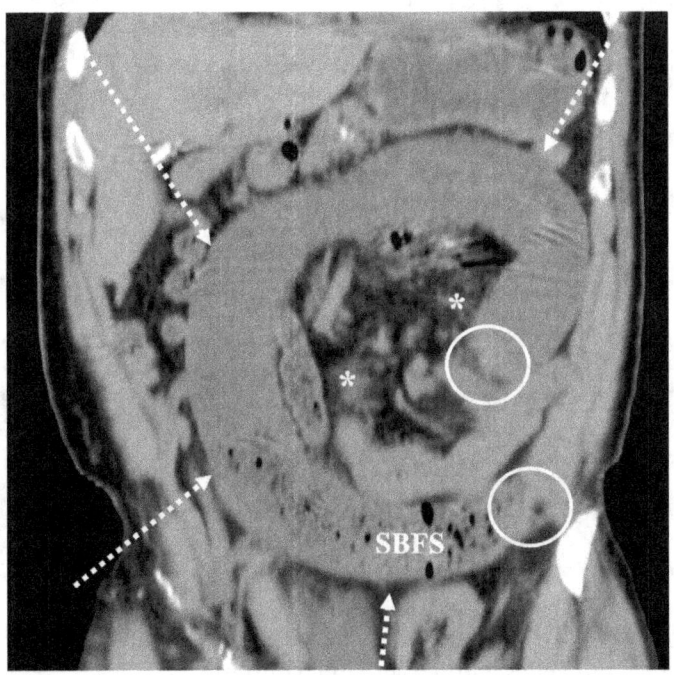

Study Above:
CT Abdomen and Pelvis with IV contrast, coronal reformat.

Radiographic findings:
Coronal image shows a "C-shaped" dilated loop of small bowel (dashed arrows) with tapering at the points of obstruction (circles). Also note that the mesentery has a mildly congested appearance from dilated vessels and lymphatics (asterisks).

Small bowel feces sign (SBFS) can be helpful in localizing the site of obstruction as it is often found just proximal to the transition point.

Tips
Coronal and sagittal images may be beneficial in diagnosis of closed-loop obstruction.

CT findings associated with strangulation (ischemia) include: bowel wall thickening (> 3 mm), mesenteric edema, decreased bowel wall enhancement, and tapering of the mesenteric vessels to a central point.

Presence of pneumatosis and portal venous or mesenteric gas is a late finding in the setting of ischemia.

Further Reading
Paulson, Erik K., and William M. Thompson. "Review of Small-Bowel Obstruction: The Diagnosis and When to Worry." *Radiology* (2015).

CASE 82

CASE AUTHOR: Rocky Saenz

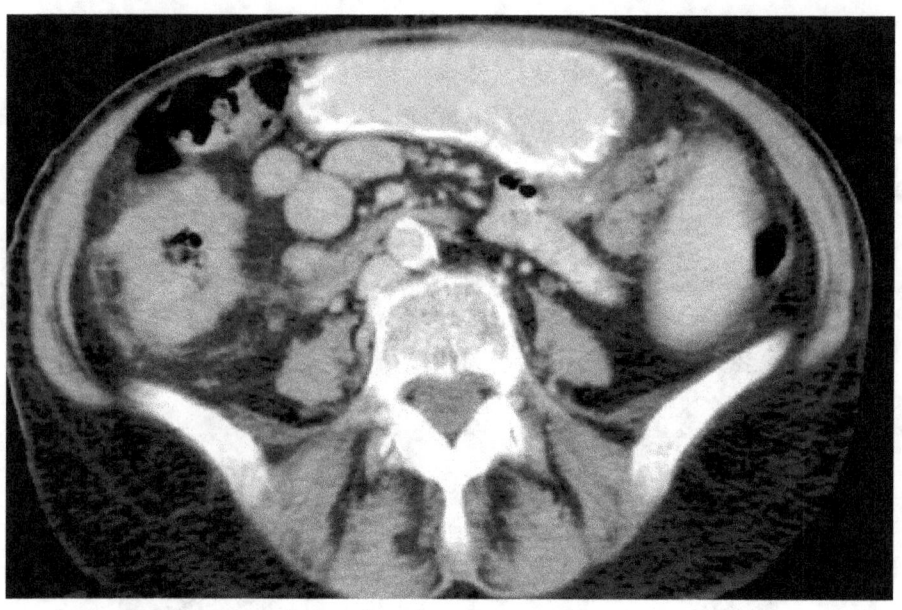

Best CT Study for Diagnosis:
CT Abdomen and Pelvis with IV and oral contrast

Key to DX
Focal thick and irregular appearance to the bowel wall.

Facts
Patients may present with rectal bleeding, pain, or thin caliber stools.
The most common primary colon tumor is adenocarcinoma.
It is usually associated with an elevated serum CEA.

TX
Colonoscopy for tumor sampling and body CT for staging (PET/CT also used).
Surgery for tumor resection.
Chemotherapy and radiation may be needed depending on stage.

COLONIC MASS

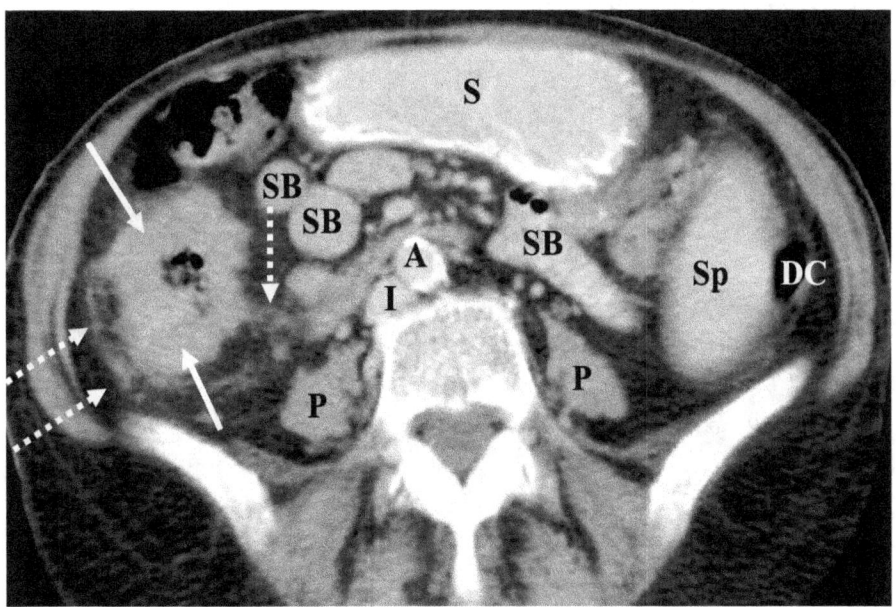

Study Above:
CT Pelvis with IV and oral contrast at the level of the upper pelvis.

Radiographic Findings:
Circumferential, irregular wall thickening of the ascending colon (arrows) resulting in luminal narrowing. Also notice that there is peripheral fat stranding (dashed arrows). Notice that the spleen is seen at the iliac crest, which indicates splenomegaly.

Tips
Colon wall should never be thicker than 3 mm (just like the small bowel).
Usually bowel wall thickening associated with malignancy is eccentric and short segment whereas infection and inflammatory etiologies are long segment (greater than 5 cm).
Scrutinize the abdomen and pelvis for adenopathy.

Normal Anatomy
S - Stomach, Sp - Spleen, A - Aorta, I - IVC, DC - Descending colon, SB - Small bowel, P - Psoas

Further Reading
Paulson, Erik K., and William M. Thompson. "Review of Small-Bowel Obstruction: The Diagnosis and When to Worry." *Radiology* (2015).

CASE 83

CASE AUTHOR: Juliann Giese

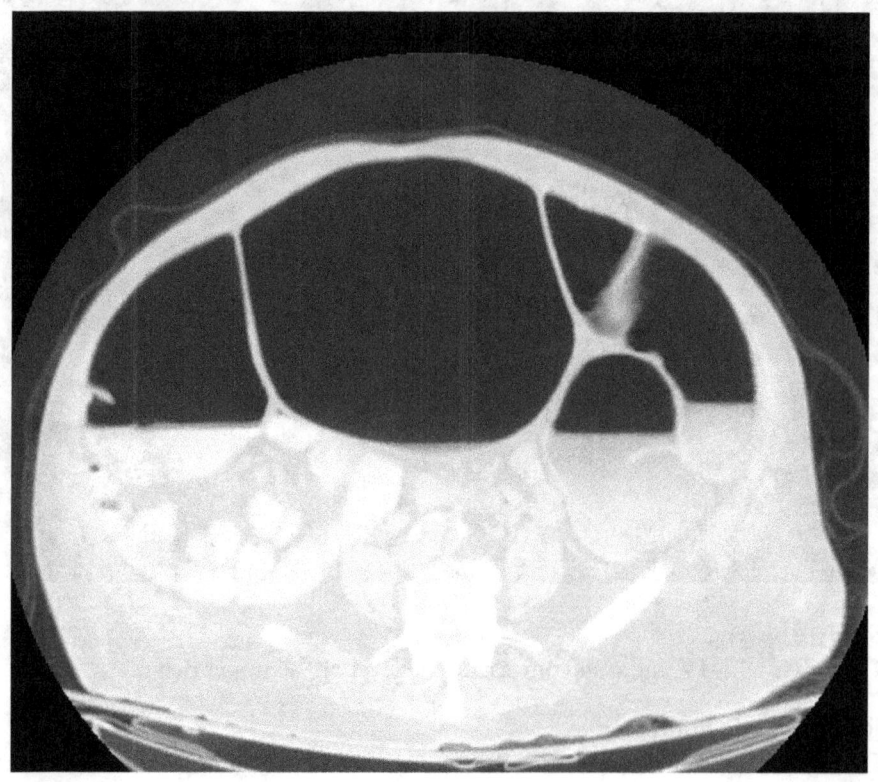

Best CT Study for Diagnosis:
CT Abdomen and Pelvis with IV and oral contrast

Key to DX
Extensive right-sided (cecal) colonic dilatation without evidence of an obstructive lesion.
Characteristic intermediate transition zone near splenic flexure.

Facts
Clinical symptoms mimic mechanical obstruction.
More common in older patients, typically greater than 60 years old.
May be acute or chronic; when chronic there is often a history of chronic constipation or cathartic abuse.
Chronic disease patients have extensive luminal distension without perforation.

TX
Acute: Supportive therapy (NGT, neostigmine, possible decompression) with potential surgical intervention if symptoms progress.
Chronic: No effective medical treatment.

COLONIC PSEUDO-OBSTRUCTION (OGILVIE'S)

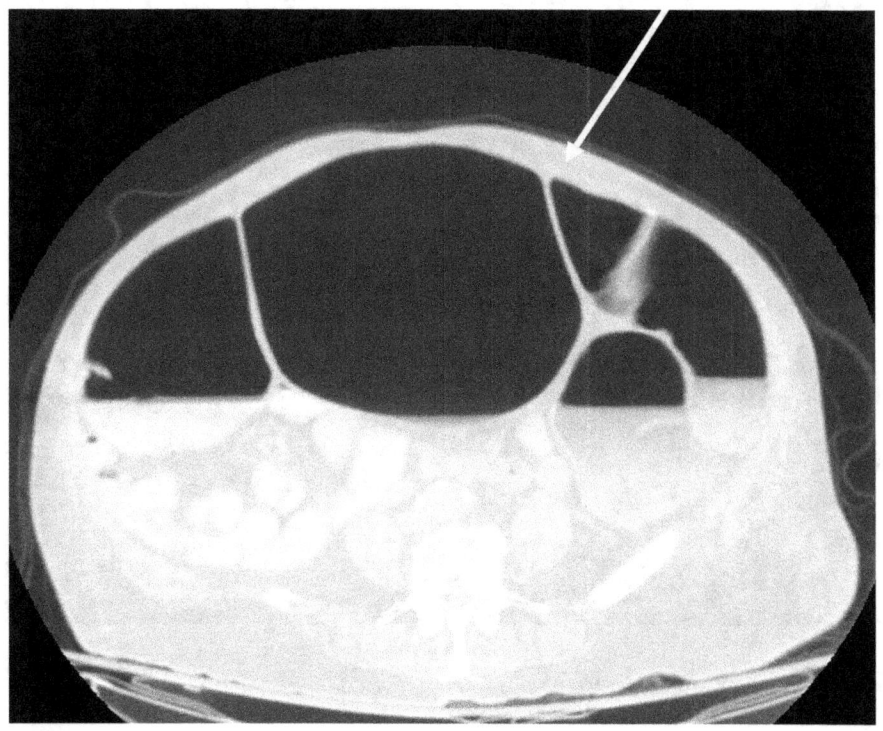

Study Above:
CT Abdomen with oral contrast at the level of the pelvis (wide or lung window).

Radiographic findings:
Extensive proximal (right-sided) colonic dilatation measuring > 8 cm without evidence of perforation. There is gradual tapering of the bowel noted within the transverse colon (arrow), compatible with pseudo-obstruction (Ogilvie's syndrome).

Tips
Rule-out the presence of an underlying obstructive mass.
Use a wide window (as above) in order to exclude pneumoperitoneum.
The transition zone at the splenic flexure/transverse colon allows ileus to be excluded.
It is important to make the proper diagnosis to avoid unnecessary surgery.

Further Reading
Choi, Ji Soo, et al. "Colonic pseudoobstruction: CT findings." American Journal of Roentgenology 190.6 (2008): 1521-1526.

CASE 84

CASE AUTHOR: Zophia Martinez

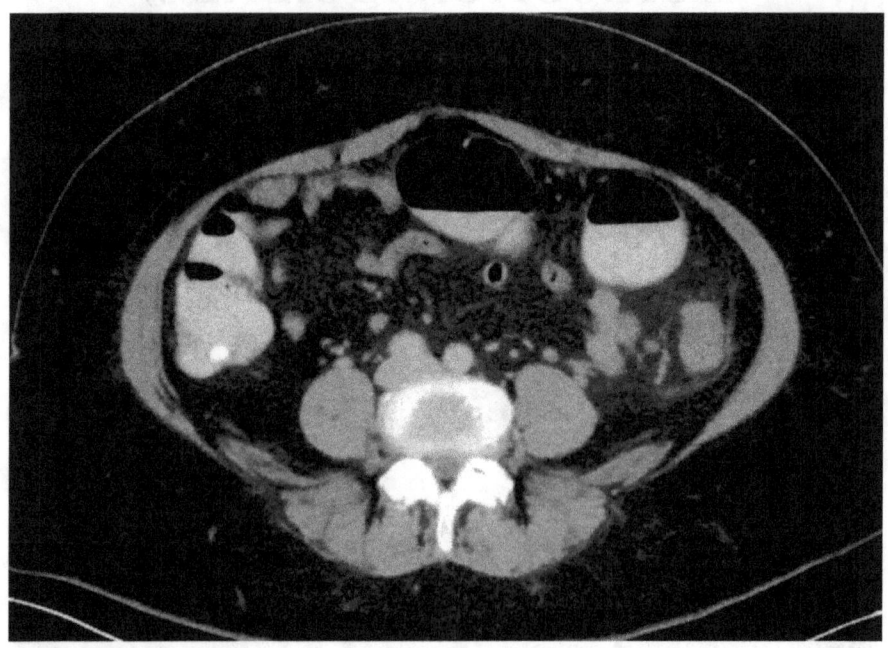

Best CT Study for Diagnosis:
CT Abdomen and Pelvis with IV and oral contrast

Key to DX
Dilated large bowel with associated air-fluid levels.

Facts
Presentation is often acute and symptoms may include abdominal pain, constipation/obstipation, and abdominal distension.
Large bowel obstruction (LBO) is much less common than small bowel obstruction.
In the US, colonic malignancy is the most common cause of LBO in adults.
Other less common causes include volvulus, diverticulitis, fecal impaction, hernias, adhesions, and inflammatory bowel disease.
Acute large bowel obstruction is an abdominal emergency with high rates of morbidity/mortality if left untreated.

TX
Emergency surgery or colonoscopy is usually required to relieve the obstruction.

LARGE BOWEL OBSTRUCTION

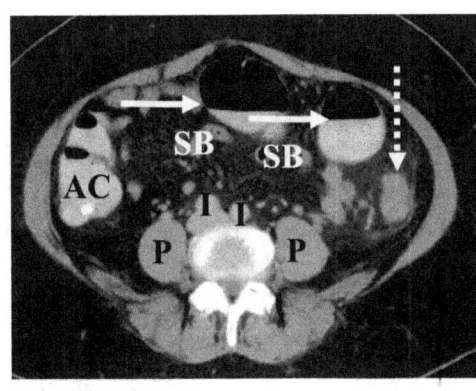
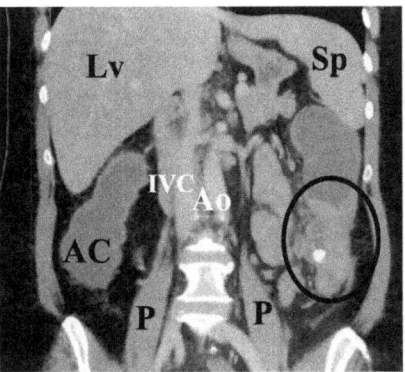

Study Above:
CT Abdomen pelvis with IV and oral contrast at the level of the mid abdomen and coronal reformat (right).

Radiographic Findings:
The large bowel is dilated with air-fluid levels (arrows). The left colon is decompressed with surrounding fat stranding (dashed arrow). In this case, there is an obstructing mass in the descending colon (black circle).

Tips
Look for dilated large bowel proximal to a transition point and decompressed bowel distal to the obstruction.
Check non-dependent portions of the abdomen and pelvis for free air.
Possible signs of associated bowel ischemia on CT include wall thickening, abnormal bowel wall enhancement, pneumatosis, free peritoneal fluid, and mesenteric fat stranding.

Normal Anatomy
AC- Ascending colon, Ao – Aorta, IVC – Inferior vena cava, Lv - Liver, SB – Small bowel, Sp - Spleen, P - Psoas, I - Iliac arteries

Further Reading
Choi, Ji Soo, et al. "Colonic pseudoobstruction: CT findings." American Journal of Roentgenology 190.6 (2008): 1521-1526.

CASE 85

CASE AUTHOR: Juliann Giese

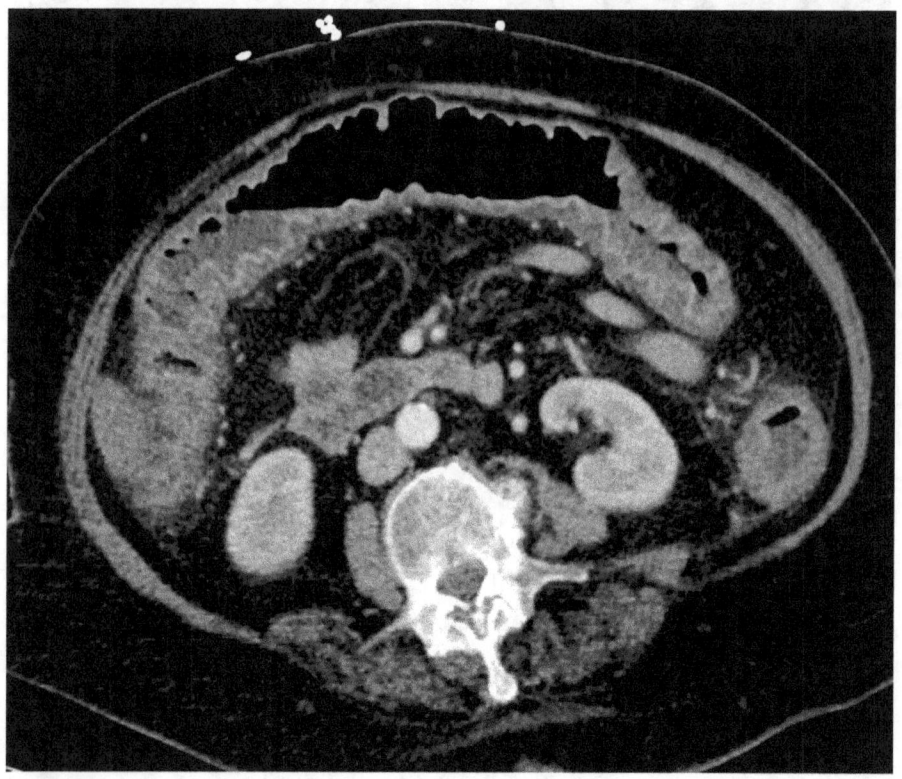

Best CT Study for Diagnosis:
CT Abdomen and Pelvis with IV contrast

Key to DX
Circumferential colonic wall thickening (> 3 mm) with mucosal hyperenhancement.

Facts
Most common cause in industrialized countries is bacterial infection.
Most common causes in the U.S. are *C. diff, Salmonella, Campylobacter,* and *E. coli.*
Most common cause in underdeveloped countries is parasitic infection.
Medical history and clinical findings are extremely helpful.
Possible complications include perforation, pericolonic abscess, fistula, peritonitis, ischemia, and obstruction (usually from stricture).

TX
Organism dependent therapy.

INFECTIOUS COLITIS

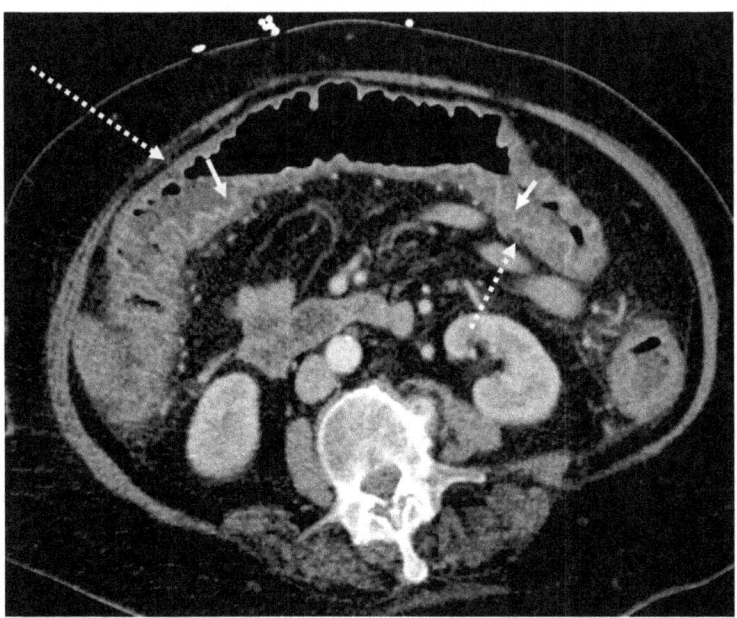

Study Above:
CT Pelvis with IV and oral contrast at the level of the lower pelvis.

Radiographic findings:
Long-segment, circumferential wall thickening of the transverse colon (dashed arrows) with mucosal hyperemia (arrows) characteristic of the "accordion sign."

Tips
Bowel wall thickening is the most common imaging finding (> 3 mm).
Differential diagnosis for colon wall thickening includes infection, inflammatory (ulcerative colitis and Crohn's), ischemia, and carcinoma (3 I's and don't forget C).
Determine whether long vs short segment involvement (long favors infection).
Determine whether concentric or eccentric wall thickening (carcinoma usually eccentric).
A single vascular distribution of colon favors ischemia.
Limited right-sided colitis may be seen with *TB, Yersinia, Amebiasis,* and *Salmonella*.
Limited left-sided colitis may be due to *Shigella* and *Schistosomiasis*.
Diffuse colonic involvement may be seen with pseudomembranous colitis (*Clostridium difficile*).

Further Reading
Maddu, Kiran K., et al. "Colorectal Emergencies and Related Complications: A Comprehensive Imaging Review—Noninfectious and Noninflammatory Emergencies of Colon." *American Journal of Roentgenology* 203.6 (2014): 1217-1229.

CASE 86

CASE AUTHOR: Jordan Verlare

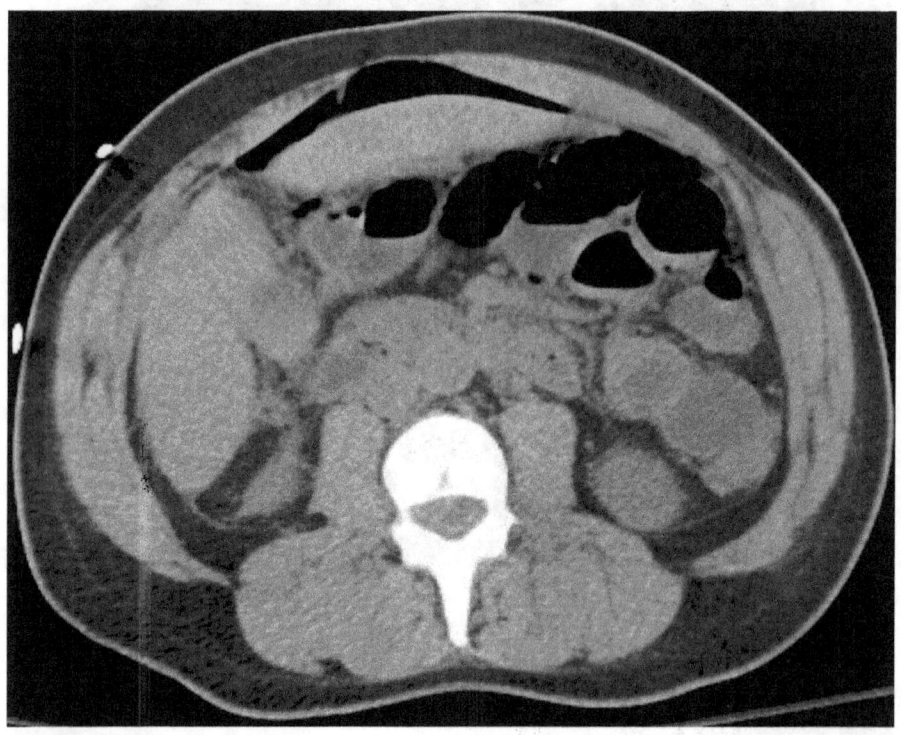

Best CT Study for Diagnosis:
CT Abdomen without contrast

Key to DX
Air that is not in a bowel loop.

Facts
Patients will usually present with abdominal pain.
This finding is a surgical emergency!
Pneumoperitoneum most commonly occurs due to a perforated hollow viscous within the abdomen; in adults, this is most frequently from a perforating ulcer and in children, most frequently from necrotizing enterocolitis in the neonate.

TX
Immediate surgical consultation needed for bowel repair.

FREE AIR, PNEUMOPERITONEUM

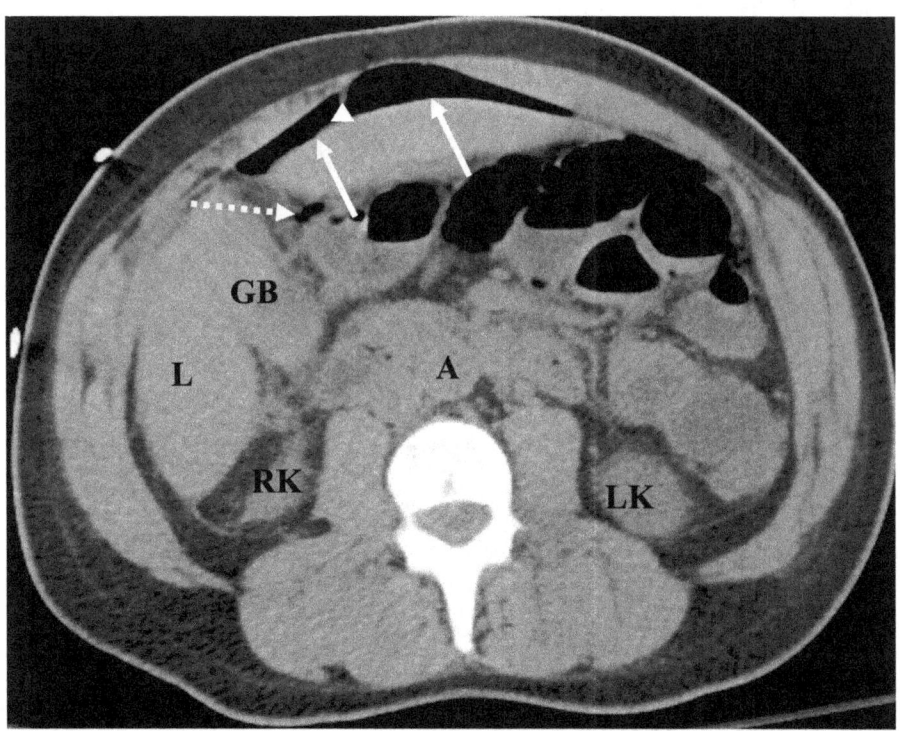

Study Above:
CT Abdomen without contrast from the level of the mid abdomen.

Radiographic Findings:
Air outside of the bowel lumen (arrows) is between the liver and the anterior abdominal wall and can be seen outlining the falciform ligament (arrowhead). Small punctate foci of air can also be seen outside the bowel lumen (dashed arrow).

Tips
Try to identify the ruptured viscus (wide windows are helpful).
Check for fat stranding (may help identify the source).
It is difficult to define the source when there is a large amount of free air.

Normal Anatomy
A - Aorta, L - Liver, RK - Right kidney, LK - Left kidney, GB - Gallbladder

Further Reading
Maddu, Kiran K., et al. "Colorectal Emergencies and Related Complications: A Comprehensive Imaging Review—Noninfectious and Noninflammatory Emergencies of Colon." *American Journal of Roentgenology* 203.6 (2014): 1217-1229.

CASE 87

CASE AUTHOR: Juliann Giese

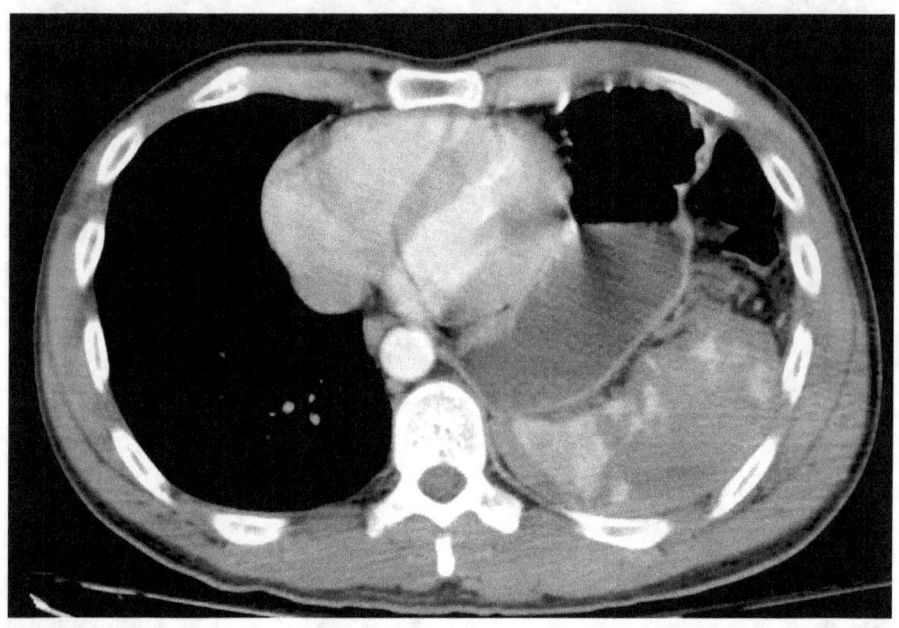

Best CT Study for Diagnosis:
CT Abdomen without contrast

Key to DX
Herniation of air-filled stomach/bowel into the lower chest.

Facts
Most common cause is blunt trauma (MVA).
Prevalence of 5% following blunt trauma.
Most common location: posterolateral aspect of the left hemidiaphragm.
Waist like narrowing of bowel or liver (collar sign): 70% seen on sagittal images.
Herniated abdominal contents abutting the posterior ribs (dependent viscera sign): 90%.
Left sided: Stomach > colon > spleen most commonly herniate.
Right sided: Upper one third of the liver most commonly herniates.

TX
Surgical repair is usually needed.

DIAPHRAGMATIC RUPTURE

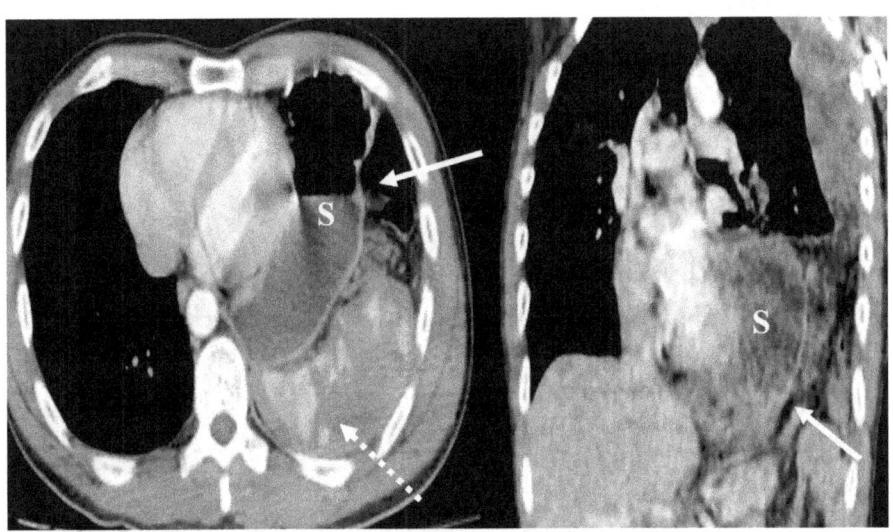

Study Above:
CT Abdomen with IV contrast at the level of the diaphragm, axial and coronal reformat (right).

Radiographic findings:
Axial image shows a large air-fluid level within the herniated stomach (S) in the left lower chest (arrow). Dependent-viscera sign is present with the lacerated spleen abutting the posterior ribs (dashed arrow). The coronal reformat demonstrates a left-sided diaphragmatic defect with intrathoracic herniation of the stomach (arrow).

Tips
Evaluate for associated abnormalities such as rib fractures (90%), liver/splenic laceration (60%), pelvic fracture (50%), and aortic injury (5%).
Use reformats; best seen on sagittal (sagittal > coronal > axial).
Latent rupture: may occur later, especially when weaning from the ventilator.
Must have a high index of suspicion; if diagnosis is missed, intrathoracic visceral herniation may occur with eventual strangulation and morbidity/mortality rate of 50%.
Differential diagnosis for an air-fluid level in the chest includes bowel (from hernia or diaphragm rupture), abscess, and pneumatocele.

Further Reading
Maddu, Kiran K., et al. "Colorectal Emergencies and Related Complications: A Comprehensive Imaging Review—Noninfectious and Noninflammatory Emergencies of Colon." *American Journal of Roentgenology* 203.6 (2014): 1217-1229.

CASE 88

CASE AUTHOR: Rocky Saenz

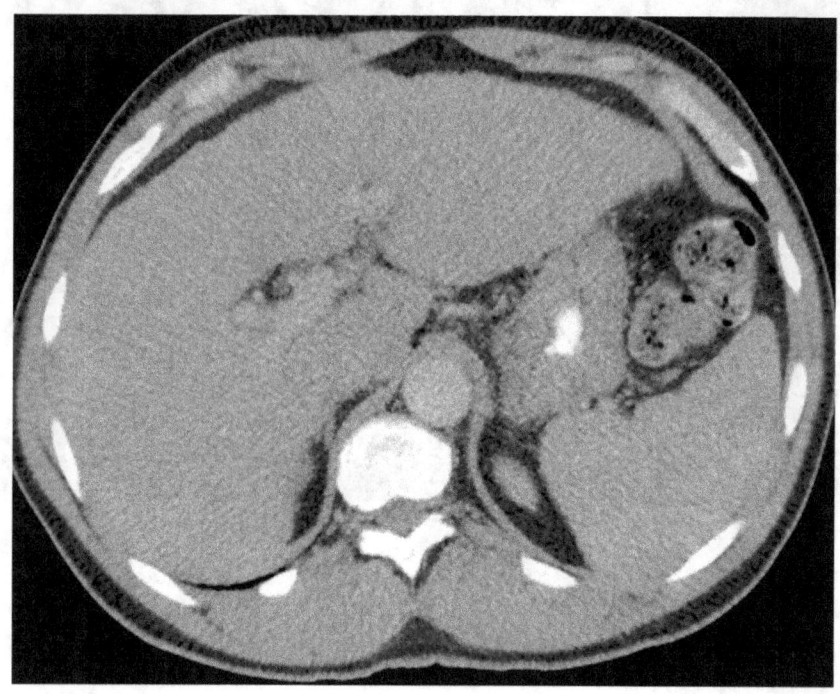

Best CT Study for Diagnosis:
CT Abdomen IV contrast, dynamic multi-phase protocol

Key to DX
Nodular contour to the liver with a heterogeneous appearance to the parenchyma.

Facts
Commonly associated with alcohol consumption.
The cirrhotic nodules may become dysplastic leading to hepatocellular carcinoma (HCC).
Correlation with serum alpha-fetoprotein is useful for detecting HCC conversion.
Evaluation with a dynamic CT of the liver is needed to exclude an HCC focus.

TX
Supportive care.
An HCC focus needs resection vs. CT guided ablation and potentially transplant.

CIRRHOSIS

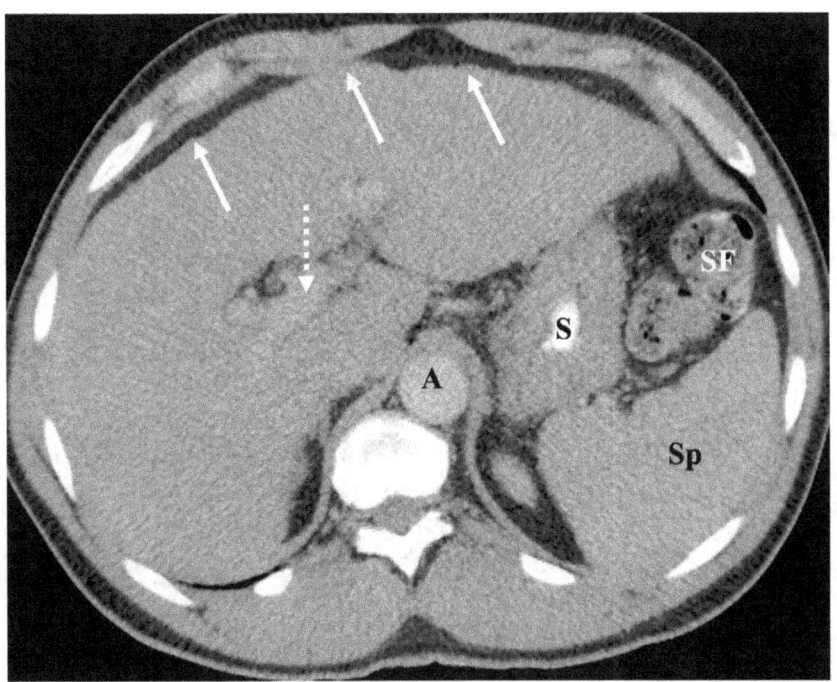

Study Above:
CT Abdomen with IV and oral contrast at the level of the upper abdomen.

Radiographic Findings:
Nodular contour to the liver margin (arrows). The portal vein is enlarged (dashed arrow).

Tips
Check for varices (an indicator of portal hypertension).
Portal hypertension on CT equals splenomegaly with an enlarged portal vein (> 14 mm).
Alcoholic liver cirrhosis is the most common cause of splenomegaly in the USA.
Multiphase/dynamic liver CT is needed to exclude arterial enhancing lesions (HCC).

Normal Anatomy
S - Stomach, Sp - Spleen, A - Aorta, SF – Splenic flexure

Further Reading
Maddu, Kiran K., et al. "Colorectal Emergencies and Related Complications: A Comprehensive Imaging Review—Noninfectious and Noninflammatory Emergencies of Colon." *American Journal of Roentgenology* 203.6 (2014): 1217-1229.

CASE 89

CASE AUTHOR: Rocky Saenz

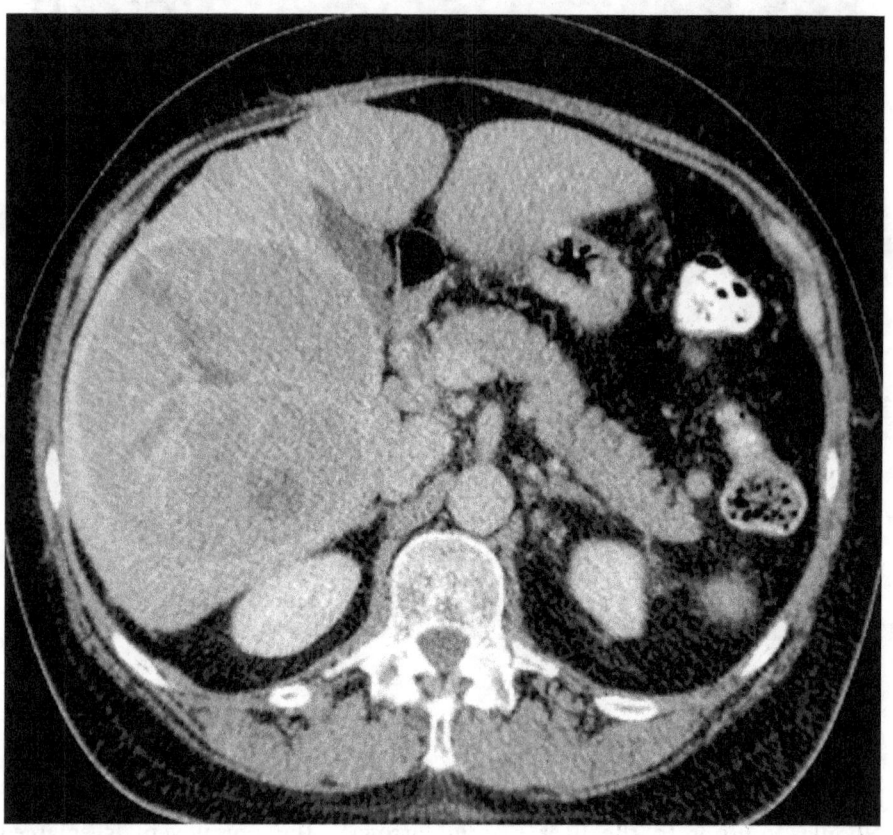

Best CT Study for Diagnosis:
CT Abdomen with IV contrast, dynamic multi-phase protocol

Key to DX
Focal soft tissue lesion within the liver parenchyma.

Facts
A focal liver lesion could represent a benign or malignant mass.
Most common benign lesion in the liver is a hemangioma.
Most common malignant liver lesion is a metastatic lesion.
Dynamic multiphase CT of the liver is necessary to categorize a liver lesion.

TX
Tissue type can be obtained with CT guided sampling.
Underlying etiology must be addressed.

LIVER MASS, HCC

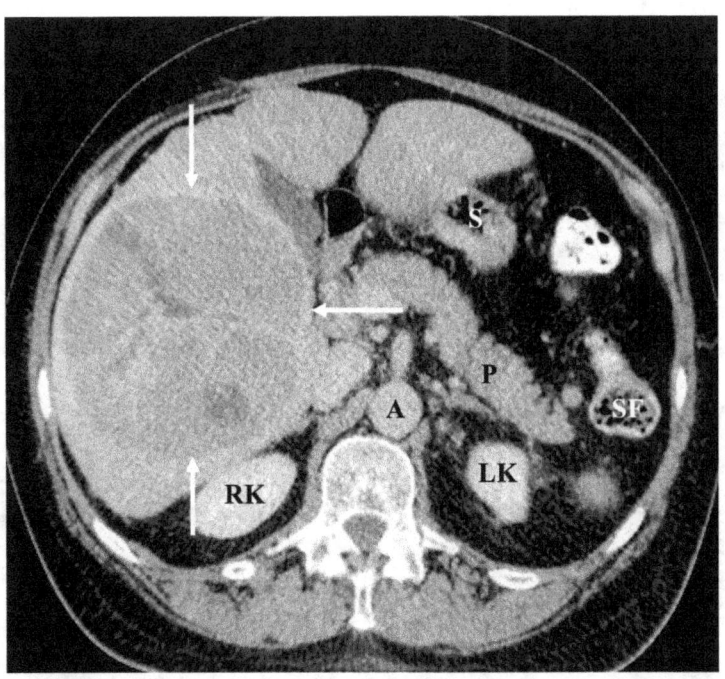

Study Above:
CT Abdomen with IV contrast at the level of the upper abdomen.

Radiographic Findings:
Large heterogeneous mass within the liver with an enhancing capsule (arrows).

Tips
Hepatocellular carcinoma (HCC) usually shows arterial enhancement with washout on delayed phase.
If CT liver dynamic study is equivocal, then consider MRI with gadoxetate disodium.
If HCC is suspected, correlate with serum alpha-fetoprotein which should be positive.
LI-RADS is an ACR reporting system used for liver lesions.

Normal Anatomy
S - Stomach, P - Pancreas, A - Aorta, SF - Splenic flexure of the colon, RK – Right kidney, LK - Left kidney

Further Reading
Maddu, Kiran K., et al. "Colorectal Emergencies and Related Complications: A Comprehensive Imaging Review—Noninfectious and Noninflammatory Emergencies of Colon." *American Journal of Roentgenology* 203.6 (2014): 1217-1229.

CASE 90

CASE AUTHOR: Michael Legacy

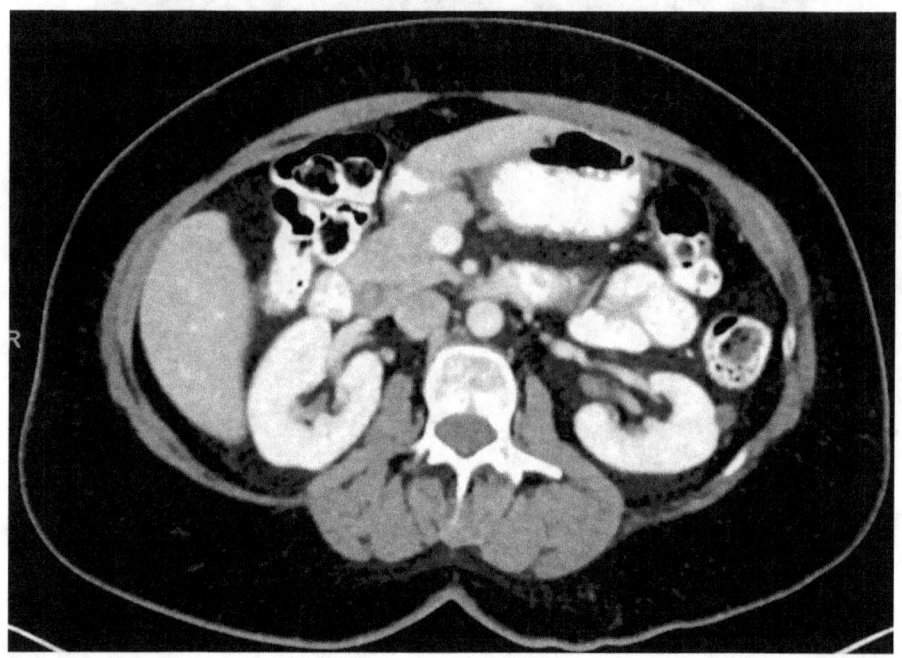

Best CT Study for Diagnosis:
CT Abdomen with IV contrast (when ultrasound is not available)

Key to DX
Focal increased attenuation within the common bile duct.

Facts
Patients may present with jaundice and acute RUQ abdominal pain.
The stones cause biliary obstruction which leads to pancreatitis or cholangitis.
The majority of gallstones and choledocholiths are non-calcified. Therefore, the detection rate by radiograph and CT is poor.
Elevated alkaline phosphatase and direct bilirubin.
The diagnosis usually requires ultrasound or magnetic resonance cholangiopancreatography (MRCP).

TX
The biliary obstruction must be decompressed. Temporary decompression can be performed with percutaneous CT catheter placement after failed ERCP.
Size of choledocholith determines treatment: < 3 mm will pass spontaneously, 3-10 mm endoscopic sphincterotomy, > 10-15 mm requires lithotripsy.

CHOLEDOCHOLITHIASIS

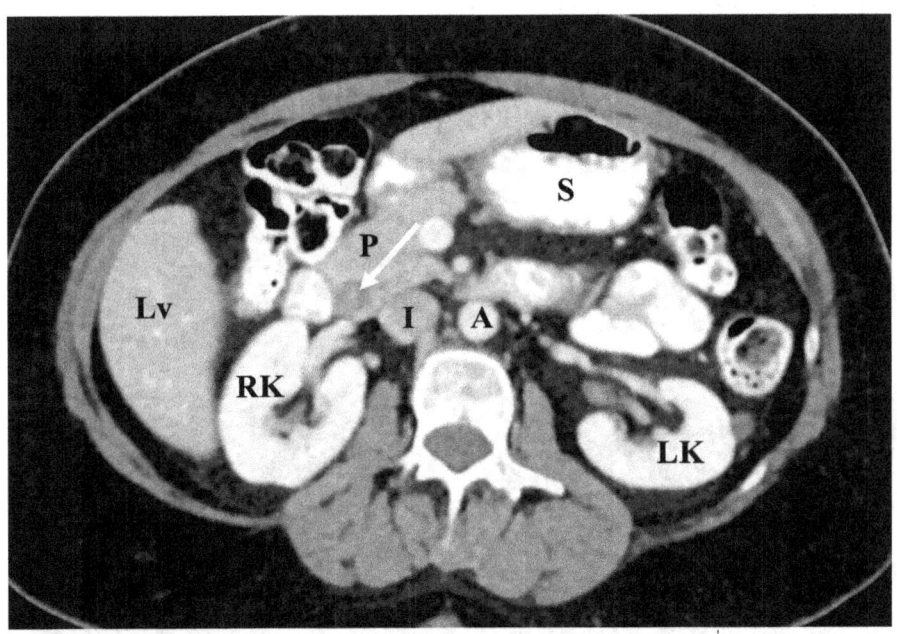

Study Above:
CT Abdomen with IV and oral contrast at the level of the mid abdomen.

Radiographic Findings:
Focal increased attenuation within the common bile duct (arrow). The common bile duct is dilated.

Tips
Narrow windows or a "liver window" may enhance visualization of stones. When gallstones or ductal stones are suspected but not seen on CT, US should be performed. If the US is negative, MRCP is warranted (usually only 20% are seen on CT).

Normal Anatomy
Lv - Liver, P - Pancreas, S - Stomach, A - Aorta, I - Inferior vena cava, RK - Right kidney, LK - Left kidney

Further Reading
Imaging of Biliary Tract Disease, Owen J. O'Connor, Siobhan O'Neill, and Michael M. Maher *American Journal of Roentgenology* 2011 197:4, W551-W558

Percutaneous Transcholecystic Management of Choledocholithiasis: A Next Horizon for Interventional Radiologists? vanSonnenberg E, Panchanathan R., Radiology. 2019 Jan;290(1):244-245. doi: 10.1148/radiol.2018181942. Epub 2018 Sep 18. PMID: 30226458.

CASE 91

CASE AUTHOR: Rocky Saenz

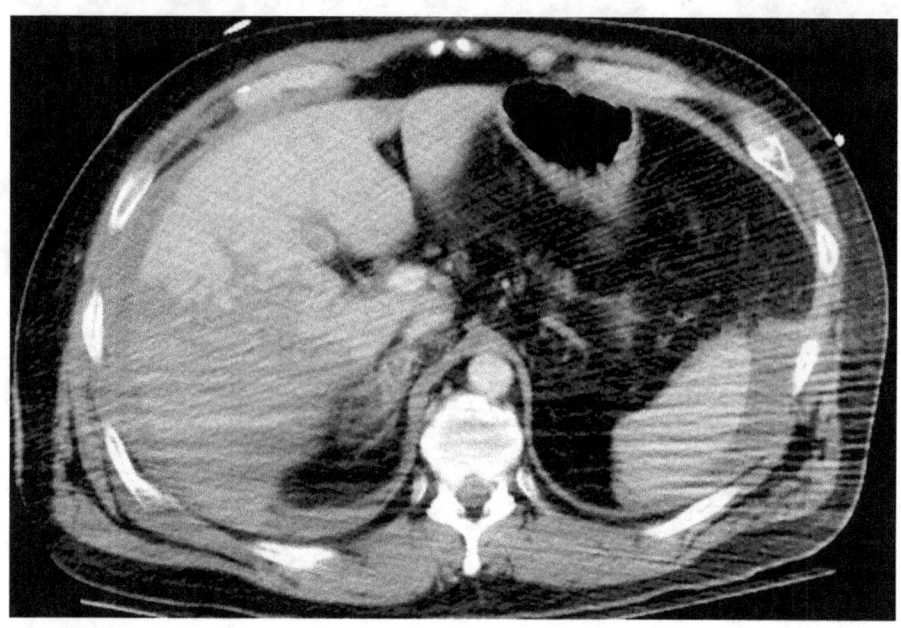

Best CT Study for Diagnosis:
CT Abdomen with IV contrast

Key to DX
Wedge shaped low density involving the liver parenchyma.

Facts
Patients may be asymptomatic or present with right upper quadrant pain.
Large infarcts will present with liver dysfunction.
Liver infarcts are uncommon because of dual blood supply.
Etiologies include trauma, intragenic, hypercoagulable states, and infections.

TX
Small infarcts typically only need supportive care, while large regions may require revascularization.
Etiology must be addressed (thrombus is the most common).

LIVER INFARCTION

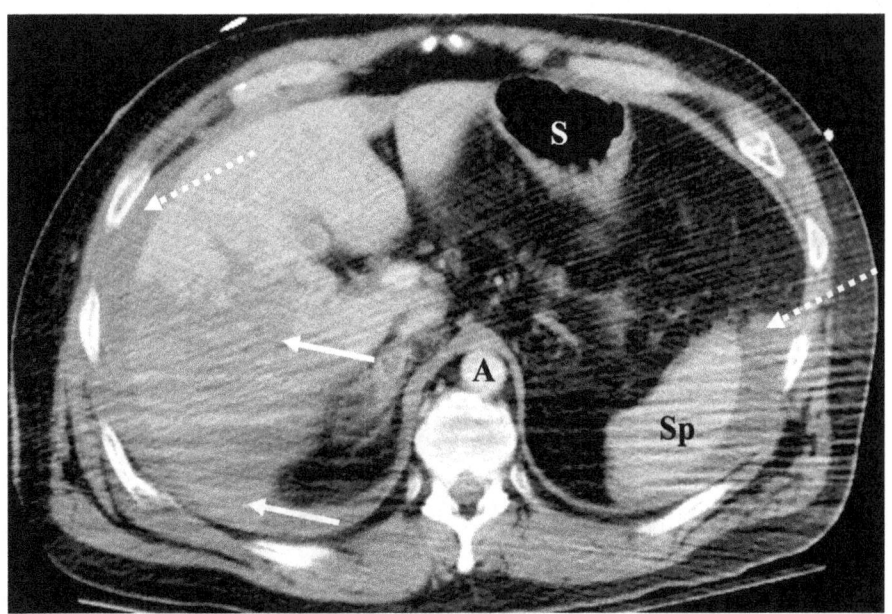

Study Above:
CT Abdomen with IV contrast at the level of the upper abdomen.

Radiographic Findings
Large wedge shaped area of hypoattenuation involving a large portion of the right lobe of the liver (white arrows). Free fluid is seen in both upper quadrants (dashed arrows).

Tips
Multiphase dynamic CT may be helpful to asses parenchymal enhancement.
Interrogate the vessels to exclude vascular injury which can be fatal!.
Exclude possible vascular thrombus.

Normal Anatomy
S - Stomach, Sp - Spleen, A - Aorta

Further Reading
Imaging of Biliary Tract Disease, Owen J. O'Connor, Siobhan O'Neill, and Michael M. Maher *American Journal of Roentgenology* 2011 197:4, W551-W558

Percutaneous Transcholecystic Management of Choledocholithiasis: A Next Horizon for Interventional Radiologists? vanSonnenberg E, Panchanathan R., Radiology. 2019 Jan;290(1):244-245. doi: 10.1148/radiol.2018181942. Epub 2018 Sep 18. PMID: 30226458.

CASE 92

CASE AUTHOR: Rocky Saenz

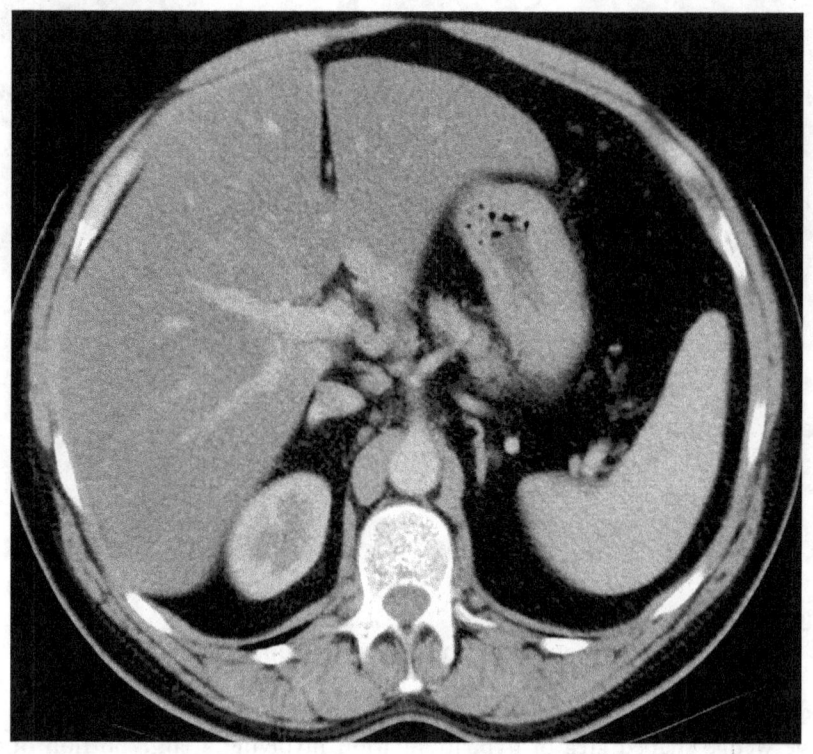

Best CT Study for Diagnosis:
CT Abdomen without IV contrast

Key to DX
Global low attenuation of the liver parenchyma.

Facts
Usually asymptomatic but may be associated with elevated liver function tests.
Common causes include alcohol, diabetes mellitus, and obesity.
Hepatomegaly may also be present.
Fatty liver disease is also called hepatic steatosis.

TX
Underlying cause must be addressed.
Control diabetes. Cessation of alcohol consumption can reverse the process.

FATTY LIVER

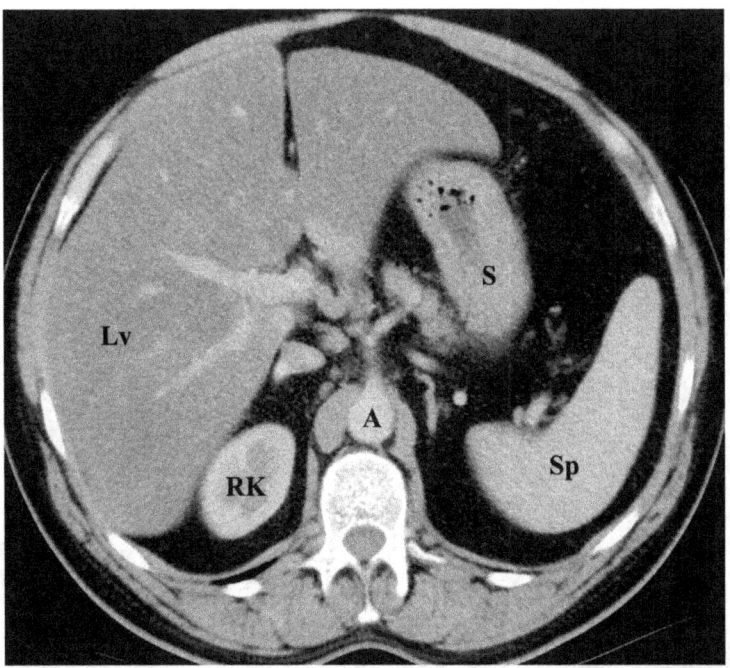

Study Above:
CT Abdomen with IV and oral contrast at the level of the upper abdomen.

Radiographic Findings:
Global hypoattenuation of the liver parenchyma (Lv).

Tips
Non-contrast CT has a higher accuracy for the diagnosis (HU less than 45).
Steatosis can be focal or global. When focal, steatosis can mimic a liver lesion.
True liver lesions have mass effect while focal fatty infiltration does not.
Focal fat is typical near the falciform ligament and is geographic in appearance.
The liver will be less dense than the spleen on portal venous phase (at least 25 HU).

Normal Anatomy
S – Stomach, Sp – Spleen, A - Aorta, RK – Right kidney

Further Reading
Imaging of Biliary Tract Disease, Owen J. O'Connor, Siobhan O'Neill, and Michael M. Maher *American Journal of Roentgenology* 2011 197:4, W551-W558

Percutaneous Transcholecystic Management of Choledocholithiasis: A Next Horizon for Interventional Radiologists? vanSonnenberg E, Panchanathan R., Radiology. 2019 Jan;290(1):244-245. doi: 10.1148/radiol.2018181942. Epub 2018 Sep 18. PMID: 30226458.

CASE 93

CASE AUTHOR: Michael Legacy

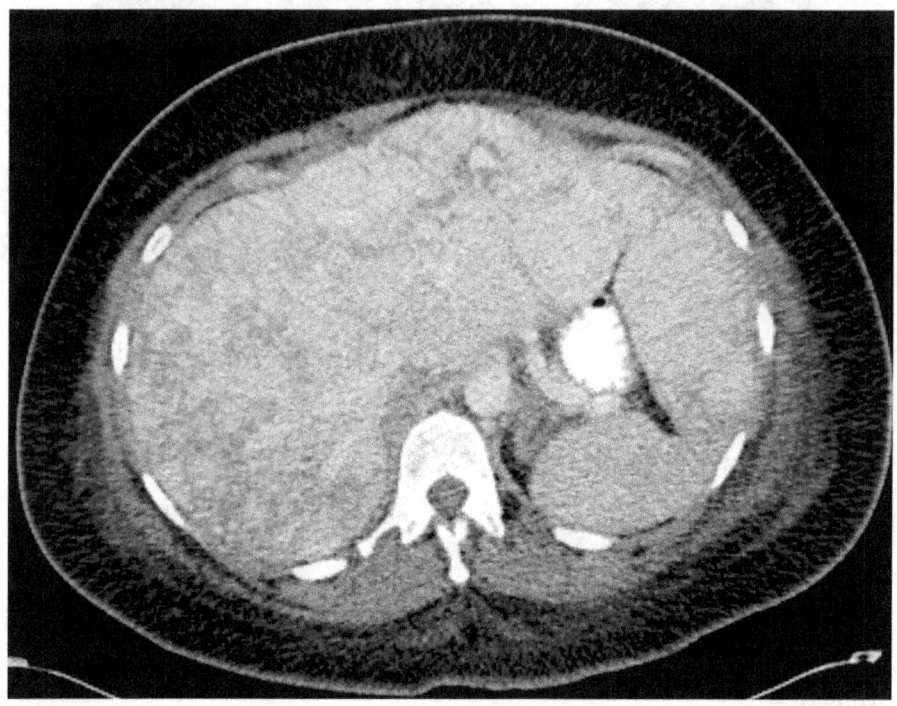

Best CT Study for Diagnosis:
CT Abdomen with IV contrast

Key to DX
Heterogeneous enhancement of the liver parenchyma.

Facts
The findings in this case are non-specific and could also represent passive venous congestion, cirrhosis, or volume overload related to resuscitation.
Hepatitis may be viral, autoimmune, or drug/alcohol induced.
Acute hepatitis may present with malaise, right upper quadrant pain, and/or elevated liver function tests.
Hepatitis C has an increased risk for hepatocellular carcinoma.

TX
No specific treatment for viral hepatitis.

ACUTE HEPATITIS

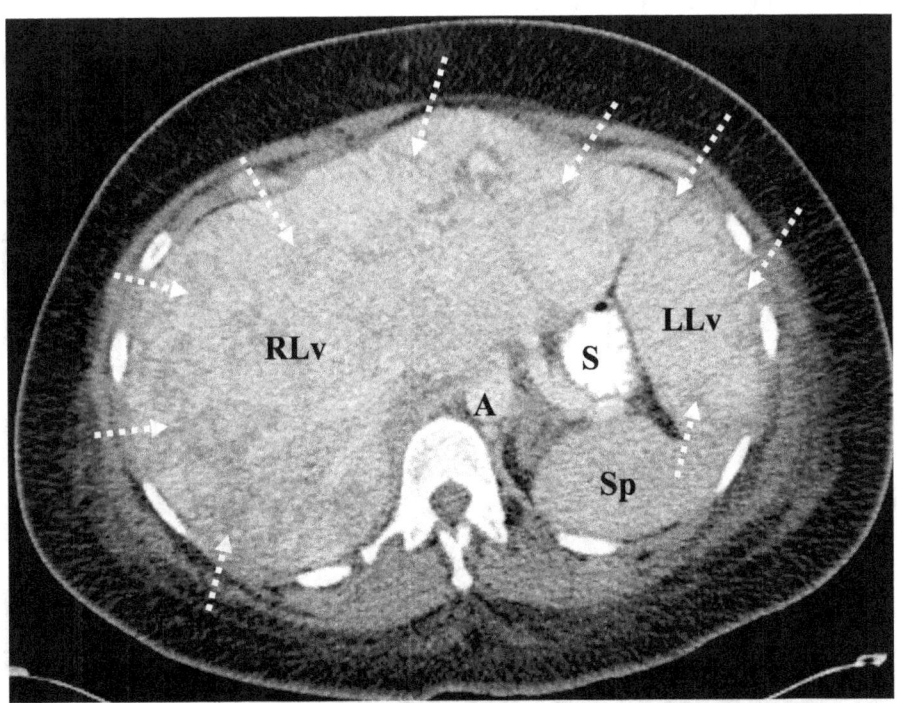

Study Above:
CT Abdomen with IV and oral contrast at the level of the upper abdomen.

Radiographic Findings:
Enlarged liver with areas of curvilinear/irregular hypoattenuation seen in the right and left hepatic lobes (dashed arrows).

Normal Anatomy
S - Stomach, LLv - Left hepatic lobe, RLv - Right hepatic lobe, Sp - Spleen,
A - Aorta,
P - Pancreas

Further Reading
Imaging of Biliary Tract Disease, Owen J. O'Connor, Siobhan O'Neill, and Michael M. Maher *American Journal of Roentgenology* 2011 197:4, W551-W558

Percutaneous Transcholecystic Management of Choledocholithiasis: A Next Horizon for Interventional Radiologists? vanSonnenberg E, Panchanathan R., Radiology. 2019 Jan;290(1):244-245. doi: 10.1148/radiol.2018181942. Epub 2018 Sep 18. PMID: 30226458.

CASE 94

CASE AUTHOR: Michael Legacy

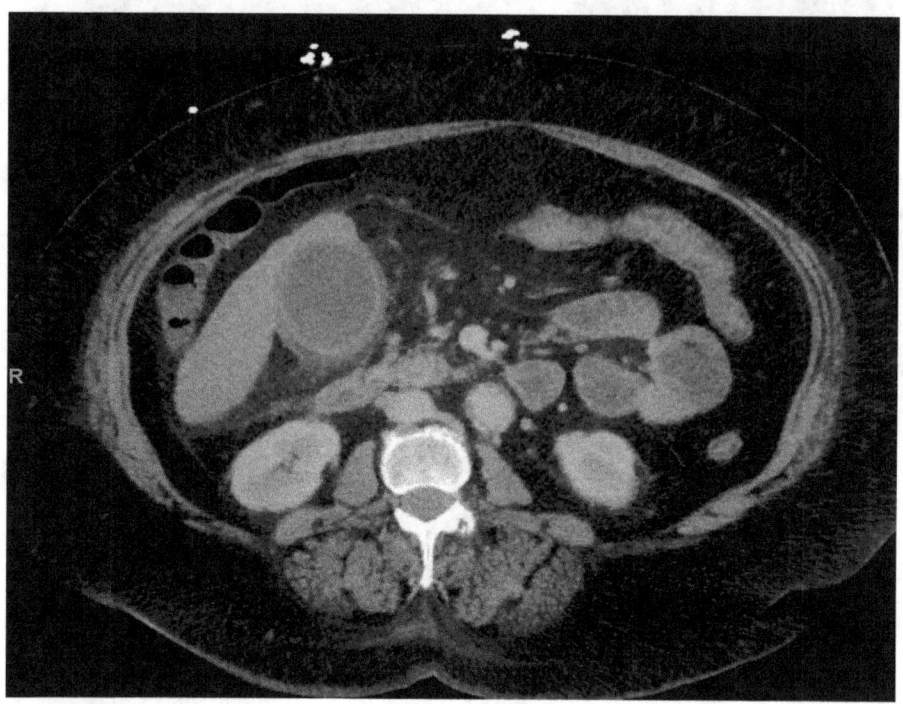

Best CT Study for Diagnosis:
CT Abdomen with IV contrast (when ultrasound is not available)

Key to DX
Gallbladder wall thickening with surrounding fat stranding.

Facts
Patients present with postprandial right upper quadrant pain.
Physical exam may elicit Murphy's Sign (pain during palpation of the right subcostal region upon inspiration).
Cholecystitis may be calculous or acalculous.
Most common in obese flatulent females in their forties (the 3 F's).

TX
Surgical gallbladder removal (cholecystectomy).

CHOLECYSTITIS

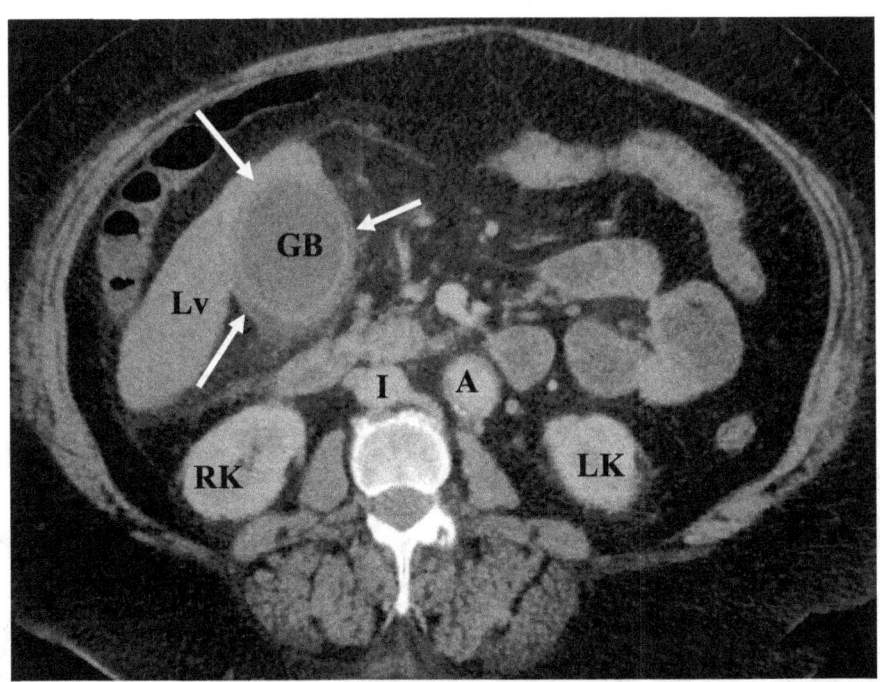

Study Above:
CT Abdomen with IV and oral contrast at the level of the mid abdomen.

Radiographic Findings:
Gallbladder wall thickening with surrounding fat stranding (arrows).

Tips
Cholelithiasis may or may not be present.
If cystic duct obstruction is of concern, consider nuclear hepatobiliary scan.
If soft tissue attenuation or eccentric gallbladder wall thickening is present, consider polyp or mass.

Normal Anatomy
GB - Gallbladder, LK - Left kidney, RK - Right kidney, I - Inferior vena cava,
A - Aorta,
Lv - Liver

Further Reading
Shakespear J.S., Shaaban A.M., and Rezvani M. CT Findings of Acute Cholecystitis and Its Complications. *American Journal of Roentgenology*. 194:6, 1523-1529; 2010.

CASE 95

CASE AUTHOR: Jordan Verlare

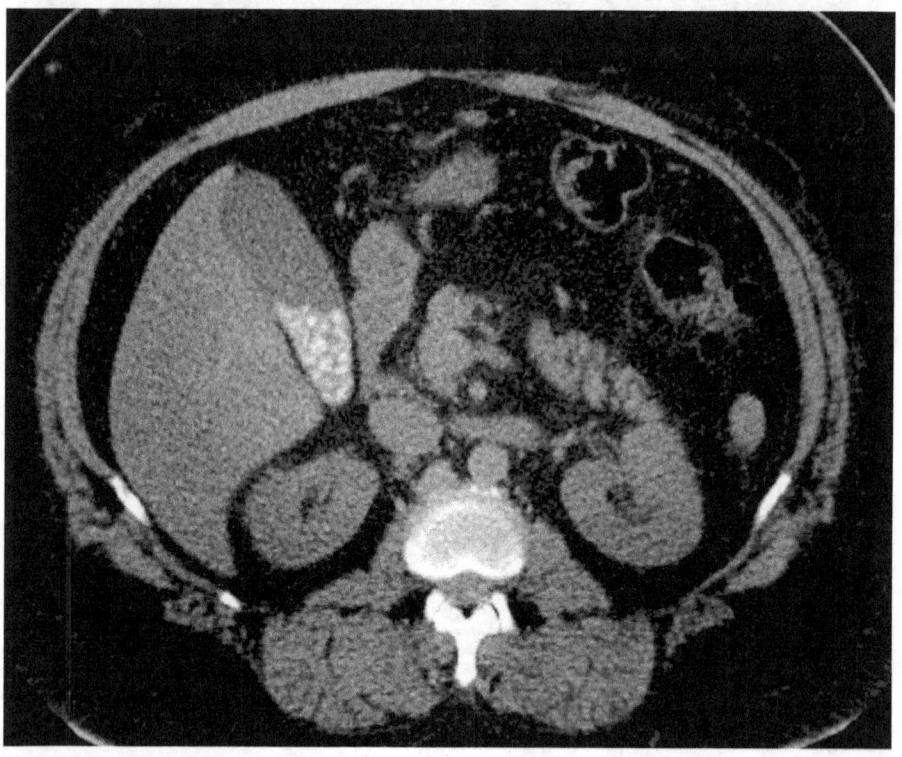

Best CT Study for Diagnosis:
CT Abdomen without contrast (if ultrasound is not available)

Key to DX
Calcific densities in the dependent portion of the gallbladder.

Facts
Patients may be asymptomatic or have postprandial right upper quadrant pain. Only 20% of gallstones are radiopaque; so, the majority are not seen on x-ray or CT. Most common in obese females in their forties.
Positive family history in a first-degree relative increases risk of gallstones by 2-fold.
Increasing ascorbic acid production boosts cholesterol catabolism, therefore a diet rich in vegetables, nuts, and coffee reduces the risk of developing gallstones.

TX
Asymptomatic gallstones require no follow-up or intervention as the risk often outweighs the benefit. Those who are symptomatic are definitively treated with cholecystectomy (gallbladder removal).

CHOLELITHIASIS

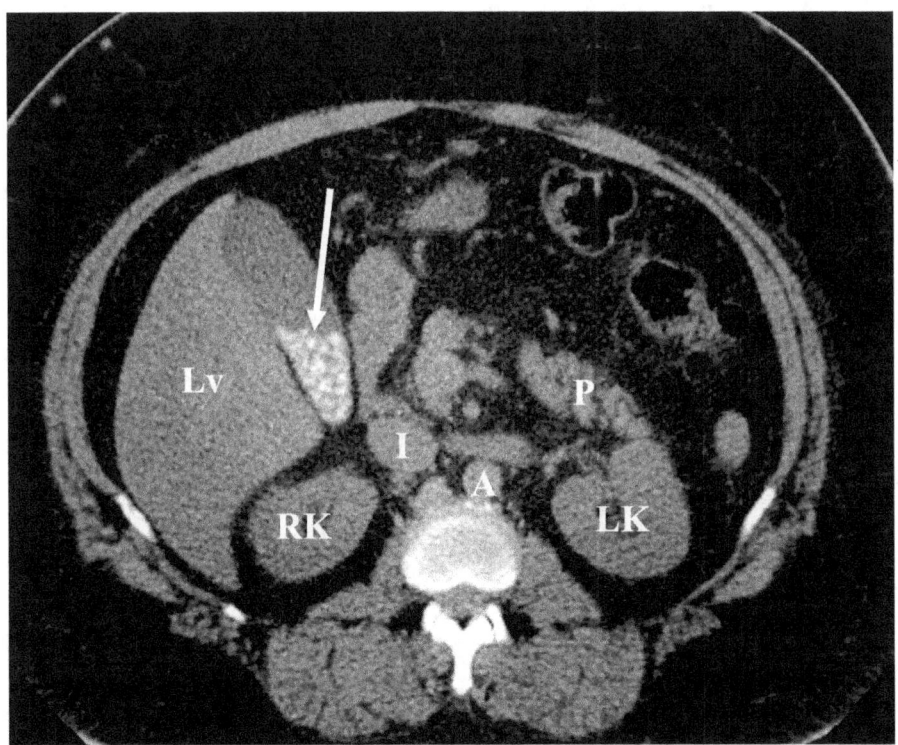

Study Above:
CT Abdomen without contrast at the level of the mid abdomen.

Radiographic Findings:
Dependent, round calcifications in the gallbladder lumen (arrow).

Tips
Gallstones should be positionally dependent. If a calcified lesion is nondependent, other diagnoses should be considered (gallbladder polyps, adenomyomatosis, or mass).
Check the common bile duct for stones.
Remember, about 20% of stones are calcified.
If cystic duct obstruction is of concern, consider nuclear hepatobiliary scan.

Normal Anatomy
P - Pancreas, LK - Left kidney, RK - Right kidney, I - Inferior vena cava, A - Aorta, Lv - Liver

Further Reading
Murphy, M.C., Gibney, B., Gillespie, C. *et al.* Gallstones top to toe: what the radiologist needs to know. *Insights Imaging.* 11, 13; 2020.

CASE 96

CASE AUTHOR: Rajeev Aravapalli

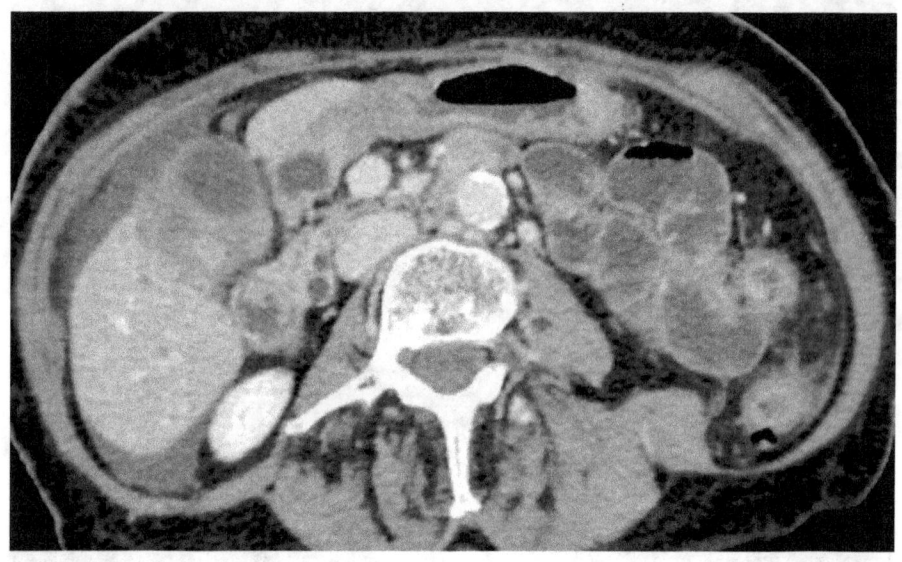

Best CT Study for Diagnosis:
CT Abdomen with IV and oral contrast

Key to DX
Soft tissue within the gallbladder.

Facts
Patients may present with right upper quadrant pain, weight loss, and/or jaundice.
Almost 90% of primary gallbladder cancer is adenocarcinoma.
There is a female predilection with a female-to-male ratio of 3:1.
Demonstrates three major patterns: a mass replacing the gallbladder, focal or diffuse gallbladder wall thickening, and an intraluminal polypoid mass.
Liver invasion is indicative of advanced disease.

TX
Surgical resection is needed.

GALLBLADDER CARCINOMA

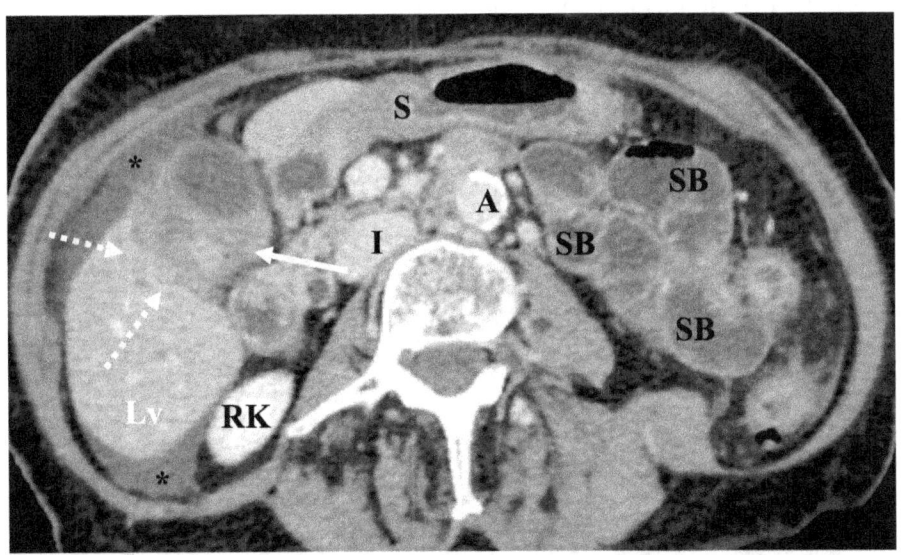

Study Above:
CT Abdomen with IV and no oral contrast at the level of the mid abdomen.

Radiographic Findings:
Irregular soft tissue attenuation within the gallbladder lumen (arrow). A patch of low attenuation is also seen in the liver parenchyma adjacent to the gallbladder (dashed arrows). This signifies liver invasion and advanced disease. Free fluid surrounding liver (asterisks).

Normal Anatomy
RK - Right kidney, S - Stomach, I - Inferior vena cava, A - Aorta, SB - Small bowel, Lv - Liver

Further Reading
Chatterjee A., Vendrami CL., Nikolaidis P., et al. Uncommon Intramural Tumors of the Gallbladder and Biliary Tract: Spectrum of Imaging Appearances. *RadioGraphics*. 39 (2): 388-412, 2019.

CASE 97

CASE AUTHOR: Gregory D. Puthoff

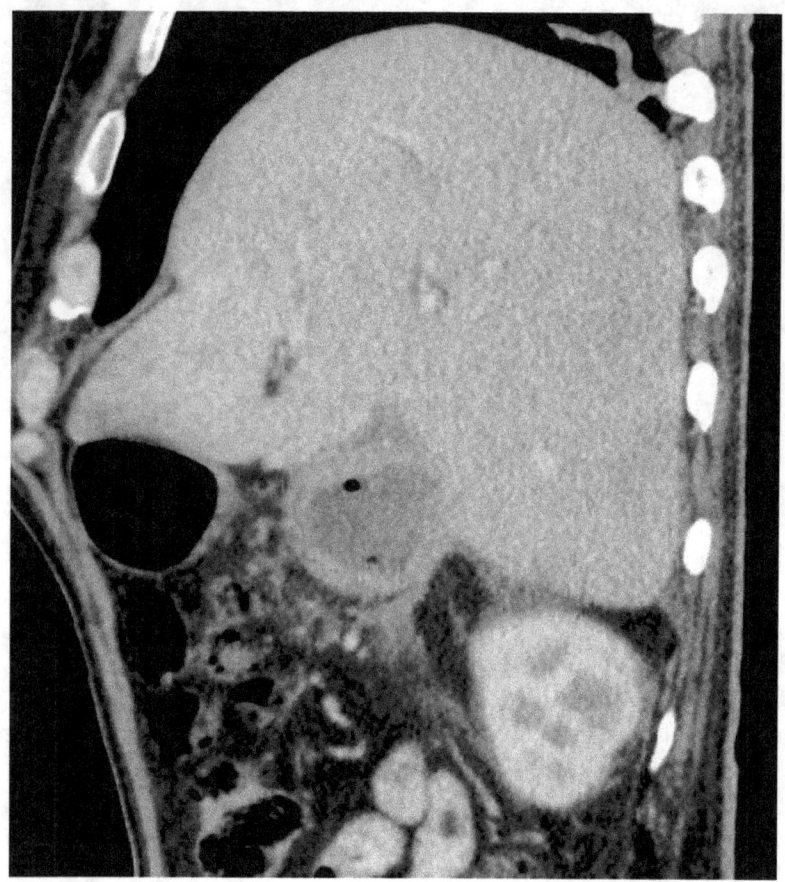

Best CT Study for Diagnosis:
CT Abdomen with IV contrast (when ultrasound is not available)

Key to DX
Intraluminal air within the gallbladder and/or air within the gallbladder wall.

Facts
Occurs when gas forming organisms such as *Clostridium perfringens, Escherichia coli,* or *Bacteroides fragilis* infect the gallbladder wall.
More likely to rupture than uncomplicated acute cholecystitis.
Men are more commonly affected.
Similar symptoms to acute cholecystitis, except many patients have non-focal pain.

TX
Emergent cholecystectomy is required. If the patient is too unstable for traditional open cholecystectomy, antibiotic therapy and percutaneous CT guided cholecystostomy tube can be utilized as a temporizing measure.

EMPHYSEMATOUS CHOLECYSTITIS

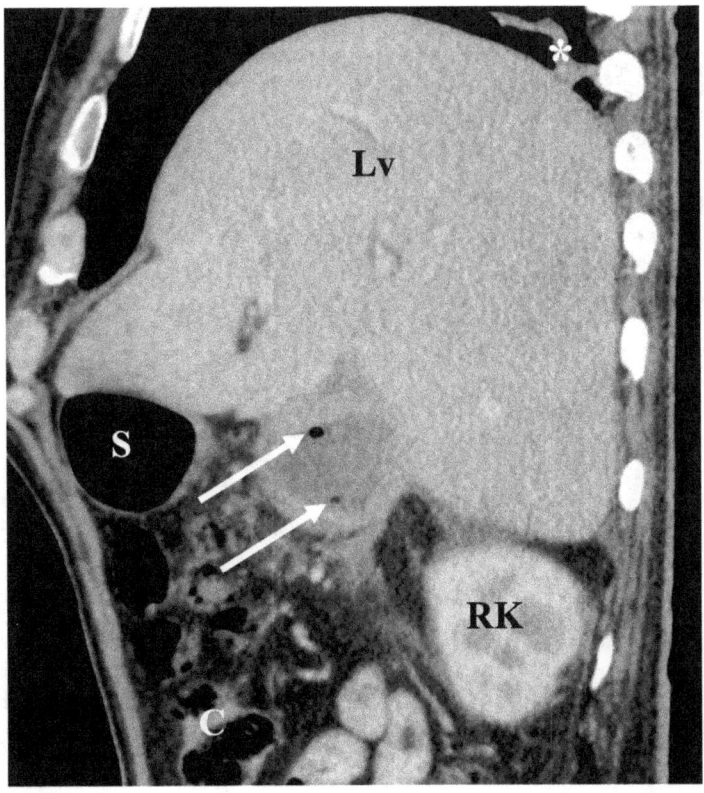

Study Above:
Ct Abdomen with IV and oral contrast, sagittal reformat of the right upper quadrant.

Radiographic findings:
Multiple foci of intraluminal air within the gallbladder (arrows). The gallbladder wall is thickened (> 3 mm) and demonstrates subtle surrounding fat stranding. Right basilar atelectasis is noted (asterisk).

Tips
Intraluminal air within the gallbladder or biliary system may be secondary to recent ERCP procedure (correlate with patient history).
Intraluminal air within the gallbladder may be easily mistaken for nitrogen filled gallstones in a contracted gallbladder or a porcelain gallbladder on ultrasound.

Normal Anatomy
S - Stomach, C - Colon, Lv - Liver, RK - Right kidney

Further Reading
Nepal P., et-al. Gas Where It Shouldn't Be! Imaging Spectrum of Emphysematous Infections in the Abdomen and Pelvis. *American Journal of Roentgenology.* 216: 812-823. 2021.

CASE 98

CASE AUTHOR: Ahmed Tahawi

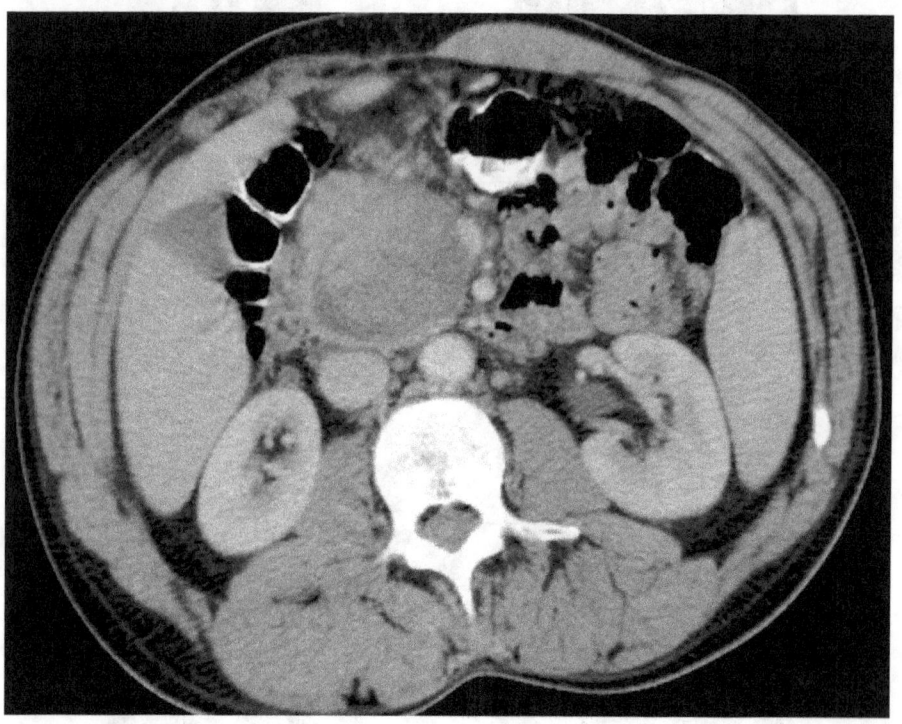

Best CT Study for Diagnosis:
CT Abdomen with IV contrast

Key to DX
Focal round or oval fluid collection with a contrast enhancing wall within the pancreatic parenchyma.

Facts
Usually arises as a complication of pancreatitis.
The most typical organism isolated is *Escherichia coli*.
Clinical presentation often includes persistent or recurrent epigastric pain.
Initial imaging should be done 5-7 days after symptom onset to assess for complications.
These collections are either fluid-filled or can contain necrotic, non-liquified debris.

TX
Conservative treatment with broad spectrum IV antibiotics in the majority of cases.
Ultrasound or CT-guided percutaneous drainage can be performed if necrosis is present.

PANCREATIC ABSCESS

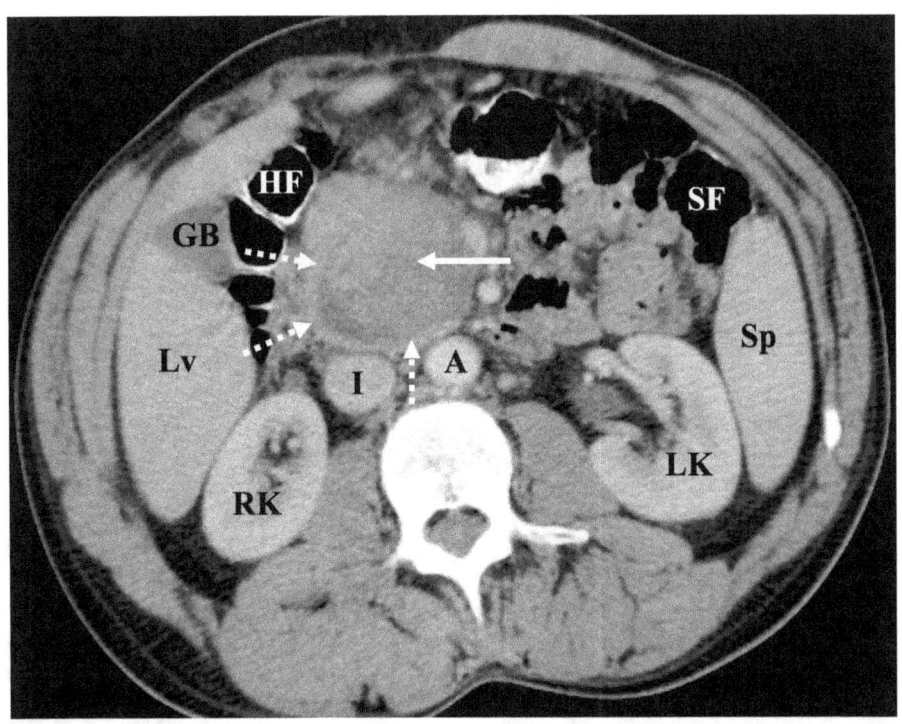

Study Above:
CT Abdomen with IV and oral contrast at the level of the upper abdomen.

Radiographic Findings:
Large, round complex fluid collection demonstrating peripheral enhancement (dashed arrows) with increased internal area of attenuation (arrow) located in the pancreatic head.

Tips
Pancreatic fluid collection with air should be considered abscess; although if air is not present, it does not exclude abscess.
Follow-up CT is recommended 4-6 weeks after treatment for re-evaluation.

Normal Anatomy
SF - Splenic flexure, HF - Hepatic flexure, Sp - Spleen, RK - Right kidney, LK - Left kidney, I - Inferior vena cava, A - Aorta, Lv - Liver, Gb – Gallbladder

Further Reading
Foster B, et al. Revised Atlanta Classification for Acute Pancreatitis: A Pictorial Essay. *RadioGraphics*. 36:675-687, 2016.

CASE 99

CASE AUTHOR: Jordan Verlare

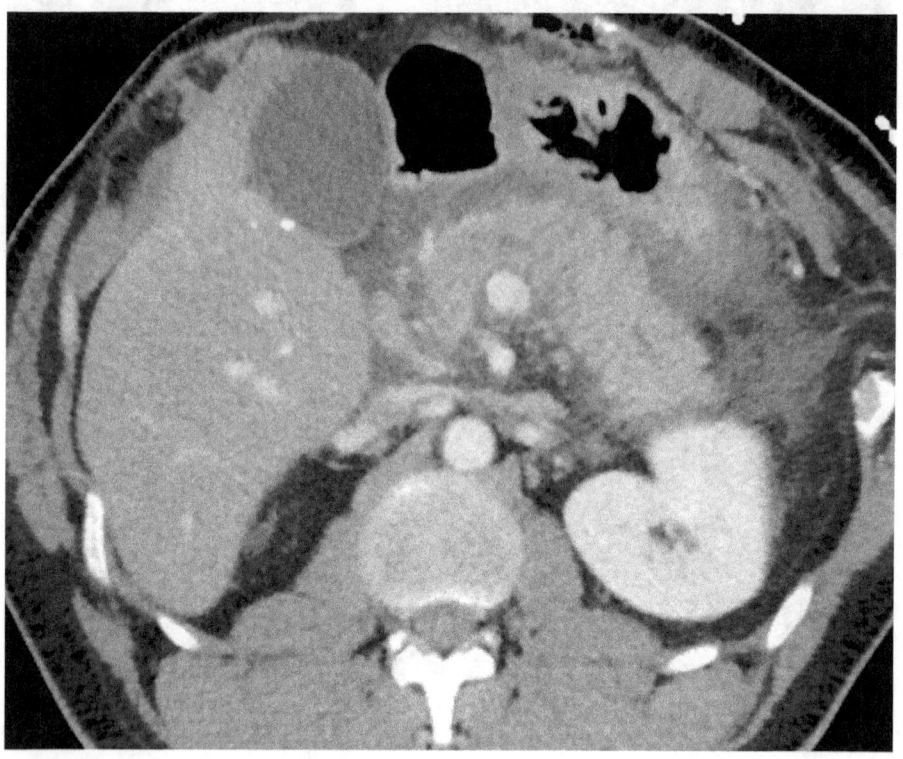

Best CT Study for Diagnosis:
CT Abdomen with IV contrast

Key to DX
Peripheral fat stranding surrounding an enlarged, edematous pancreas.

Facts
Patients usually present with epigastric pain radiating to the back. On a physical exam, may have Grey Turner sign (Case 104) or Cullen sign (infra-umbilical hematoma).
Serum amylase and lipase are typically elevated.
CT is reserved for patients with sustained or progressive symptoms more than 48 hours.
The most common cause of *acute* pancreatitis is gallstones.
The most common cause of *chronic* pancreatitis is alcohol consumption.

TX
Supportive treatment with IV hydration, NG tube, analgesics, and NPO diet.
Complex cases with necrosis require surgical intervention.

ACUTE PANCREATITIS

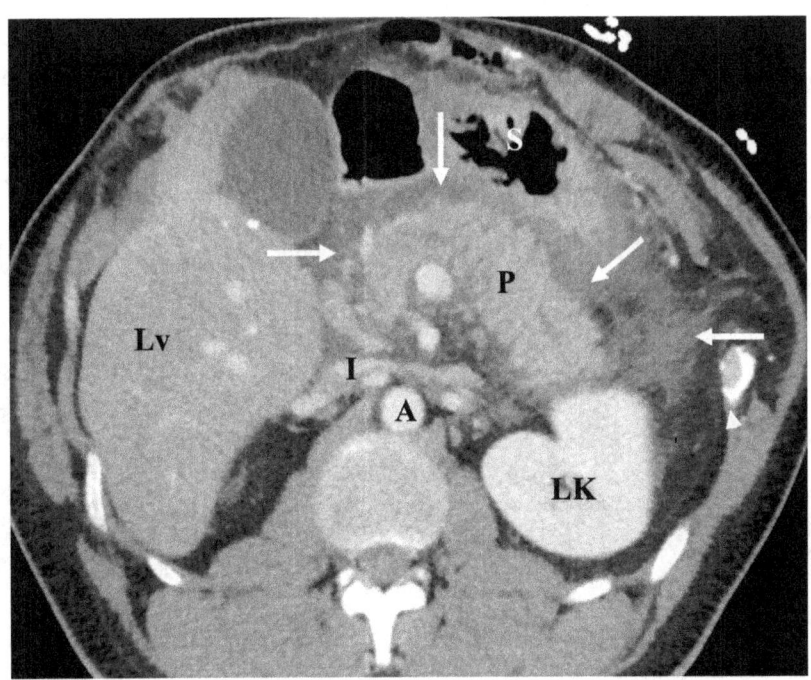

Study Above:
CT Abdomen with IV contrast and oral contrast at the level of the mid abdomen.

Radiographic Findings
Peripheral fat stranding is seen around the pancreas (arrows). Oral contrast is noted in the descending/left colon (arrowhead).

Tips
Closely interrogate the portal, splenic, and mesenteric veins for thrombosis.
Search the whole abdomen and pelvis for pseudocyst formation.
Areas of pancreatic non-enhancement signify necrosis!
Chronic pancreatitis will have 3 classic findings: parenchymal calcifications, atrophy, and ductal enlargement.
Review the 2012 Revised Atlanta Criteria (reference below) to understand the pancreatitis descriptors used by radiologists for classification, prognostic prediction, and sequelae.

Normal Anatomy
S – Stomach, P – Pancreas, LK - Left kidney, A - Aorta, I - Inferior vena cava, Lv - Liver

Further Reading
Foster B, et al. Revised Atlanta Classification for Acute Pancreatitis: A Pictorial Essay. RadioGraphics. 36:675-687, 2016.

CASE 100

CASE AUTHOR: Rajeev Aravapalli

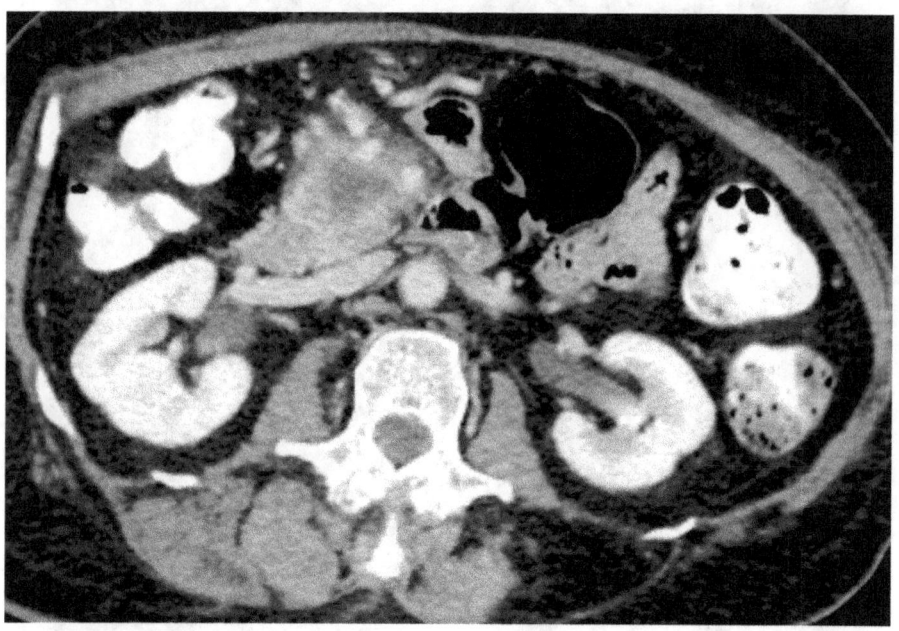

Best CT Study for Diagnosis:
CT Abdomen with IV and oral contrast

Key to DX
Focal soft tissue mass within the pancreas.

Facts
Patients may be asymptomatic when tumors are small or may present with jaundice and elevated bilirubin levels.
The most common location is the pancreatic head.
Pancreatic ductal adenocarcinoma accounts for over 90% of all pancreatic malignancies and is the second most common digestive-system cancer after colorectal cancer in the United States.
"Double-duct sign" is usually present which refers to dilation of the pancreatic and common bile duct secondary to proximal duct extrinsic compression.

TX
Standard of care is surgery followed by adjuvant chemotherapy.
Surgical removal of tumor in non-advanced cases (Whipple resection).
The majority of patients have advanced disease at time of diagnosis.

PANCREATIC CARCINOMA

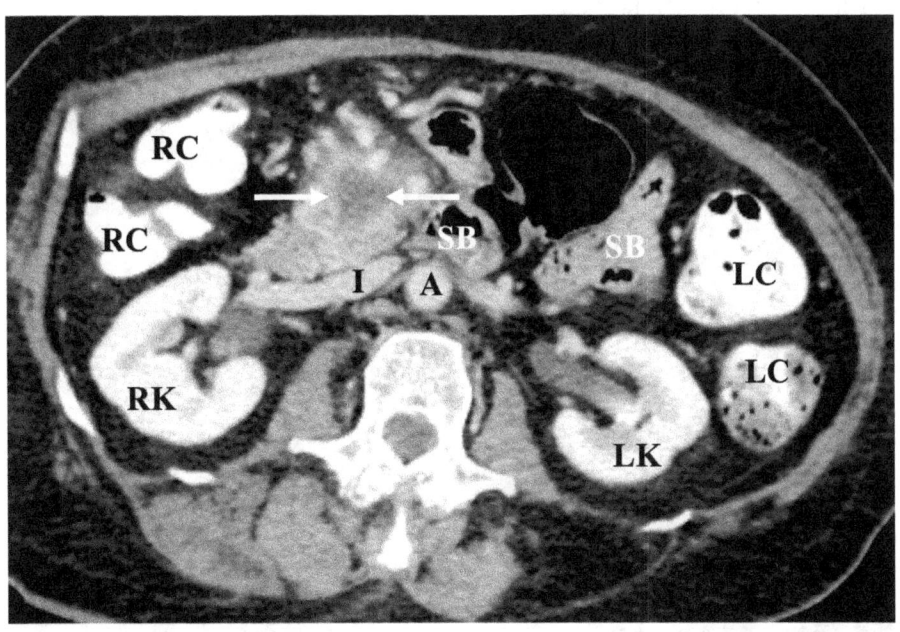

Study Above:
CT Abdomen with IV and oral contrast at the level of the mid abdomen.

Radiographic Findings:
Focal soft tissue low attenuated lesion centered in the head of the pancreas (arrows).

Tips
Majority of pancreatic adenocarcinomas have metastasis on presentation; so check for mets!
Vascular encasement of mesenteric root makes tumor non-resectable.
Serum CA 19-9 is usually elevated.

Normal Anatomy
RK - Right kidney, LK - Left kidney, RC - Right colon, SB - Small bowel, LC - Left colon, I - Inferior vena cava, A - Aorta

Further Reading
Zins M, Matos C, Cassinotto C. Pancreatic Adenocarcinoma Staging in the Era of Preoperative Chemotherapy and Radiation Therapy. *Radiology*. 287(2): 374-390; 2018.

CASE 101

CASE AUTHOR: Colby Jones

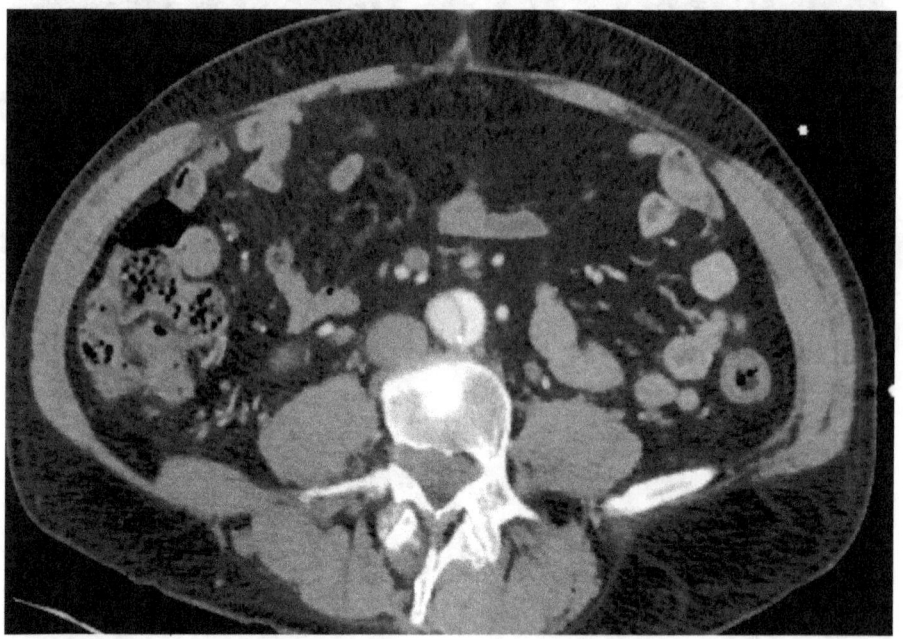

Best CT Study for Diagnosis:
CT Abdomen and Pelvis with IV contrast

Key to DX
Linear low attenuation band traversing the lumen of the aorta.

Facts
This may be asymptomatic or present with acute tearing pain.
It is most common in elderly hypertensive patients or in patients with underlying connective tissue disorders.
Rupture may occur, which is usually due to expansion of the false lumen.
If an aneurysm is also present, the risk of rupture is magnified.

TX
Therapy usually depends upon severity (size, vessel branch involvement) and the presence of an underlying aneurysm).
Medical treatment and surgical reduction (both open and endovascular).

ABDOMINAL AORTIC DISSECTION

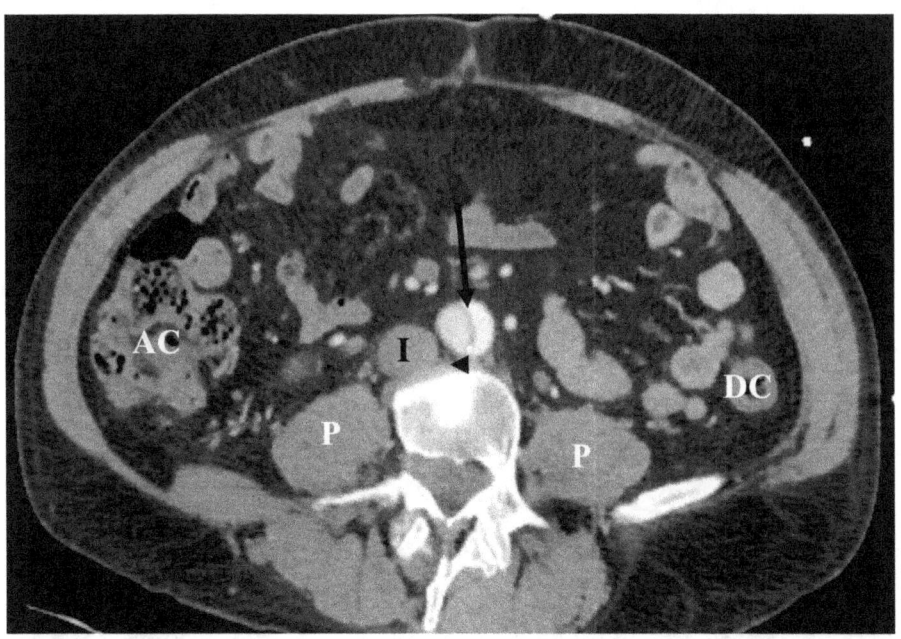

Study Above:
CT Abdomen with IV contrast at the level of the mid abdomen.

Radiographic Findings
Dual lumen appearance of the aorta with a low attenuation cleft dividing it (arrow). The cleft is the intimal flap. Also note the displacement of the intimal calcifications toward the center of the aortic lumen (arrowhead).

Tips
If a dissection is present on the first images of study, consider Chest CT with intravenous contrast because the thoracic aorta could also be involved.
Follow the dissection and report if any of the aortic branches are involved.
False lumen is typically larger and may enhance late or not at all.
Vascular dissection is not always associated with aneurysmal dilation.

Normal Anatomy
P - Psoas, DC – Descending colon, AC - Ascending colon, I - Inferior vena cava

Further Reading
Murillo, H., Molvin, L., Chin, A. S., & Fleischmann, D. Aortic Dissection and Other Acute Aortic Syndromes. *RadioGraphics*. 2021. 41(2), 425–446

CASE 102

CASE AUTHOR: Matt Waldrop

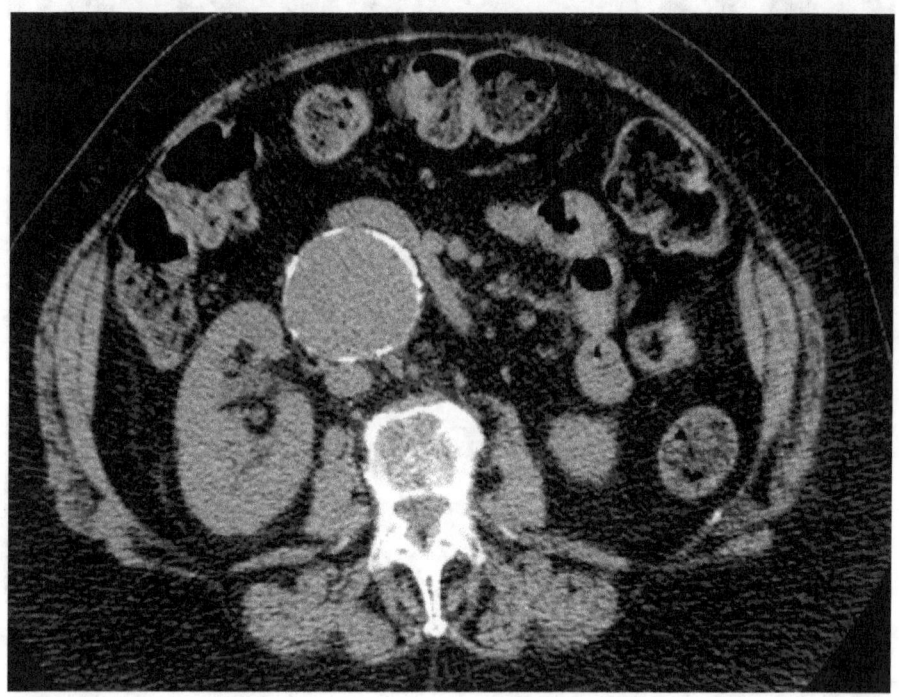

Best CT Study for Diagnosis:
CT Abdomen and Pelvis without contrast

Key to DX
Abdominal aortic diameter larger than 3 centimeters.

Facts
Patients are typically asymptomatic.
Suspected on physical exam when there is a large pulsating abdominal mass.
The larger an aneurysm, the more likely it is to rupture.
Most common in elderly males.
Risk factors include smoking, hypertension, and hypercholesterolemia.

TX
Must consider the patient's hemodynamic stability.
Vascular surgical consultation for repair.
Open surgical repair with graft or endovascular graft.
Elective repair mortality 5%.

ABDOMINAL AORTIC ANEURYSM

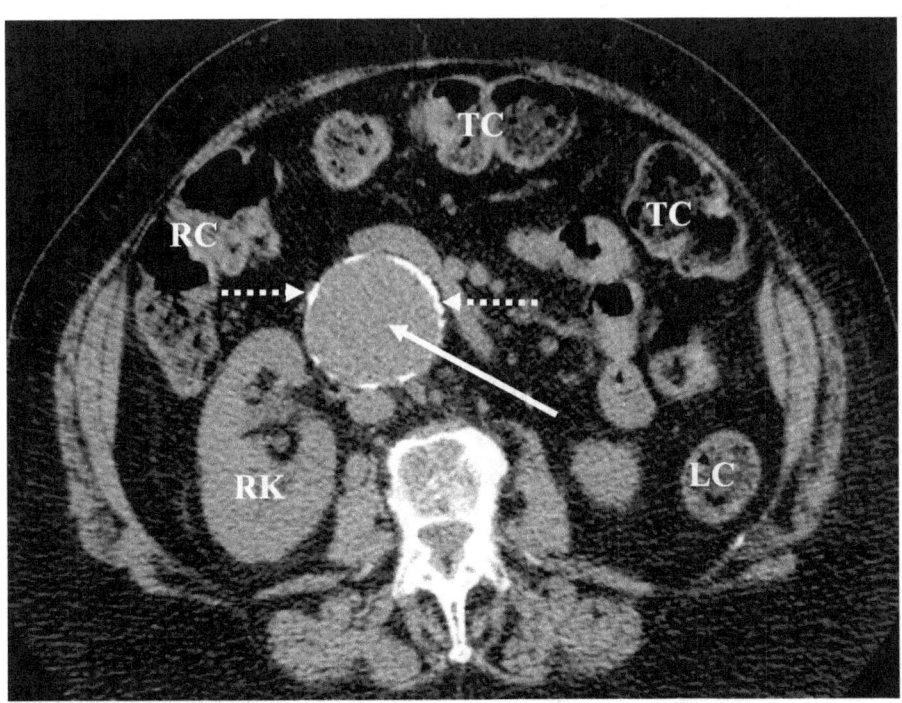

Study Above:
CT Abdomen without contrast at the level of the kidneys (left kidney not fully seen on this image).

Radiographic Findings
Enlargement of the diameter of the abdominal aorta (solid arrow). Notice there are peripheral calcifications of the aortic wall (dashed arrows). Mural thrombus formation is seen along the left aspect where low attenuation is present.

Tips
The aorta should never be larger than a vertebral body.
Aortic dissection can only be excluded with IV contrast.

Normal Anatomy
RK – Right kidney, RC - Right colon, TC - Transverse colon, LC - Left colon

Further Reading
Wadgaonkar AD, Black JH, 3rd, Weihe EK, et al. Abdominal Aortic Aneurysms Revisited: MDCT with Multiplanar Reconstructions for Identifying Indicators of Instability in the Pre- and Postoperative Patient. *Radiographics*. 35:254-68, 2015.

CASE 103

CASE AUTHOR: Matt Waldrop

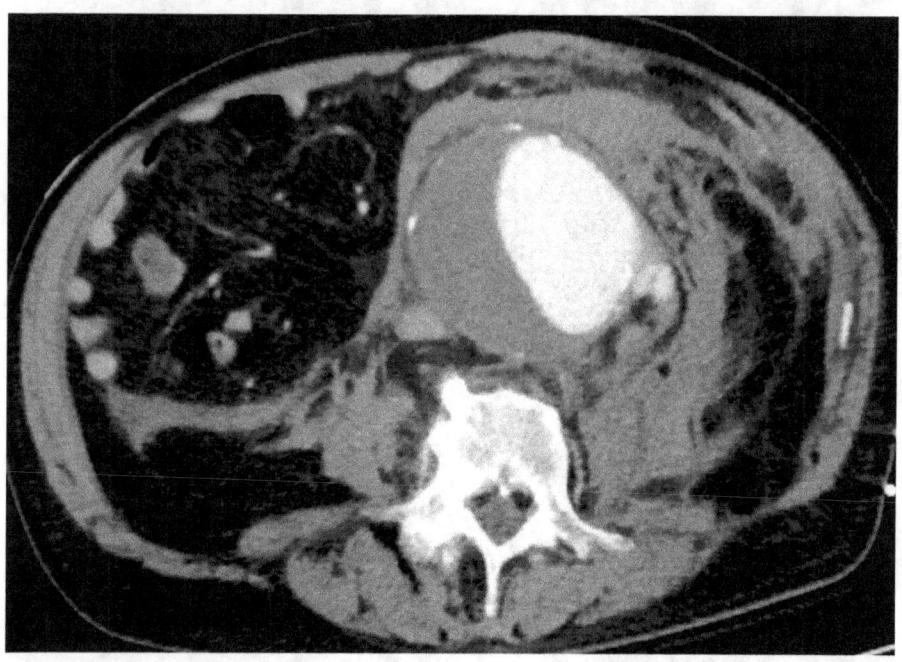

Best CT Study for Diagnosis:
CT Abdomen and Pelvis without IV contrast

Key to DX
Enlarged aorta with associated adjacent irregular intermediate attenuation within the retroperitoneum.

Facts
Patients commonly present with acute abdominal pain which may radiate down the flank or into the groin (secondary to mass effect from the retroperitoneal hematoma).
Significant hypotension may be seen.
The diagnosis of aneurysm can be made without IV contrast, but dissection and active extravasation need IV contrast!

TX
Must consider the patient's hemodynamic stability.
Emergent consultation with vascular surgery needed.
Surgical reduction (open or intravascular).
Emergent operative mortality rate is greater than 50%.

ABDOMINAL AORTIC ANEURYSM RUPTURE

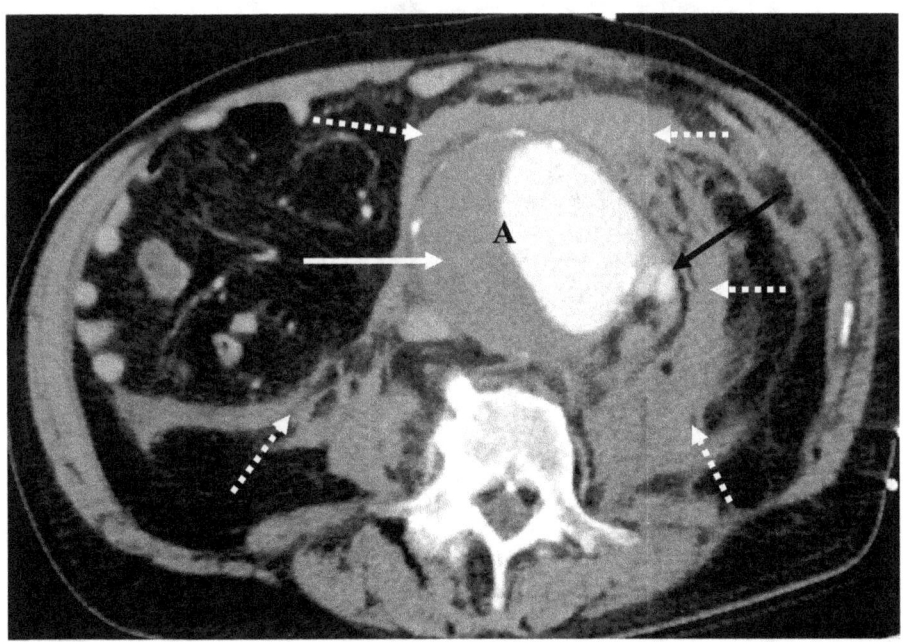

Study Above:
CT Abdomen with IV contrast at the level of the lower abdomen.

Radiographic Findings:
Infrarenal abdominal aortic aneurysm with peripheral calcifications (A). There is non-enhancement along the right lumen within the aorta representing mural thrombus (white arrow). There is an amorphous attenuation surrounding the aorta (dashed arrows). Intravenous contrast is seen actively extravasating through the ruptured aorta (black arrow) leading to a retroperitoneal hematoma (dashed arrows).

Tips
Must define the extent of the aneurysm with regards to location (is it above or below the renal arteries, does it involve the iliac arteries) and size.
If aortic rupture cannot be excluded on non-contrast CT, administer IV contrast (to accurately examine for extravasation).

Further Reading
Sever A, Rheinboldt M. Unstable abdominal aortic aneurysms: a review of MDCT imaging features. Emerg Radiol. 23(2):187–96; 2016.

CASE 104

CASE AUTHOR: Colby Jones

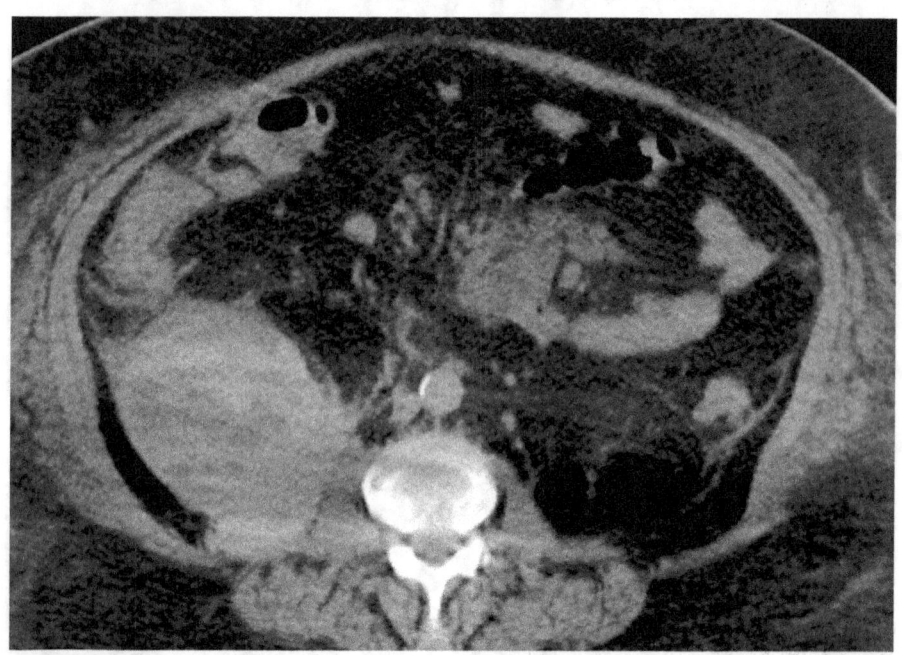

Best CT Study for Diagnosis:
CT Abdomen and Pelvis without contrast

Key to DX
Irregular intermediate attenuation within the retroperitoneum.

Facts
Patients present with flank pain that may radiate inferiorly.
May see discoloration of the flank (Grey Turner's Sign)
The most common cause is coagulopathy.
Other common causes include tumor and aneurysm rupture.
May cause displacement or compression of retroperitoneal organs.

TX
Must address patient's underlying coagulopathy
Since this is usually iatrogenic, hold anticoagulants and consider protamine.
When related to aneurysm rupture, must seek emergent vascular surgical consultation.

RETROPERITONEAL HEMORRHAGE

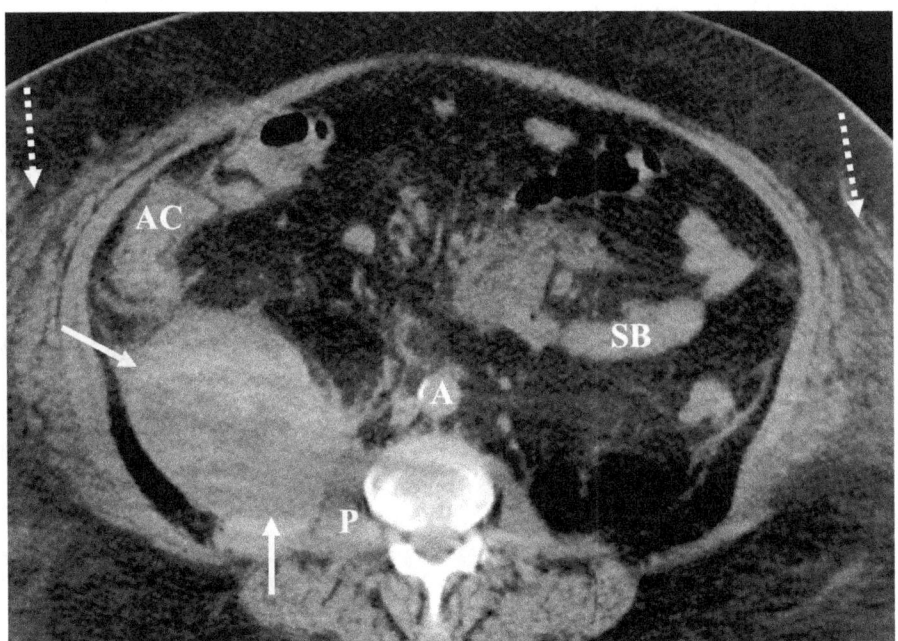

Study Above:
CT Abdomen without IV contrast with oral contrast at the level of the lower abdomen.

Radiographic Findings
Intermediate and heterogeneous attenuation within the right retroperitoneum (arrows). Notice there is some mass effect on the anterior loops of bowel in the region. Bilateral flank subcutaneous fat stranding related to hemorrhage, Grey Turner's Sign (dashed arrows).

Tips
IV contrast is not needed to diagnose retroperitoneal hematoma.
These bleeds are almost always venous (don't consult for radiology intervention). Always check the psoas muscles for symmetry, when one is enlarged and of increased density compared to the other, its likely retroperitoneal hematoma.

Normal Anatomy
AC- Ascending colon, P – Psoas, SB – Small bowel, A - Aorta

Further Reading
Smillie, R. P., Shetty, M., Boyer, A. C., Madrazo, B., & Jafri, S. Z. Imaging Evaluation of the Inferior Vena Cava. *RadioGraphics*. 35(2), 578–592; 2015.

CASE 105

CASE AUTHOR: Colby Jones

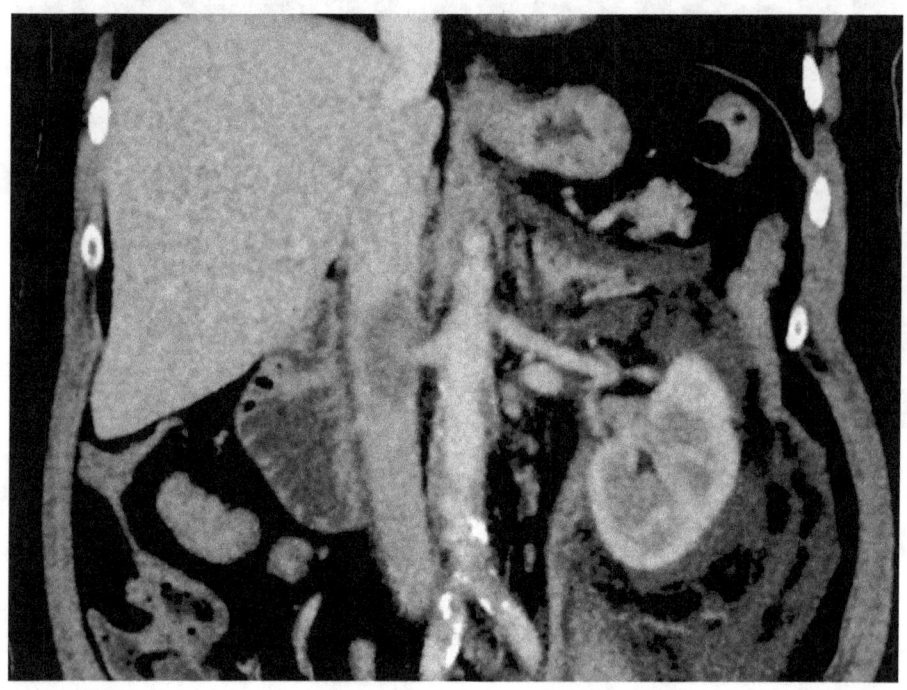

Best CT Study for Diagnosis:
CT Abdomen and Pelvis with IV contrast

Key to DX
Focal low attenuation within the inferior vena cava (IVC) lumen.

Facts
Patients may present with venous stasis issues including pain of lower extremities, leg edema, and leg ulcers.
Etiologies include trauma, tumor, and hypercoagulable states.
Patients are at risk for organ infarction and pulmonary embolism.
About 15% of patients will also have a DVT.

TX
Must address the patient's underlying coagulopathy.
Consider IVC filter placement to prevent pulmonary embolism.

INFERIOR VENA CAVA THROMBOSIS

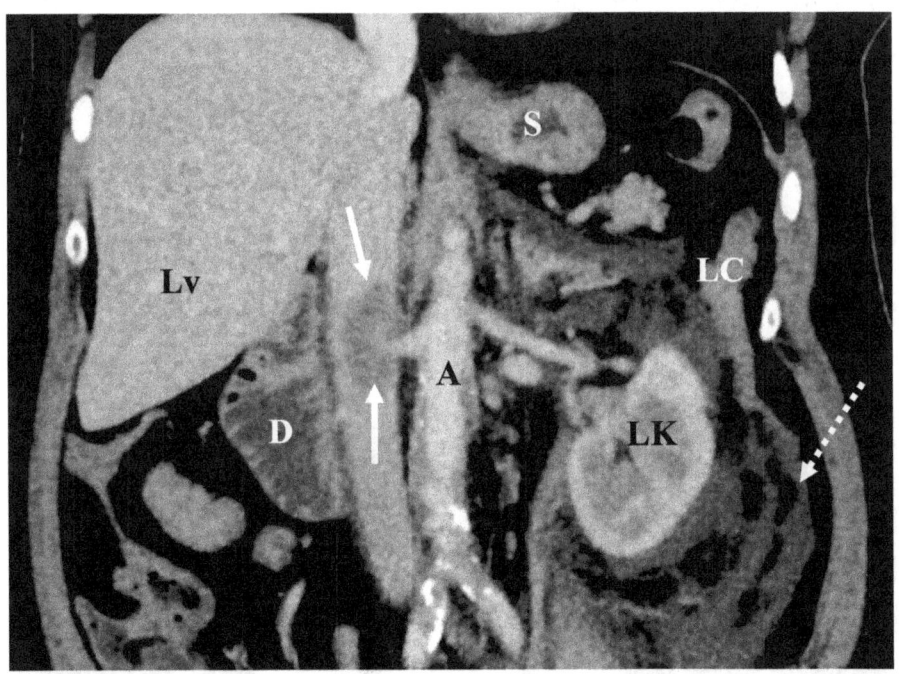

Study Above:
CT Abdomen with IV contrast, coronal reformat.

Radiographic Findings:
Hypoattenuated filling defect in the lumen of the IVC (arrows). Also note increased attenuation surrounding the left kidney (dashed arrow) secondary to edema from the clot extending into the left renal vein (not shown).

Tips
Scrutinize the venous system for other sites of thrombus formation.
Portal venous phase and delayed imaging at 3 minutes is ideal.
Beware of artifacts on arterial phase imaging which appear as pseudo filling defects due to mixing of contrast enhanced blood with non-contrast enhanced blood.

Normal Anatomy
LK - Left kidney, D – Duodenum, S - Stomach, LC - Left colon, A - Aorta, Lv - Liver

Further Reading
Smillie, R. P., Shetty, M., Boyer, A. C., Madrazo, B., & Jafri, S. Z. Imaging Evaluation of the Inferior Vena Cava. *RadioGraphics*. 35(2), 578–592; 2015.

CASE 106

CASE AUTHOR: Lauren Corley

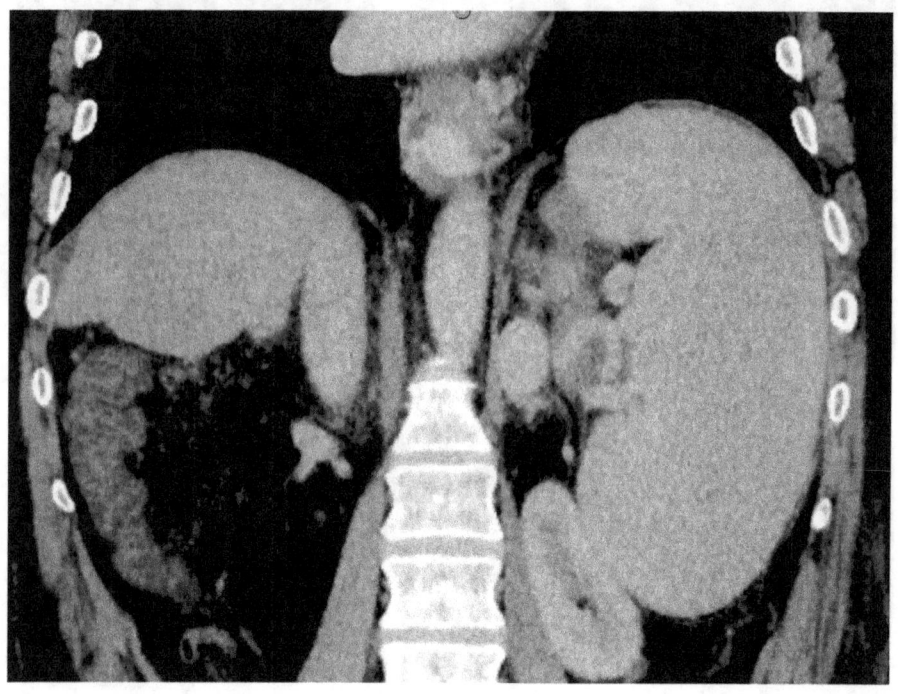

Best CT Study for Diagnosis:
CT Abdomen without IV contrast

Key to DX
Spleen larger than 14 centimeters in any dimension.

Facts
The most common etiologies include infection (mononucleosis classically), portal venous hypertension (secondary to cirrhosis), metastatic disease, and profound anemia.
May cause compression of neighboring organs (note the mass effect on the left kidney).
Enlargement can be self-limiting, such as in cases of infection.

TX
May improve with the treatment of the underlying etiology.

SPLENOMEGALY

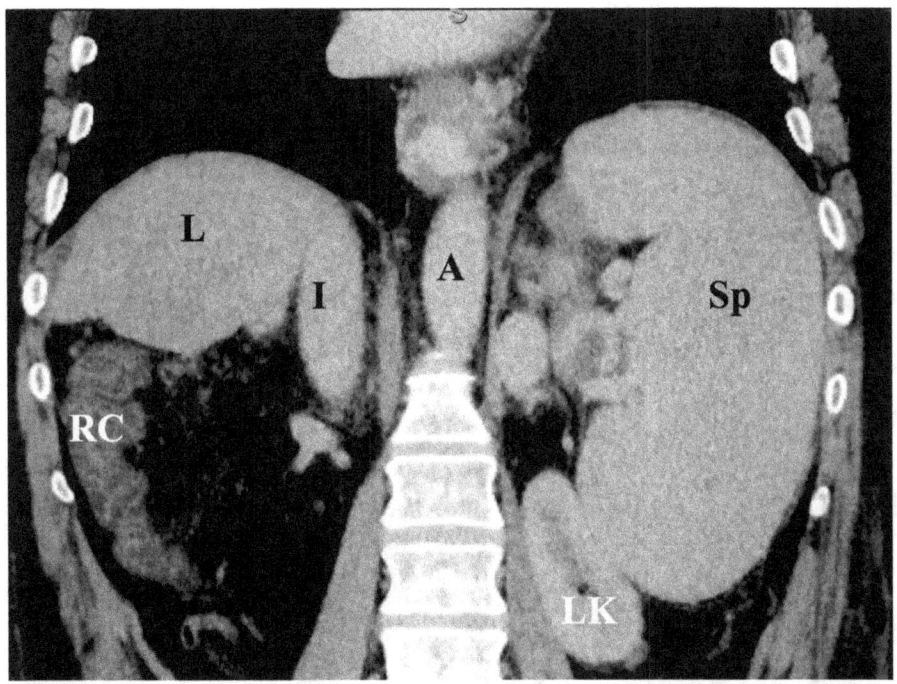

Study Above:
CT Abdomen with IV contrast, coronal reformat.

Radiographic Findings:
Marked enlargement of the spleen (Sp) at 20 cm in craniocaudal dimension. The left kidney (LK) is being compressed by the spleen.

Normal Anatomy
L - Liver, RC - Right colon, I - Inferior vena cava, A - Aorta

Further Reading

Sjoberg, B., Menias, C., Lubner, M., et al. Splenomegaly. *Radiologic Gastrointestinal Imaging.* 3, Vol. 47, 643–666; 2018.

CASE 107

CASE AUTHOR: Lauren Corley

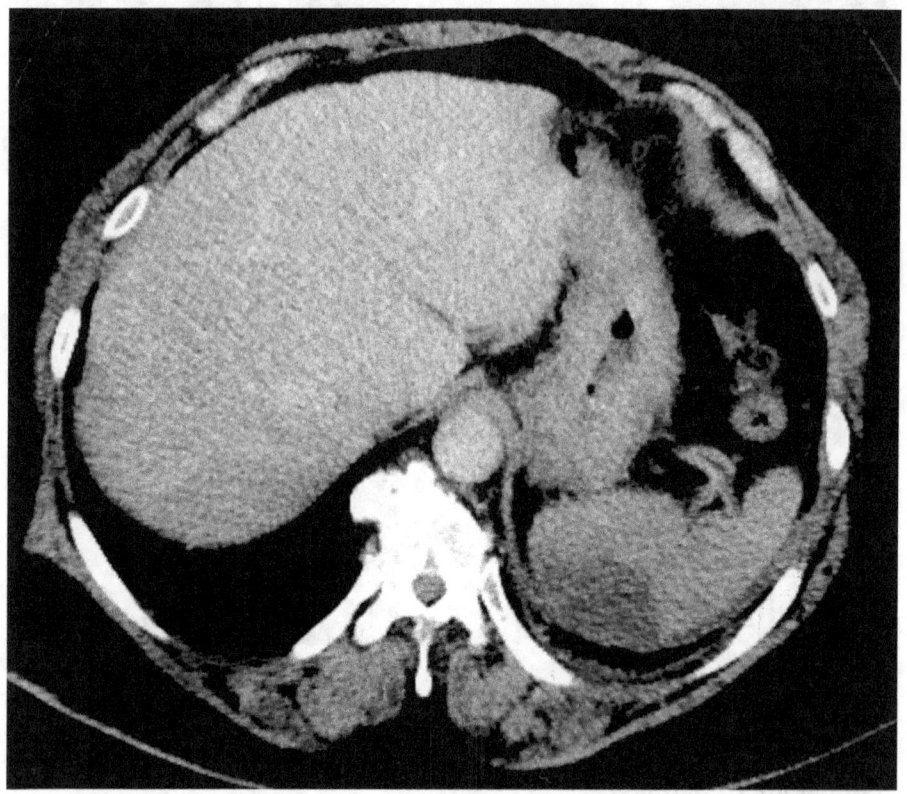

Best CT Study for Diagnosis:
CT Abdomen with IV contrast

Key to DX
Wedge shaped area of low attenuation involving the splenic parenchyma extending towards the periphery.

Facts
Typical symptoms include left upper quadrant pain, fever, and leukocytosis.
Additional infarcts in other organs may be present.
Differential for a "wedge" shaped splenic lesion includes infarct, trauma, or malignancy.
Therefore, history for these patients is essential.

TX
Evaluate origin and extent of coagulopathy, such as lower extremity venous ultrasound.
Generally treated with supportive care and anti-coagulants.

SPLENIC INFARCT

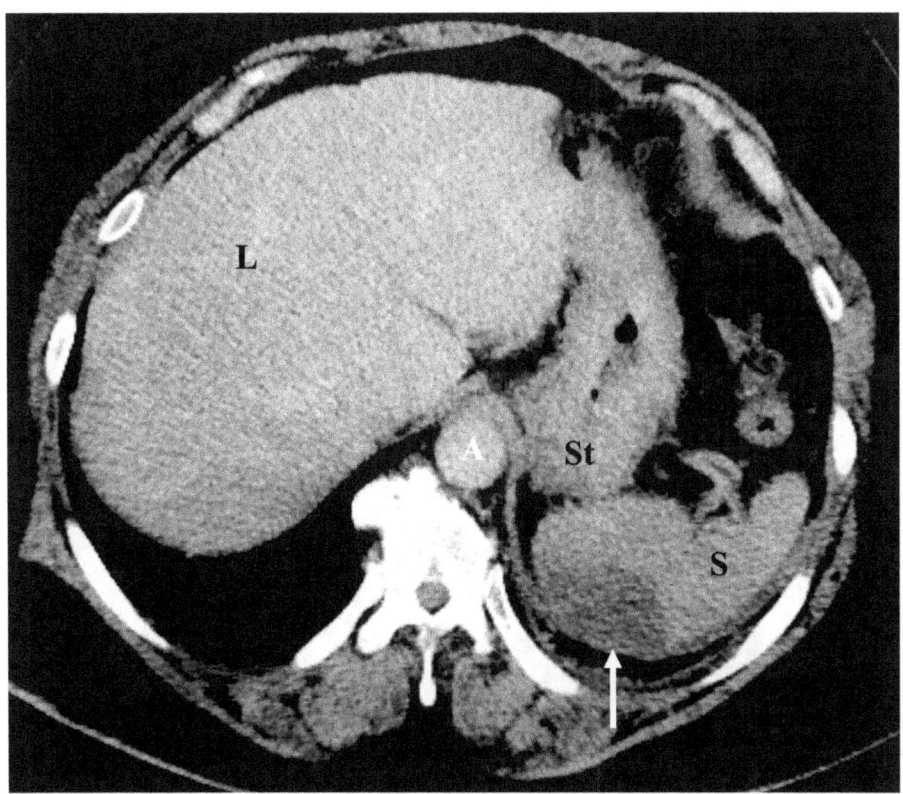

Study Above:
CT Abdomen with IV contrast at the level of the upper abdomen.

Radiographic Findings:
Wedge shaped area of low attenuation involving the splenic parenchyma extending to the periphery (arrow).

Tips
Critically evaluate adjacent organs (liver and kidneys) for areas of additional infarcts.
Scrutinize arterial and venous vasculature for thrombus.
Infarct may demonstrate preservation of peripheral enhancement (cortical rim sign).

Normal Anatomy
St – Stomach, S- Spleen, L - Liver, A - Aorta

Further Reading
Unal, E., Onur, M.R., Akpinar, E., et al. Imaging Findings of Splenic Emergencies: a Pictorial Review. *Insights into Imaging.* 7 (2), 215–222; 2016.

CASE 108

CASE AUTHOR: Lauren Corley

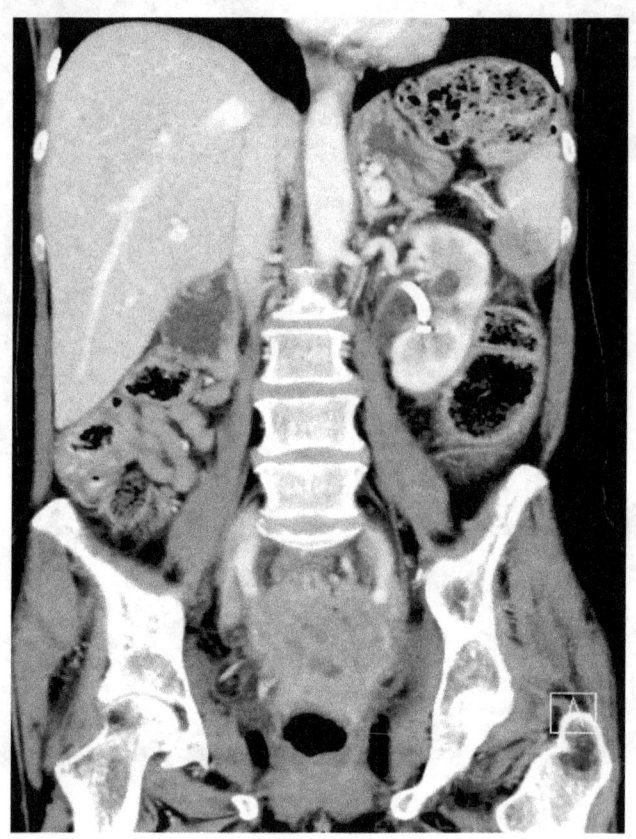

Best CT Study for Diagnosis:
CT Abdomen with IV contrast

Key to DX
Focal heterogeneous attenuation in the spleen.

Facts
The most common splenic lesion is metastasis, and the most common benign lesion is a hemangioma.
Primary splenic carcinomas are rare with the most common being angiosarcoma. Diagnosis of lymphoma is favored when there is concurrent mesenteric or retroperitoneal adenopathy. Splenic lymphoma is almost always secondary not primary malignancy.

TX
Depends upon etiology of the lesion.

SPLENIC MASS

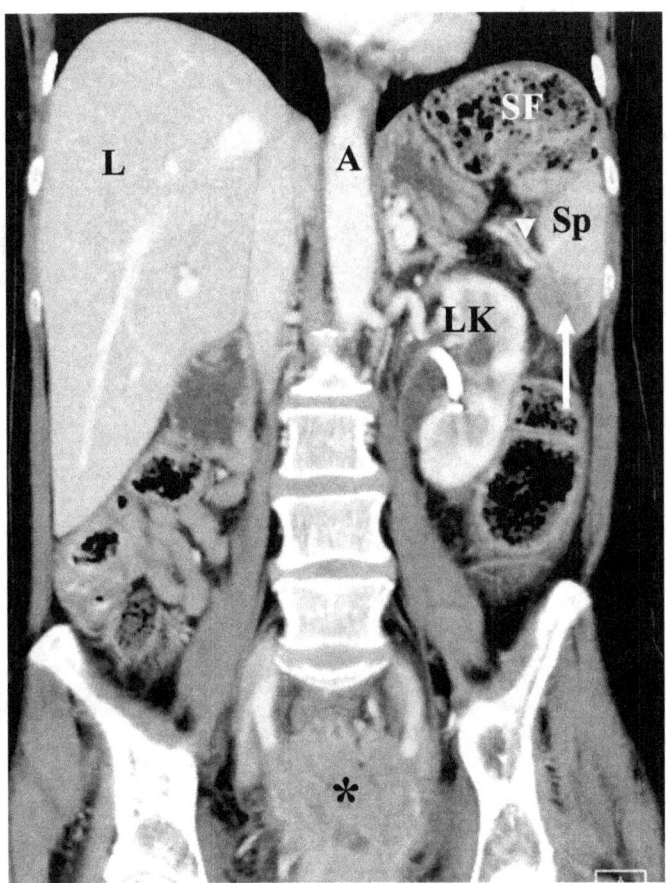

Study Above:
CT Abdomen with IV contrast, coronal reformat.

Radiographic Findings:
Round, low attenuated lesion within the spleen (white arrow). Tumor thrombus extends into the splenic artery (arrowhead). Within the pelvis, there is a heterogeneous pelvic mass (black asterisk). Splenic lesion in this case was metastasis from cervical cancer.

Normal Anatomy
LK - Left kidney, SF - Splenic flexure of the colon, Sp - Spleen, A - Aorta, L – Liver

Further Reading
Kim N, et al. Algorithmic Approach to the Splenic Lesion Based on Radiologic-Pathologic Correlation. *RadioGraphics* 2022.

CASE 109

CASE AUTHOR: Rocky Saenz

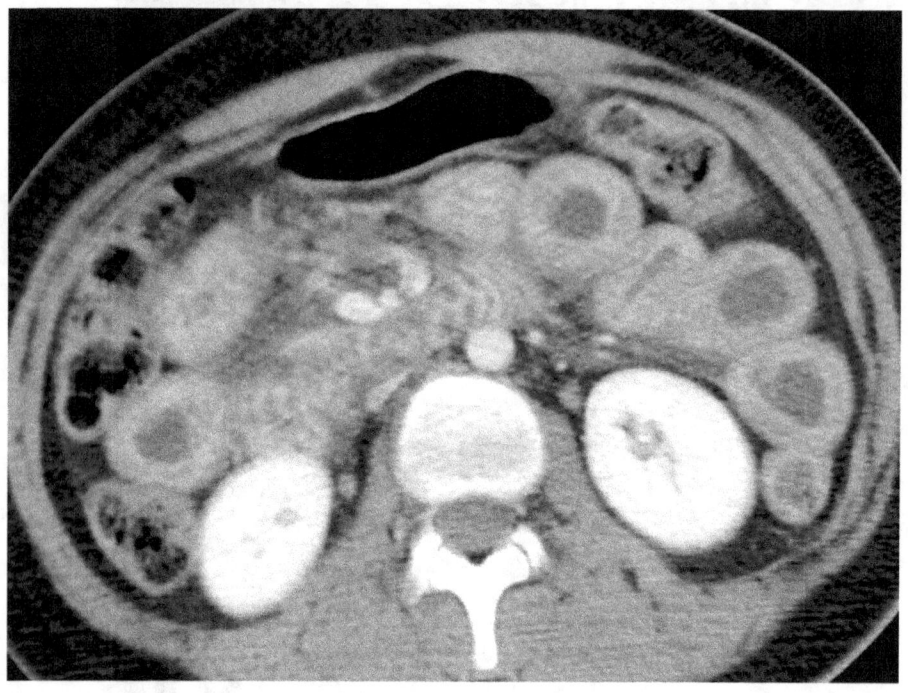

Best CT Study for Diagnosis:
CT Abdomen with IV contrast

Key to DX
Marked small bowel wall thickening with increased enhancement and a flat inferior vena cava.

Facts
This is also known as the "hypoperfusion complex."
The etiology is significant blood loss from acute trauma.
The small bowel wall should never be thicker than 3 millimeters.
There is an associated high mortality rate of 70%.

TX
Treat the source of blood loss (stop the bleeding)!
Volume replacement is needed emergently (IV fluids fully open, Stat).

SHOCK BOWEL

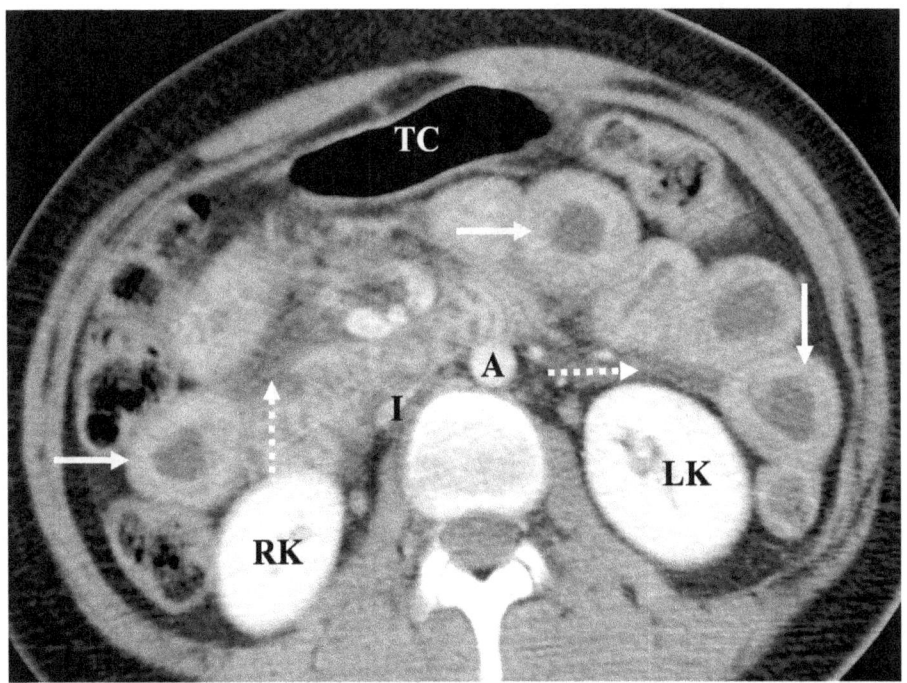

Study Above:
CT Abdomen with IV contrast from the level of the mid abdomen.

Radiographic Findings:
Marked bowel wall thickening of the small bowel loops is noted (arrows). Free fluid is seen in the abdomen (dashed arrows). Also note the inferior vena cava is flattened in AP dimension (I).

Tips
Scrutinize the bowel for non-enhanced segments, which may represent ischemia.
Check the density of free fluid when present as it may represent hemoperitoneum.
With shock bowel, the pancreas and spleen are typically hypoattenuated secondary to splanchnic vasoconstriction.
"Flat IVC" is an AP dimension less than 9 mm (can be normal in elderly females).

Normal Anatomy
RK - Right kidney, LK - Left kidney, TC - Transverse colon, A - Aorta

Further Reading
Ames JT, Federle MP. CT hypotension complex (shock bowel) is not always due to traumatic hypovolemic shock.. *AJR*.192(5):W230-5; 2009.

CASE 110

CASE AUTHOR: Ahmed Tahawi

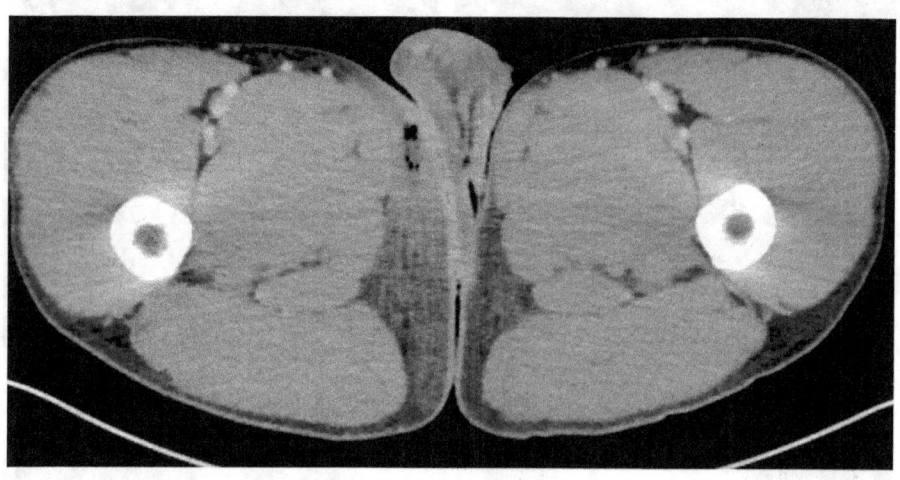

Best CT Study for Diagnosis:
CT Pelvis without IV contrast

Key to DX
Air within the subcutaneous tissues of the perineum.

Facts
Patients present with severe perineal pain, fever, and leukocytosis.
There may be palpable crepitus involving the scrotum and/or the perineum.
Typically arises from localized infection spread along the fascial planes of the perineum.
Risk factors include diabetes, chronic alcohol use, and immunosuppression.
This more commonly occurs in older men with diabetes.
It is a polymicrobial infection with *Escherichia coli* being the predominant aerobe.
If diagnosis and management is delayed, patients can exhibit impotence or incontinence.

TX
Urological emergency requiring broad-spectrum intravenous antibiotics and aggressive surgical debridement of necrotic tissue.

FOURNIER'S GANGRENE

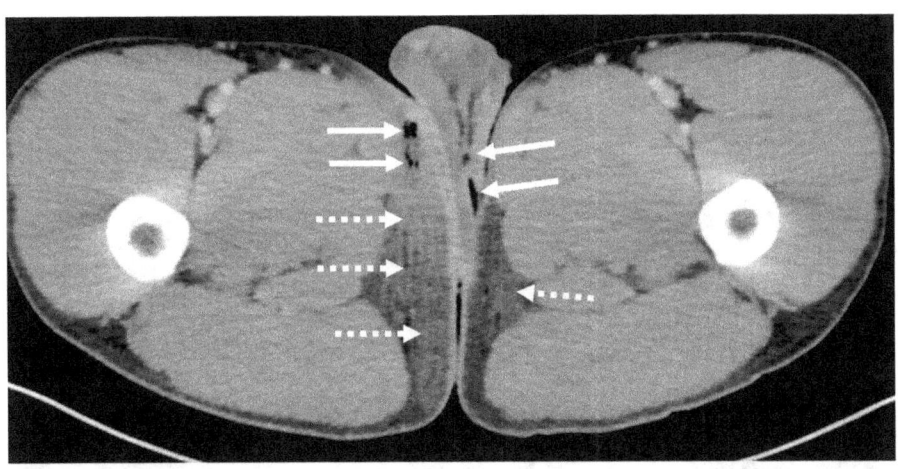

Study Above:
CT Pelvis with IV contrast at the level of the perineum.

Radiographic Findings:
Punctate pockets of gas are present within the subcutaneous fat of the perineum (arrows). Also note the extensive soft tissue fat stranding (dashed arrows).

Tips
Always describe the extent of tissue involvement.
Air within the subcutaneous tissues is never a normal finding!
If air is seen in the perineum, it is an advanced infection and necrotizing until proven otherwise.
Search the perineum for discrete fluid collections in order to exclude abscess formation (helpful for surgical planning and pathologic specimen sampling).
CT Tip: As stated earlier, fat stranding is non-specific. It may represent an acute or chronic process (fibrosis). The main differential to consider is: inflammation, infection, infiltration by tumor, or trauma.

Further Reading
Choe J, et al. Imaging of Acute Conditions of the Perineum. *RadioGraphics*. 1111-1130; 2018.

CASE 111

CASE AUTHOR: Zachary Franks

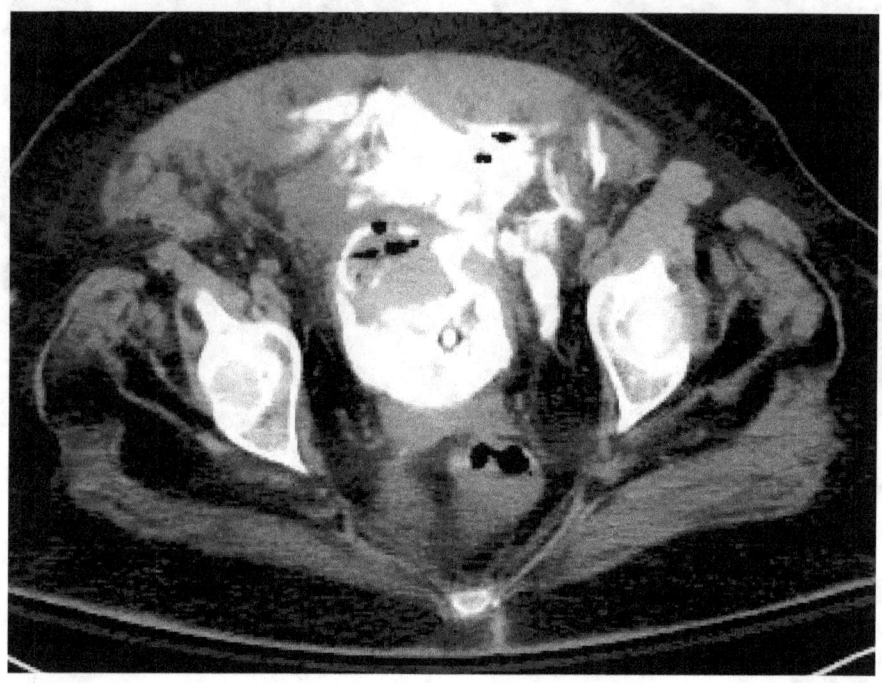

Best CT Study for Diagnosis:
CT Pelvis cystogram

Key to DX
Extravasated contrast seen within the extraperitoneal space.

Facts
Patients present with pelvic pain and hematuria after blunt trauma.
Urinary bladder rupture may be intraperitoneal or extraperitoneal.
The chance of an injury is directly related to the degree of urinary bladder distention.
An intraperitoneal rupture results when the bladder dome is injured.
Extraperitoneal injury is from compromise of the bladder base.
Delay in diagnosis can result in a 10-22% increase in morbidity and mortality.

TX
The treatment depends on the site of rupture. If the injury is intraperitoneal, the treatment is typically surgical.

URINARY BLADDER RUPTURE

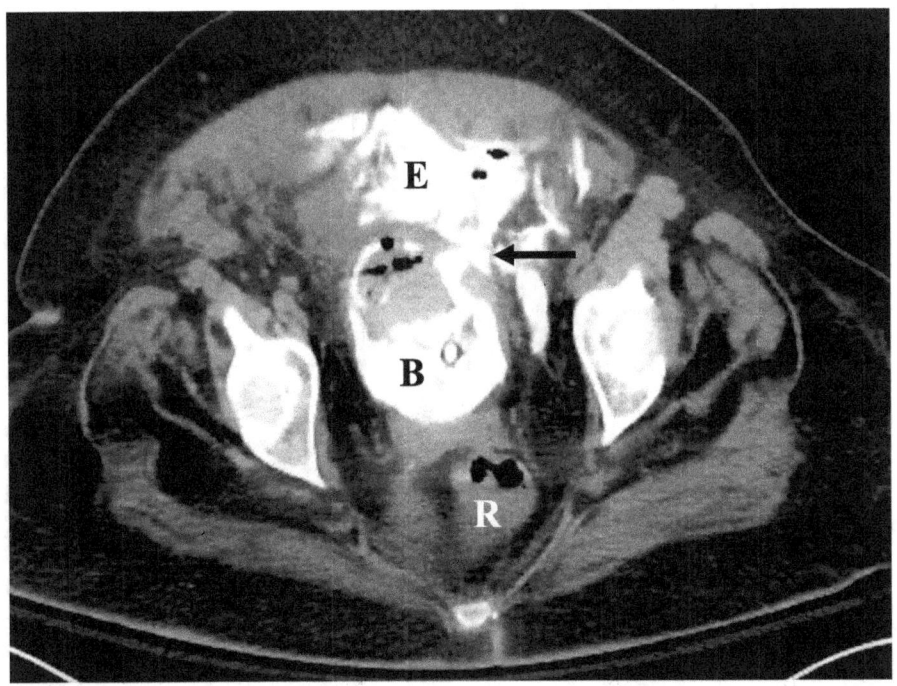

Study Above:
CT Pelvis cystogram (contrast inserted into the urinary bladder via catheter).

Radiographic Findings:
Contrast is seen within the extraperitoneal space (E) with a defect in the left anterolateral urinary bladder wall (arrow).

Tips
The urinary bladder injury is intraperitoneal if contrast is seen layering along the paracolic gutters, peritoneum, or cul-de-sac.
Extraperitoneal rupture is present when contrast leakage is retained anterior to the urinary bladder into the perivesical space or into the pelvic soft tissues.
Contrast outlining bowel loops is pathognomonic for intraperitoneal rupture.
Extraperitoneal injury is typically seen with pelvic fractures.

Normal Anatomy
E - Extraperitoneal space, B - Urinary bladder, R - Rectum

Further Reading
Fouladi DF., Shayesteh S., Fishman EK. *et al.* Imaging of urinary bladder injury: the role of CT cystography. *Emerg Radiol* 27, 87–95; 2020. https://doi.org/10.1007/s10140-019-01739-3

CASE 112

CASE AUTHOR: Zachary Franks

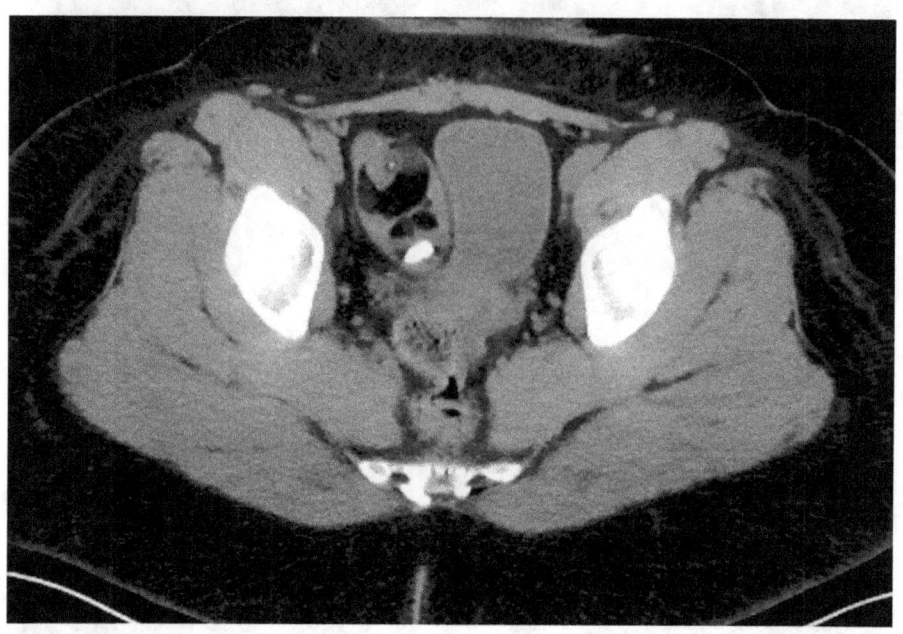

Best CT Study for Diagnosis:
CT Pelvis with IV contrast (when ultrasound is not available)

Key to DX
An adnexal lesion with fat, soft tissue density, and calcification.

Facts
Most patients are asymptomatic, although they can present with pelvic pain.
It is also known as a mature cystic teratoma and made of at least two of the three germ cell layers.
Dermoids are the most common ovarian mass.
These lesions are commonly seen in women with a mean age of 30.
Dermoids are bilateral in 10% of patients.

TX
The treatment depends on size. Lesions larger than 6 centimeters are removed surgically.

OVARIAN DERMOID

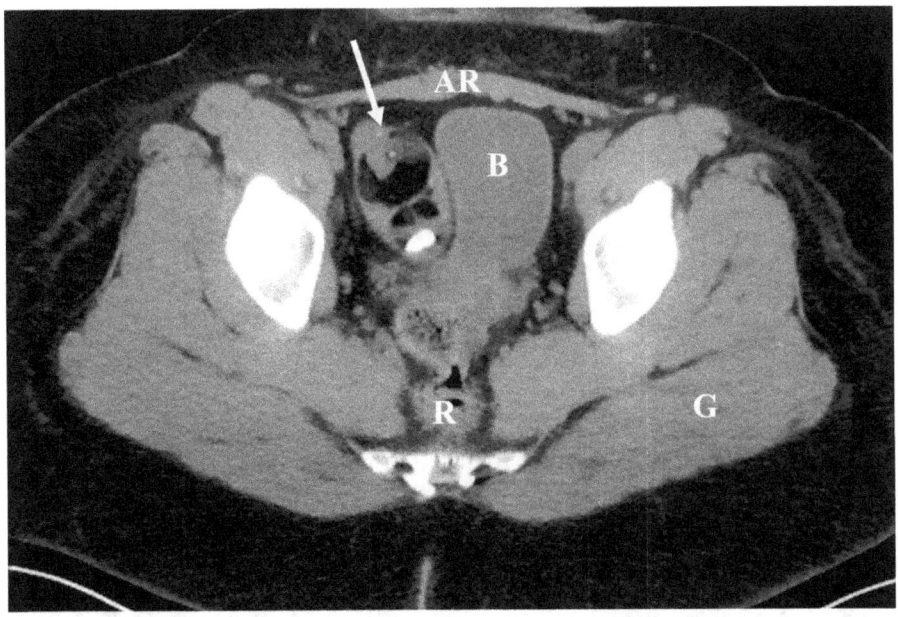

Study Above:
CT Pelvis with IV and oral contrast at the level of the right ovary.

Radiographic Findings:
A well circumscribed right adnexal mass is seen (arrow). Notice that this mass has an abundance of fat density! Note the calcification as well.

Tips
Fat attenuation is seen in greater than 90% of cases.
The density of the lesion should be similar to the subcutaneous fat.
A rare complication is peritonitis from dermoid rupture.
Rokitansky nodule or plug may be seen.
About 1% of cases undergo malignant degeneration.

Normal Anatomy
B - Urinary bladder, R - Rectum, AR - Abdominus rectus, G - Gluteus maximus

Further Reading
Outwater EK., Siegelman ES., and Hunt JL. Ovarian Teratomas: Tumor Types and Imaging Characteristics. *RadioGraphics*. 21:2, 475-490, 2001.

CASE 113

CASE AUTHOR: Zachary Franks

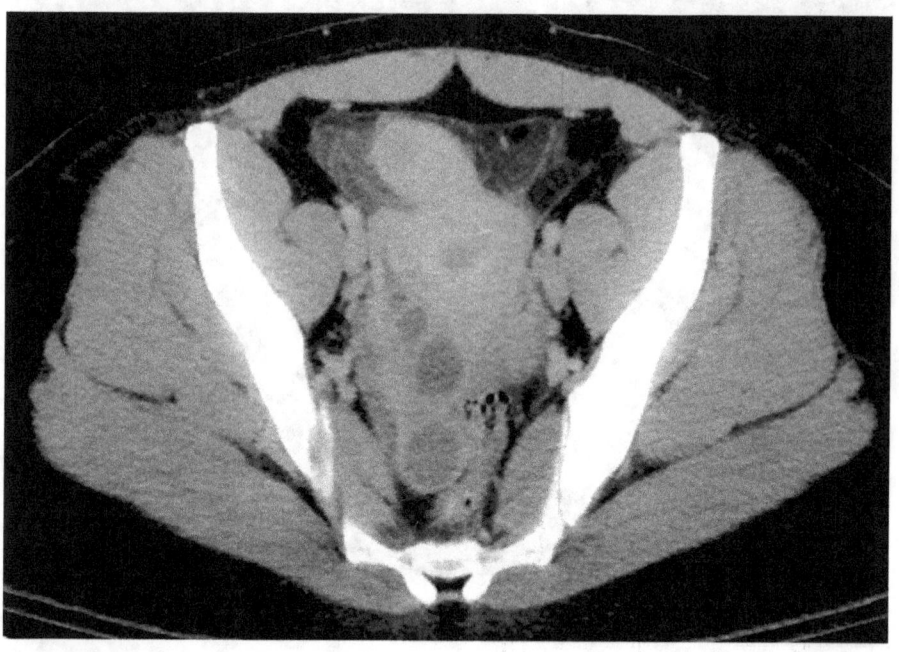

Best CT Study for Diagnosis:
CT Pelvis with IV and oral contrast (when ultrasound is not available)

Key to DX
Tubular fluid attenuated lesions within the adnexa with fat stranding.

Facts
Patients present with pelvic pain, vaginal discharge, or vaginal bleeding.
Physical exam yields a positive chandelier sign (cervical motion tenderness) and purulent fluid emanating from the cervix.
This entity typically occurs in young women < 35.
Risk factors include prior sexually transmitted disease and multiple or new sex partners.
Complications include tubo-ovarian abscess, ectopic pregnancy, Fitz-Hugh Curtis syndrome, and chronic pain.
Neisseria gonorrhoea and *Chlamydia* are commonly the culprits.

TX
The treatment is antibiotics.

PELVIC INFLAMMATORY DISEASE

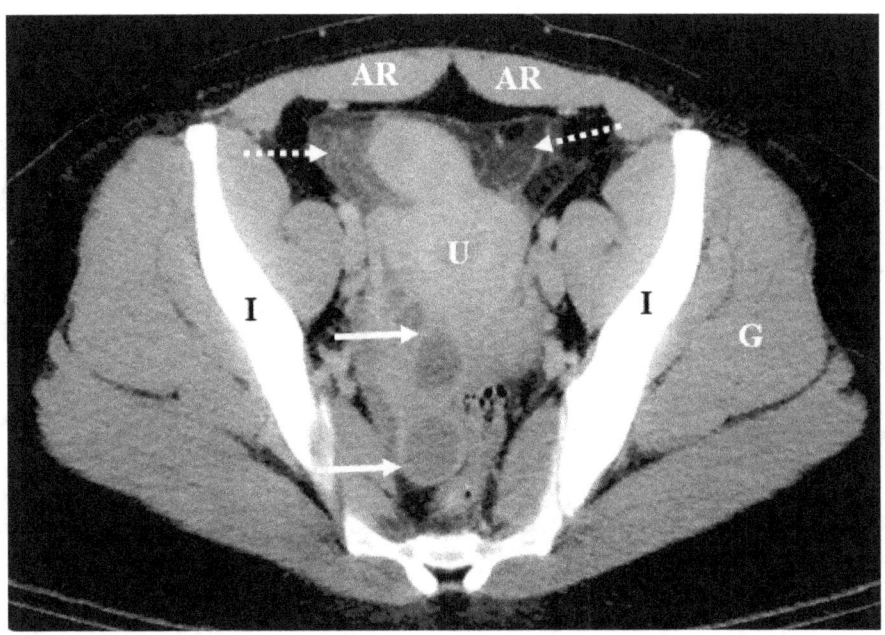

CT Pelvis with IV and oral contrast at the level of the adnexa.

Radiographic Findings:
Right lateral tubular adnexal structure is seen representing a dilated fallopian tube (arrows). Fat stranding is seen anterior to the uterus (dashed arrows).

Tips
Small nodules are seen along the lumen of the fallopian tubes on CT and US termed mural excrescences (arrows). This is helpful to confirm a tubal origin. Reformatted images may be helpful to see the serpiginous morphology of the tubes.
Ultrasound with vaginal probe imaging is more sensitive.

Normal Anatomy
I – Iliac bone, AR – Abdominus rectus, G – Gluteus medius, U – Uterus

Further Reading
Revzin MV., Mahan M., Haatal DB, et al. Pelvic Inflammatory Disease: Multimodality Imaging Approach with Clinical-Pathologic Correlation. *RadioGraphics*. 36:5, 1579-1596; 2016.

CASE 114

CASE AUTHOR: Rajeev Aravapalli

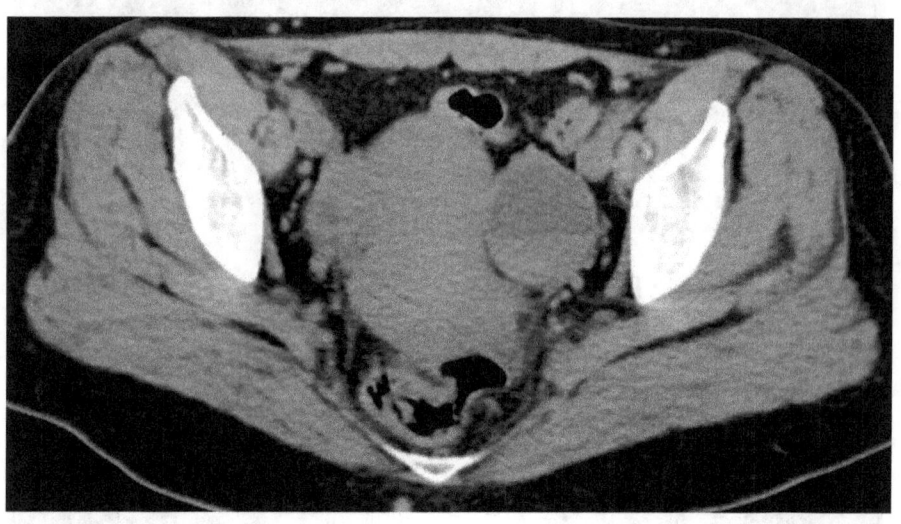

Best CT Study for Diagnosis:
CT Pelvis without IV and oral contrast (when ultrasound is not available)

Key to DX
A fluid-fluid level within a cystic pelvic lesion in a female.

Facts
Patients present with dull to sharp pelvic pain. This can be masked by Mittelschmerz.
Mittelschmerz is pelvic pain associated with ovulation mid cycle.
If the cyst ruptures, it may cause peritonitis.
Patients may present with severe pelvic pain if ovarian torsion occurs.
Cysts less than 5 centimeters typically resolve.

TX
The treatment depends on size. Cysts greater than 5 centimeters should be followed with a pelvic ultrasound in 6-8 weeks. Although cyst rupture may cause hemoperitoneum, most patients can be followed with conservative treatment unless they are unstable. If the cysts do not resolve or cause significant clinical symptoms, surgical removal may be needed.

HEMMORHAGIC OVARIAN CYST

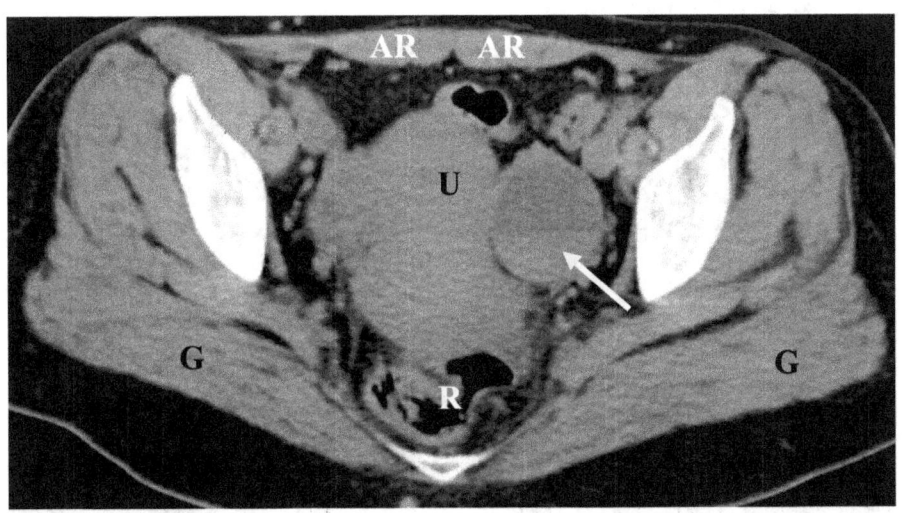

Study Above:
CT Pelvis without contrast at the level of the lower pelvis.

Radiographic Findings:
A cystic lesion is seen with a fluid-fluid level in the left adnexa (arrow). The high density is dependent (represents blood products).

Tips
Check for complex free fluid in the pelvis which can represent hemoperitoneum in acute cyst rupture.
Ultrasound via vaginal probe imaging is more accurate and should be done to better characterize the lesion.

Normal Anatomy
R - Rectum, U - Uterus, AR - Abdominus rectus, G - Gluteal muscle group

Further Reading
Iraha Y, Okada M, Iraha R., et al. CT and MR imaging of gynecologic emergencies. *Radiographics* 37:1569–1586; 2017.

CASE 115

CASE AUTHOR: Matt Waldrop

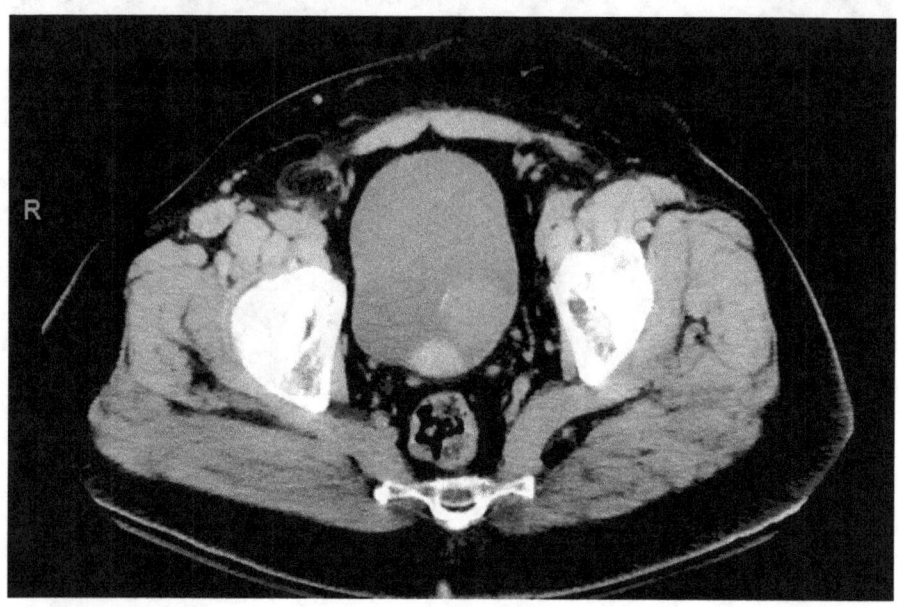

Best CT Study for Diagnosis:
CT Pelvis with IV contrast

Key to DX
A soft tissue mass within the urinary bladder.

Facts
Patients present with dull pelvic pain and hematuria.
Urinary bladder cancer is most common in Caucasian males.
Urinary bladder cancer is the fourth most common cancer in men.
More than 50% of cases are associated with smoking.
The most common type is transitional cell carcinoma.
Direct visualization with cystoscopy and sampling is needed for diagnosis.

TX
The treatment depends on the tumor stage. A combination of surgery, fulguration (electric current applied through a needle device to remove the lesion), intravesical therapy (BCG), and/or chemotherapy are utilized.

URINARY BLADDER CARCINOMA

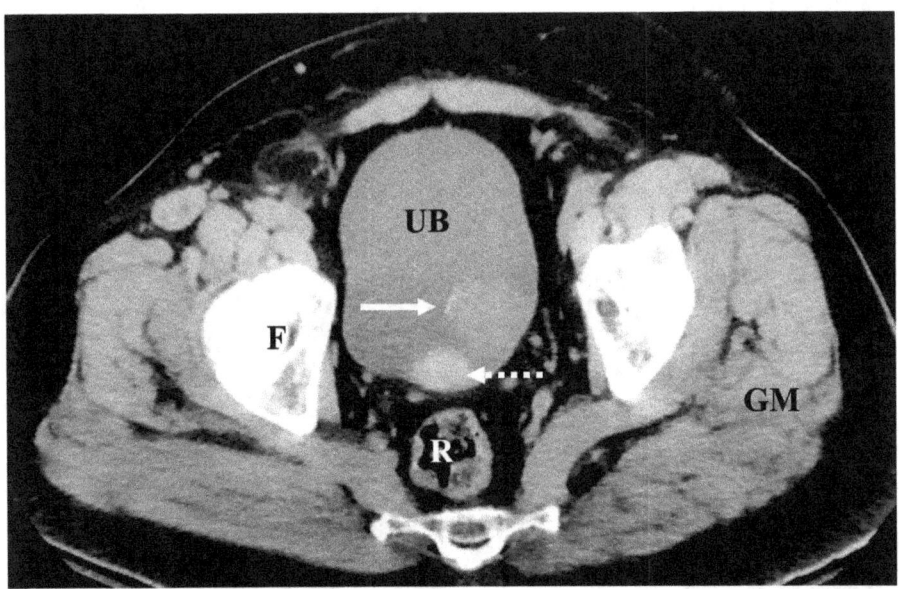

Study Above:
CT Pelvis with IV contrast at the level of the lower pelvis.

Radiographic Findings:
A lobulated soft tissue mass of low attenuation with peripheral calcification is seen projecting off the posterior left wall of the urinary bladder (arrow). An additional enhancing mass is seen posteriorly (dashed arrow).

Tips
Delayed imaging may be helpful to fill the urinary bladder with contrast to observe a filling defect.
Check the pelvis for adenopathy.
Examine the surrounding soft tissues for direct invasion.
Check the ureters and renal pelves for lesions as the urinary bladder mass could be a "drop" metastatic deposit.

Normal Anatomy
F – Femur, R – Rectum, UB – Urinary bladder, GM – Gluteus maximus

Further Reading
Lee CH, Tan CH, Faria SC, Kundra V. Role of imaging in the local staging of urothelial carcinoma of the bladder. *AJR Am J Roentgenol.* 208(6):1193–1205; 2017.

CASE 116

CASE AUTHOR: Rocky Saenz

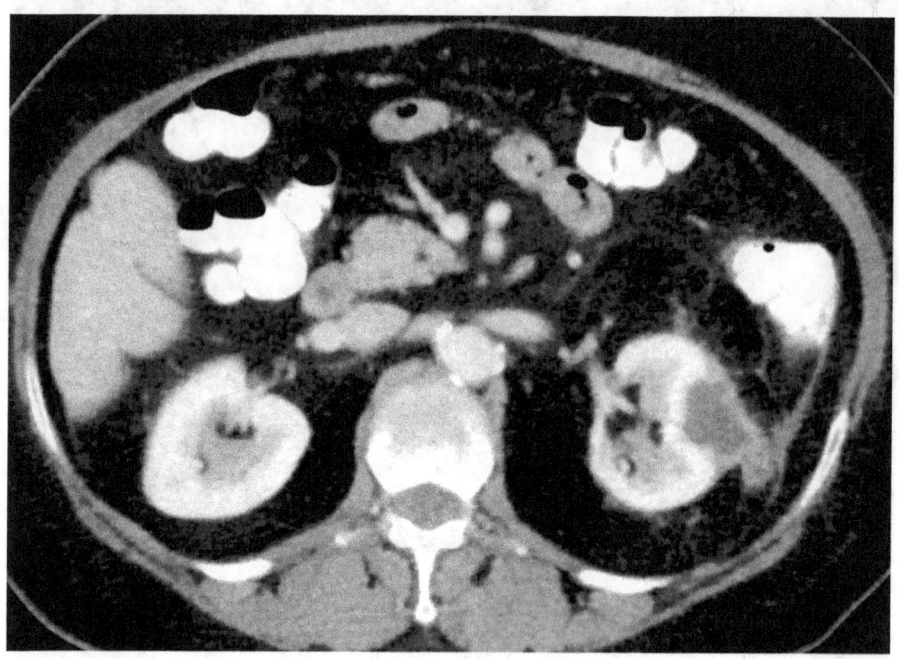

Best CT Study for Diagnosis:
CT Abdomen with IV contrast

Key to DX
A well circumscribed fluid density lesion with a contrast enhancing border.

Facts
Patients present with flank pain, fever, and leukocytosis.
Risk factors include immunocompromised, vesicoureteral reflux, diabetes, and chronic infections.
The most common organism is *Escherichia coli*.
Patients are at risk for developing urosepsis.
More than 50% of patients are diabetic.

TX
Intravenous antibiotics and abscess removal. Abscess is usually drained with percutaneous CT guided catheter placement (Radiology to the rescue, again).

RENAL ABSCESS

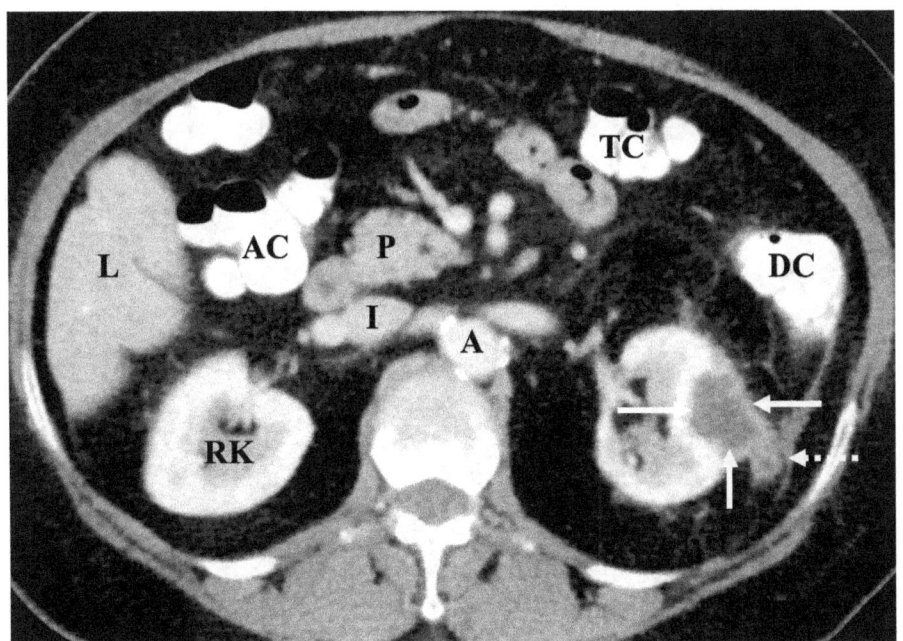

Study Above:
CT Abdomen with IV and oral contrast at the level of the kidneys.

Radiographic Findings:
A well circumscribed fluid attenuated lesion is present within the left kidney consistent with an abscess (arrows). Notice that the borders of the abscess are contrast enhancing. Adjacent fat stranding is seen in the retroperitoneum (dashed arrow).

Tips
Remember that the minority of abscesses have air.
Notice that the wall of the abscess is irregular whereas the walls of a cysts are thin and almost imperceptible.
If air is present in the renal parenchyma, emphysematous pyelonephritis must be excluded.
Examine the remaining renal cortex for other collections.

Normal Anatomy
P - Pancreas, AC - Ascending colon, TC - Transverse colon, DC - Descending colon, L - Liver, RK - Right kidney, A - Aorta, I - Inferior vena cava

Further Reading
Nepal P., et-al. Gas Where It Shouldn't Be! Imaging Spectrum of Emphysematous Infections in the Abdomen and Pelvis. *American Journal of Roentgenology.* 216: 812-823. 2021.

CASE 117

CASE AUTHOR: Maqsood Kahn

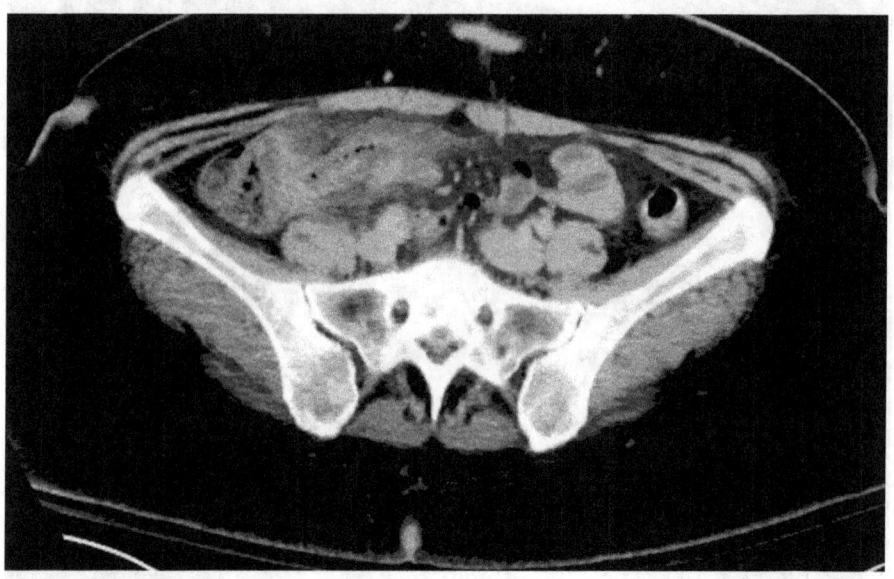

Best CT Study for Diagnosis:
CT Abdomen and Pelvis with IV and oral contrast

Key to DX
Dilated appendix with associated fat stranding.

Facts
Patients present with right lower quadrant pain, fever, and leukocytosis.
On physical exam, rebound tenderness is classically located at McBurney's point (the lateral third along the line joining the umbilicus to the anterior superior iliac spine).
Only 10-20% of cases have an appendicolith.
Patients are typically teens to early twenties but can occur at any age.
More than 50% of patients do not have the classic signs and symptoms.

TX
The treatment is typically surgical removal.
If there is an associated abscess, it can be drained via CT guidance with pigtail catheter placement.

Further Reading
Chin C, Lim K. Appendicitis: Atypical and Challenging CT Appearances: Resident and Fellow Education Feature. *Radiographics*. 2015.

APPENDICITIS

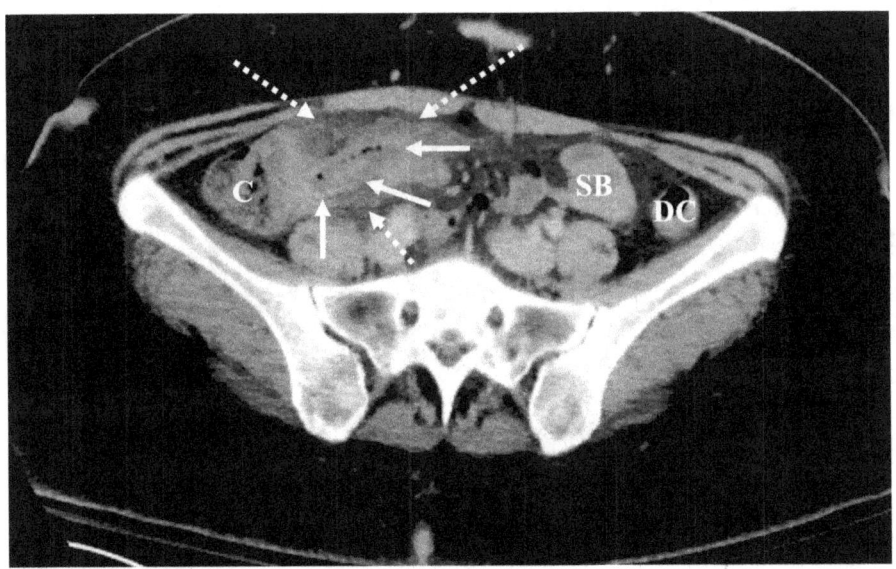

Study Above:
CT Abdomen and Pelvis with IV contrast at the level of the appendix.

Radiographic Findings:
The appendix is dilated (arrows) with surrounding fat stranding (dashed arrows). Notice that the walls of the appendix are contrast enhancing indicating hyperemia.

Tips
A non-contrast filled appendix should not be wider than 6 millimeters.
To find the appendix: typically just inferior to the ileocecal valve.
Evaluate the surrounding soft tissues for adjacent abscess formation.
Examine the non-dependent portions of the abdomen and pelvis for free air.
Coronal and sagittal reformats may be helpful for appendix confirmation.
A consideration after appendectomy is stump appendicitis which is related to the appendix remnant.
Appendicitis can present in a femoral hernia, De Garengeot hernia.

Normal Anatomy
C - Cecum, DC - Descending colon, SB - Small bowel

Further Reading
Chin C, Lim K. Appendicitis: Atypical and Challenging CT Appearances: Resident and Fellow Education Feature. *Radiographics*. 2015.

CASE 118

CASE AUTHOR: Gregory D. Puthoff

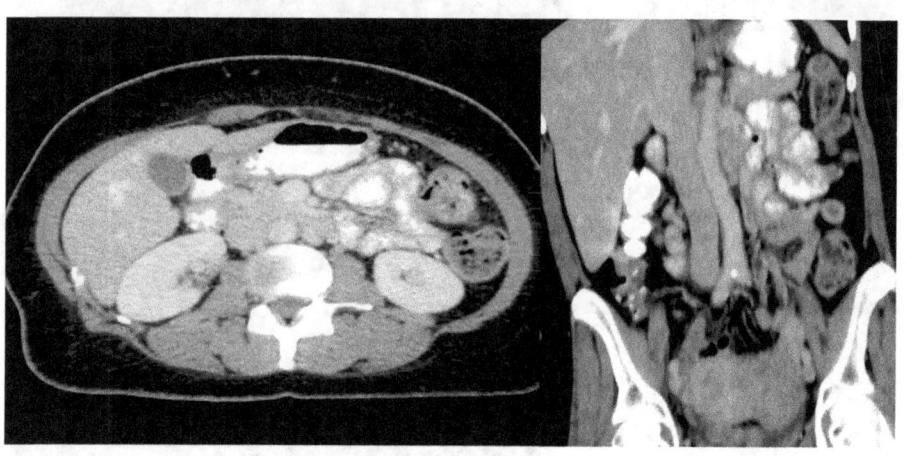

Best CT Study for Diagnosis:
CT Abdomen and Pelvis with IV and oral contrast

Key to DX
Filling defect within the ovarian vein.

Facts
Commonly encountered with pregnancy or puerperium.
May also be seen with other conditions such as: pelvic inflammatory disease, inflammatory bowel disease, oncologic patients, and pelvic surgery.
Superimposed infection may be present and represent ovarian vein thrombophlebitis.
During pregnancy, the right ovarian vein is more commonly affected.

TX
Treatment with anticoagulation and antibiotics is essential to prevent propagation of clot and ultimately pulmonary embolism.

OVARIAN VEIN THROMBOSIS

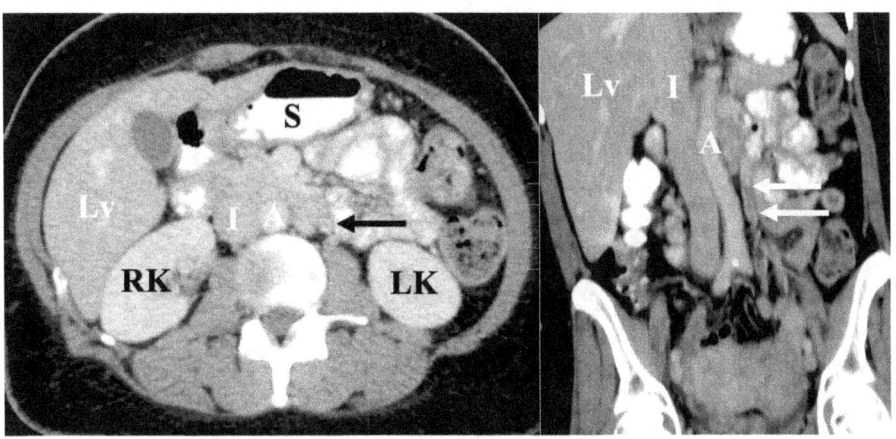

Study Above:
CT Abdomen and Pelvis with IV and oral contrast at the level of the mid abdomen, axial and coronal reformat (right).

Radiographic findings:
Peripherally enhancing left ovarian vein with a central low attenuated filling defect (arrows).

Tips
Follow the ovarian veins from their origins down into the pelvis for anatomical confirmation.
An enlarged ovarian vein (> 8 mm) may be seen with pelvic congestion syndrome.
Check the IVC and other veins for thrombus.
Consider ultrasound doppler to exclude lower extremity thrombus.

Normal Anatomy
S - Stomach, A - Aorta, I - Inferior vena cava, Lv - Liver, RK - Right kidney, LK - Left kidney

Further Reading
Puthoff G. and Saenz R. JAOCR at the Viewbox; Ovarian Vein Thrombosis. *Journal of Am Osteopath Coll Radiol. Vol. 5, Issue 2 Page 31.* 2016.

CASE 119

CASE AUTHOR: Gregory D. Puthoff

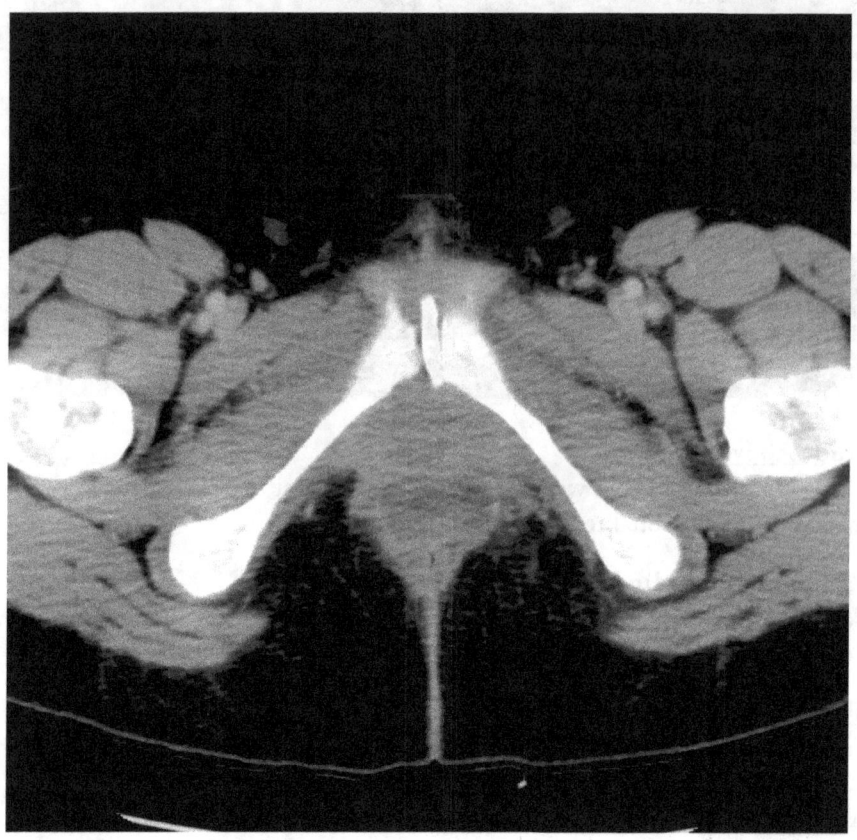

Best CT Study for Diagnosis:
CT Pelvis with IV contrast

Key to DX
Fluid attenuated peripherally enhancing perirectal fluid collection.

Facts
Typically presents clinically with perianal pain and fever.
CT with IV contrast is important to differentiate perirectal abscess from perirectal cellulitis as the treatment for abscess requires intervention.
Classified based on location: perianal, ischiorectal, intersphincteric, and supralevator.
Associated with diabetes, Crohn's disease, pelvic infections, and trauma.
Also known as perianal abscess.

TX
Surgical drainage and antibiotic therapy.

PERIRECTAL ABSCESS

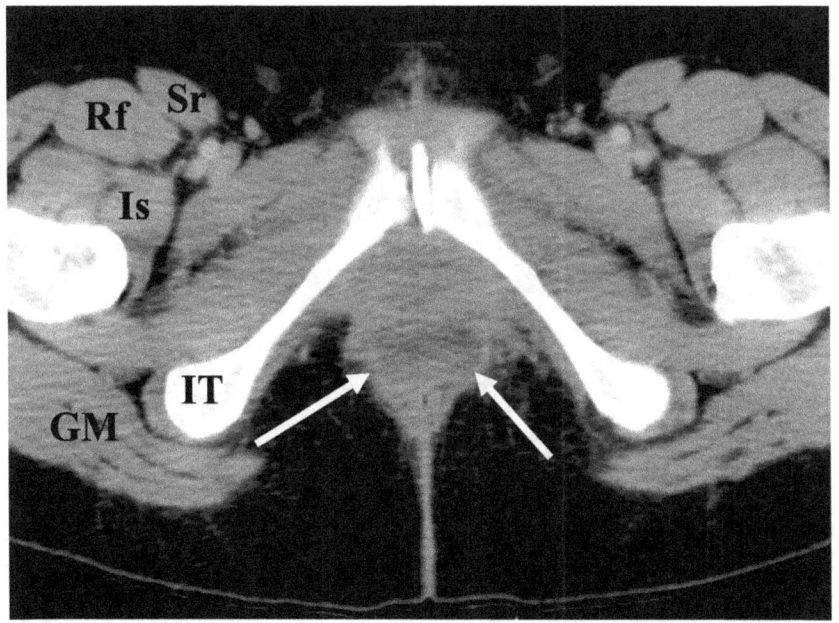

Study Above:
CT Pelvis with IV contrast at the level of the anus.

Radiographic Findings:
Peripherally enhancing perianal fluid collection with inflammatory stranding of the bilateral ischiorectal fat (arrows).

Tips
Must evaluate for possible perianal fistula, which requires MRI for definitive exclusion.
Supralevator perirectal abscess are the most difficult to diagnose secondary to obscure presentation and difficult palpation on physical examination.
Remember air is present in the minority of abscesses (hematoma may look identical).

Normal Anatomy
GM - Gluteus maximus, Is - Iliopsoas, Rf - Rectus femoris, Sr - Sartorius, IT - Ischial tuberosity

Further Reading
Saenz. Top 3 Differentials in Abdominal Radiology. Case 76. Thieme. 2019.

CASE 120

CASE AUTHOR: Juliann Giese

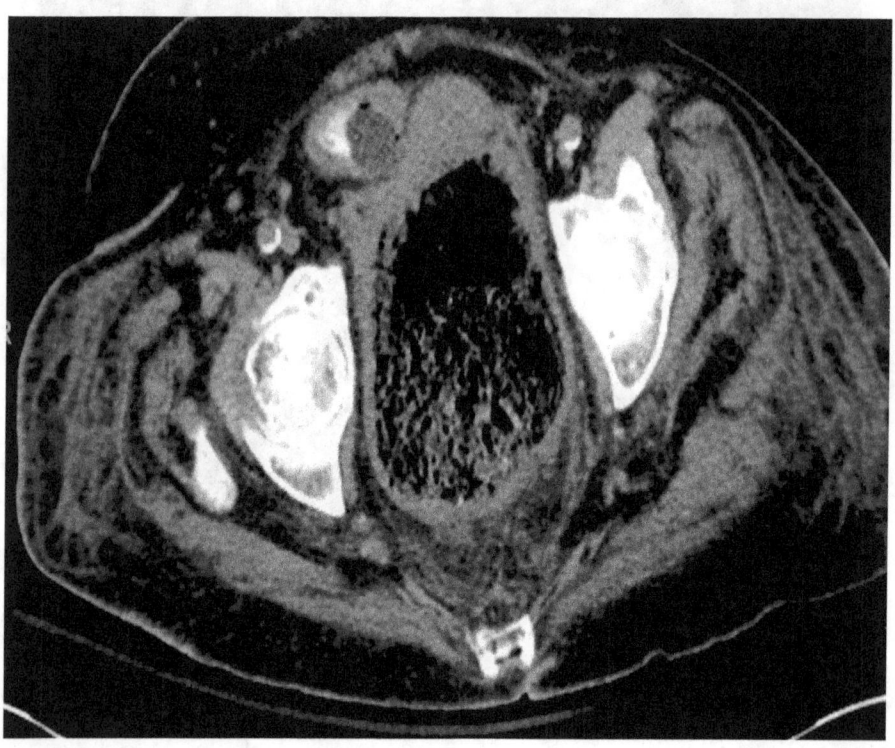

Best CT Study for Diagnosis:
CT Abdomen and Pelvis with IV and oral contrast

Key to DX
Large fecal ball with rectal wall thickening, perirectal and presacral fat stranding.

Facts
Potential surgical emergency.
Most common in elderly and debilitated patients.
Inflammatory process due to pressure necrosis caused by distension from fecal debris.
May lead to ulceration with subsequent perforation, peritonitis, and death if not urgently treated.
Mortality rate if untreated (35%).

TX
Manual disimpaction (medical students be sure to double glove!).

STERCORAL COLITIS

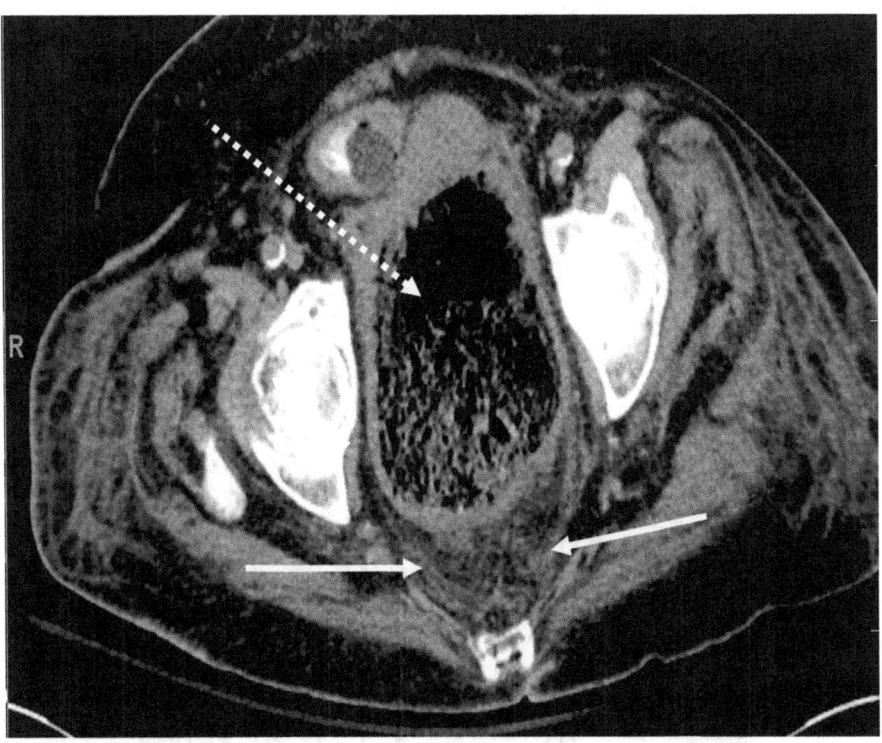

Study Above:
CT Abdomen and Pelvis without contrast at the level of the lower pelvis.

Radiographic findings:
Dilated rectum with impacted fecal ball/fecaloma (dashed arrow) and adjacent presacral edema/perirectal fat stranding (arrows).

Tips
If fecal impaction is identified, check for pericolonic fat stranding and bowel wall thickening to assess for possibility of stercoral colitis.
Colon is considered dilated if measures > 6 cm.
Colonic wall is considered thickened if measures > 3 mm.
Check for additional signs of ischemia (pneumatosis coli and portal venous gas).
Evaluate for underlying rupture by assessing for extraluminal air or abscess formation.
Most cases of uncomplicated stercoral colitis are managed effectively with manual disimpaction.

Further Reading
Ünal, E., et al. Stercoral colitis: diagnostic value of CT findings. *Diagnostic and Interventional Radiology.* 23.1, 5; 2017.

CASE 121

CASE AUTHOR: Juliann Giese

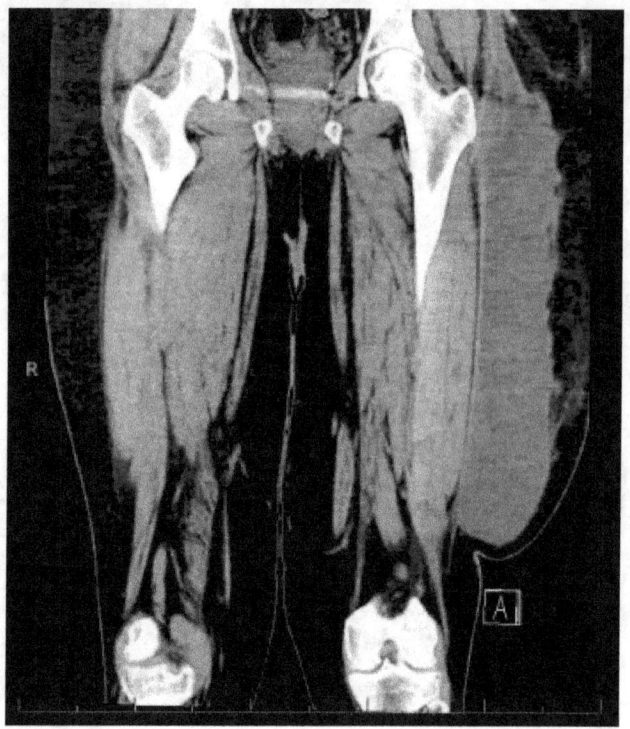

Best CT Study for Diagnosis:
CT Hip or Pelvis with IV contrast

Key to DX
Lateral fluid collection along the myofascial plane adjacent to the proximal to mid thigh.

Facts
Traumatic soft tissue closed degloving injury.
Clinically it will mimic a mass, but the clue is a prior history of trauma.
Severe shearing injury disrupts the fascial plane resulting in blood and lymph collection.
The fluid collection forms between fascia and subcutaneous tissues.
Most common location: anterolateral thigh adjacent to greater trochanter.
May become painful and increase in size over time.

TX
Acute: Percutaneous drainage to prevent infection.
Chronic: Complete surgical excision including the pseudocapsule due to recurrence.

MOREL-LAVALLEE LESION

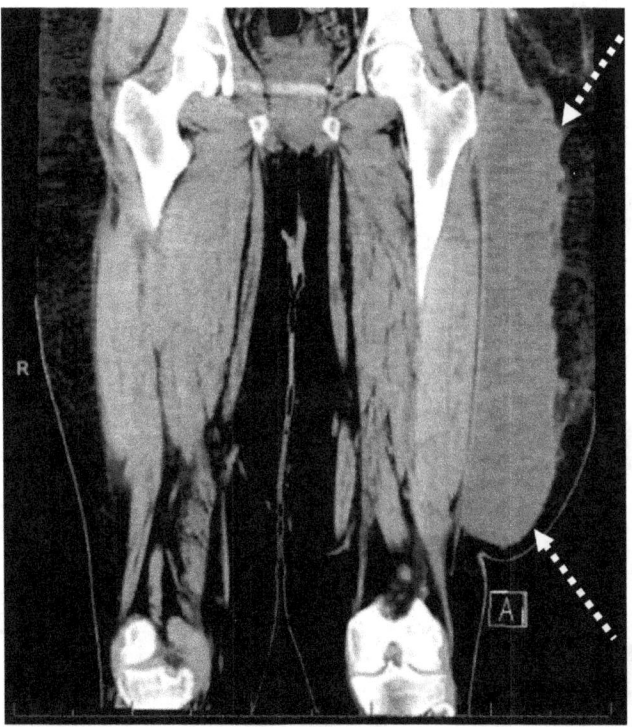

Study Above:
CT Bilateral Femurs without contrast, coronal reformat.

Radiographic findings:
An oval hypodense, well-marginated fluid collection is noted superficial to the muscles along the fascial plane within the anterolateral thigh (dashed arrows).

Tips
Differential diagnosis for soft tissue mass: hematoma, infection, and tumor (HIT).
If the lesion shows internal enhancement, strongly consider a tumor.
If there is air in the lesion, infection must be excluded.
If chronic, may be confused with soft tissue tumor due to tendency to expand.
The Morel-Lavellee lesion is superficial to the tensor fascia lata.
MRI may be helpful to make the diagnosis.
May also occur in the soft tissue anterior to the knee.

Further Reading
Zhuang, K. D., et al. "MRI features of soft-tissue lumps and bumps." *Clinical radiology* 69.12 (2014): e568-e583.

CASE 122 PEDIATRICS

CASE AUTHOR: Tammam Beydoun

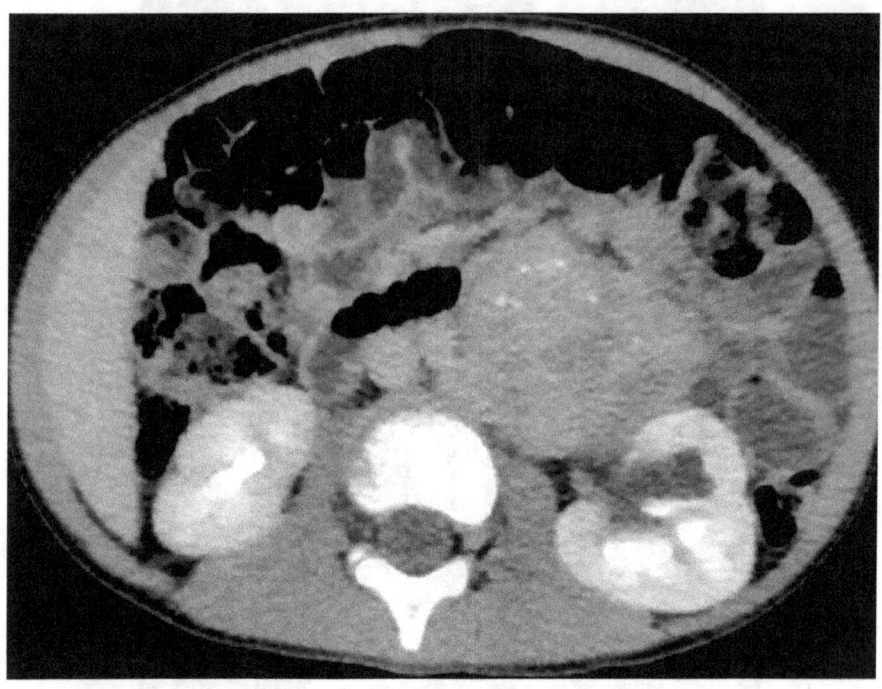

Best CT Study for Diagnosis:
CT Abdomen and Pelvis with IV contrast

Key to DX
Retroperitoneal mass with internal calcifications in a child.

Facts
Most common solid malignancy in children outside the CNS (only slightly ahead of Wilms tumor).
Most common origin is the adrenal gland, followed by extra adrenal retroperitoneal.
Originates from the primitive neural crest cells which make up the sympathetic chain and therefore can present anywhere along this path.
Metastasis is present 50-60% of the time at diagnosis.

TX
Staging and extent is the first priority requiring further imaging including MRI and nuclear medicine. In some equivocal cases, tissue biopsy may be of benefit by interventional radiology. Tissue sampling also serves for cytogenetic profiling. Once staged, treatment can include surgical intervention (which may be curative in low risk disease), chemotherapy, and/or stem cell transplant.

NEUROBLASTOMA

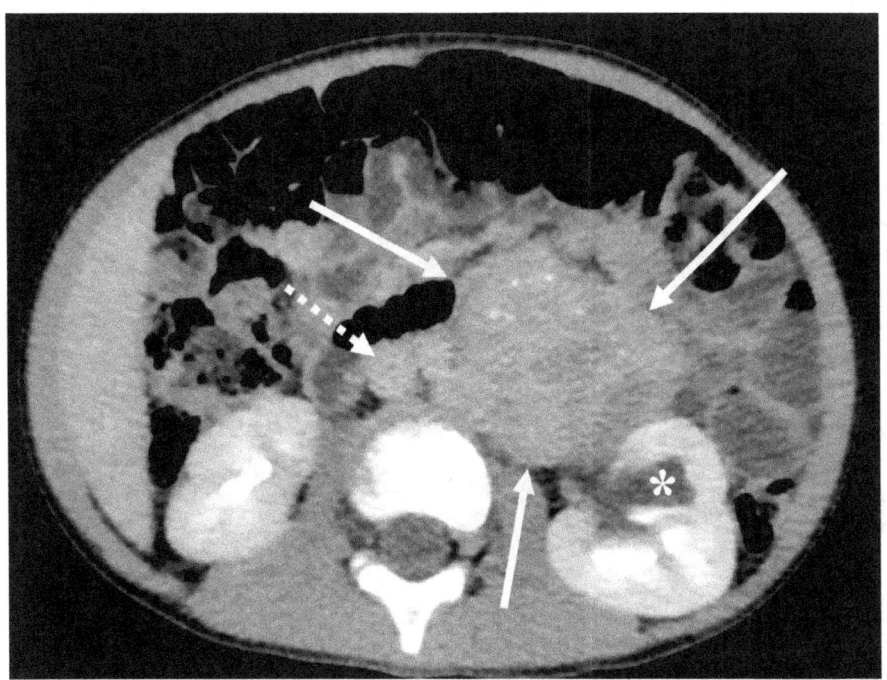

Study Above:
CT Abdomen and Pelvis with IV contrast at the level of the kidneys.

Radiographic findings:
Large, solid retroperitoneal mass (arrows) displacing the aorta anterolaterally (dashed arrow) and demonstrating internal calcifications. Fat plane between kidney and mass appears preserved. Incidental note is a moderate left hydronephrosis (asterisk) from ureteral compression by the retroperitoneal tumor

Tips
Rule out renal origin. A Wilms tumor is your first alternate diagnosis in this location.
Intratumoral foci of calcification is highly suggestive of neuroblastoma.
Neuroblastoma classically surrounds vessels instead of displacing them.
"Blueberry muffin" lesions represent skin metastases and "raccoon eyes" represent orbital metastases (often confused with trauma).
Mean age of presentation is 2 years and very unlikely in children older than 10 years of age.

Further Reading
Woodward PJ, Sohaey R, Kennedy A et-al. From the archives of the AFIP: a comprehensive review of fetal tumors with pathologic correlation. *Radiographics*. 25 (1): 215-42.

CASE 123

CASE AUTHOR: Tammam Beydoun

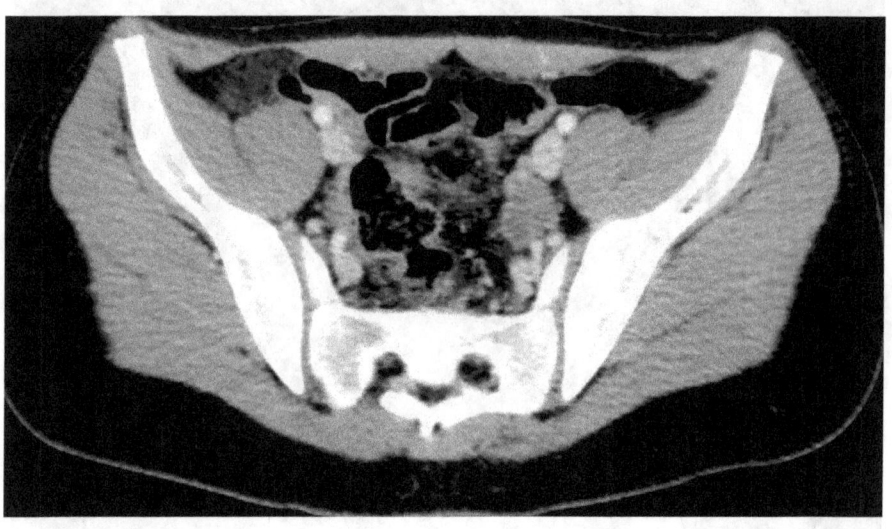

Best CT Study for Diagnosis:
CT Abdomen and Pelvis with IV contrast

Key to DX
Focus of hazy mesentery just deep to the anterior abdominal wall.

Facts
Typically patients present with sudden abdominal pain in absence of fever.
Thought to be caused by low omental blood flow or vascular occlusion and may be post-surgical.
Right lower quadrant is a common location.
May become infected forming an abscess, although rare.

TX
Self-limiting disease requiring only pain control.
Rarely surgical excision may be necessary in patients with intractable pain.

OMENTAL INFARCT

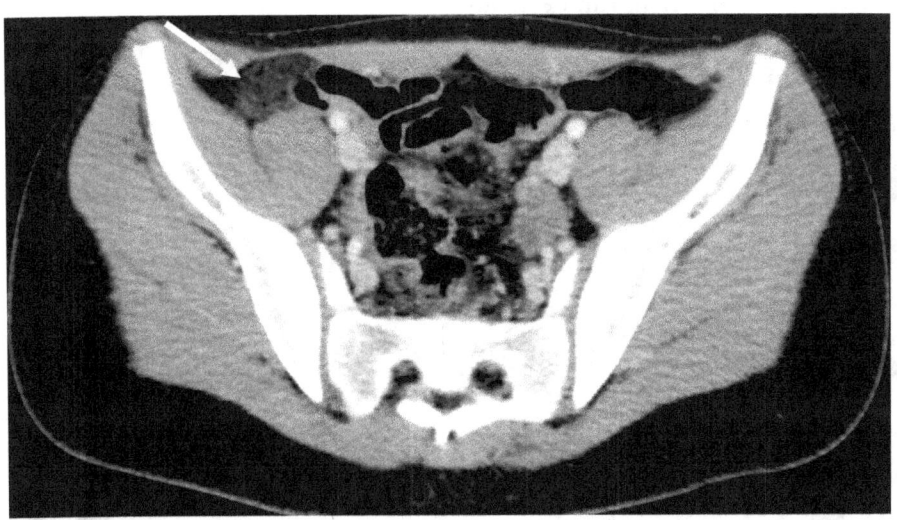

Study Above:
CT Abdomen and Pelvis with IV Contrast at the level of the lower pelvis.

Radiographic findings:
Well circumscribed area of hazy fat stranding (arrow) within the right lower quadrant. There is no free fluid nor abnormal bowel wall thickening to suggest enteric inflammation.

Tips
Rule out alternate diagnoses including appendicitis, diverticulitis and epiploic appendagitis (Cases 117, 76 and 75).
Adjacent bowel should be spared without evidence for bowel wall thickening.
More common in adults but also identified in children, especially in search of appendicitis.

Further Reading
Kamaya A, Federle MP, Desser TS. Imaging manifestations of abdominal fat necrosis and its mimics. *Radiographics*. 2011;31 (7): 2021-34.

CASE 124 PEDIATRICS
CASE AUTHOR: Tammam Beydoun

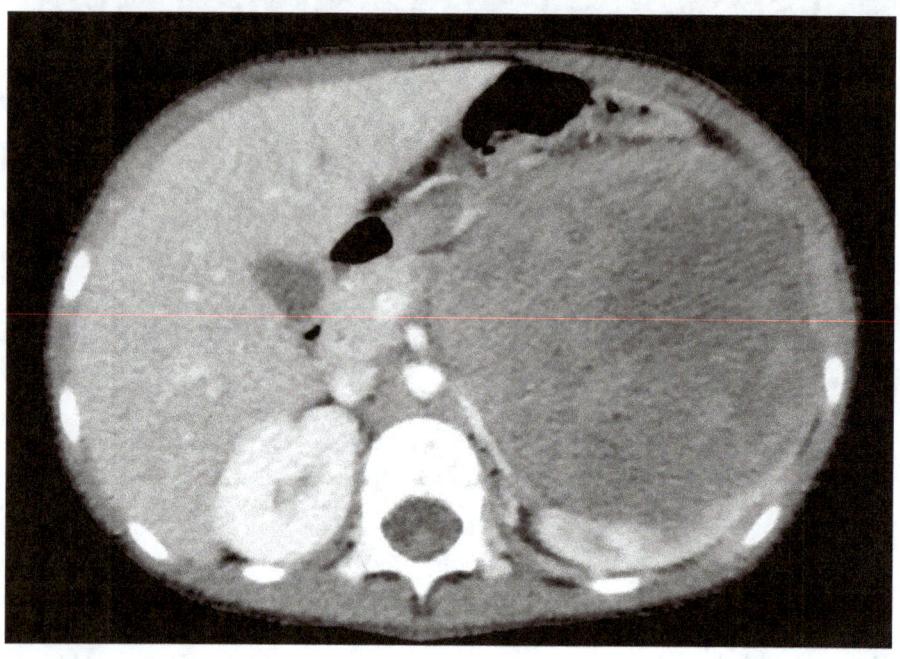

Best CT Study for Diagnosis:
CT Abdomen and Pelvis with IV contrast

Key to DX
Renal mass in a child.

Facts
Most commonly presents as palpable abdominal mass. Symptoms include hematuria, vomiting, and hypertension.
Most common pediatric renal tumor. Peaks at 3 years of age with 80% presenting before 5 years of age.
Lung metastases present in 10-20%.
Bilateral renal lesion present in 4-13%.

TX
Staging is based on tumor invasion and histology.
Most commonly treated with surgical resection of tumor followed by chemotherapy and possible radiation.
Cure rates are currently over 90%.

WILMS TUMOR

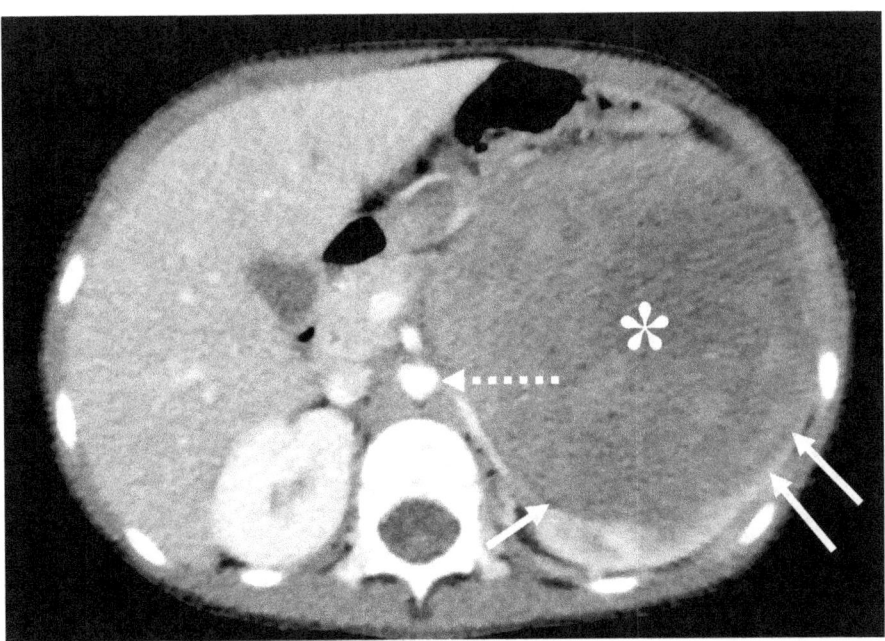

Study Above:
CT Abdomen and Pelvis with IV contrast at the level of the kidneys.

Radiographic findings:
Large heterogeneous mass (asterisk) emanating from the left kidney, as indicated by renal "claw sign" (solid arrows). Mass enhancement is less than that of renal parenchyma. Mass displaces the aorta without encasement (dashed arrow).

Tips
Evaluate for extension of tumor into the renal vein or inferior vena cava.
If the mass encases the aorta, think neuroblastoma.
Origin of large tumors can be difficult to discern (coronal images are helpful).
MRI may be required in more complex cases to evaluate tumor extension.
When Wilms is diagnosed, CT chest without IV contrast is needed to evaluate for lung metastasis.
Always scrutinize the contralateral kidney for a lesion.

Further Reading
Lowe LH, Isuani BH, Heller RM, et al. Pediatric renal masses: Wilms tumor and beyond. *Radiographics*. 2000;20(6):1585.

www.ingramcontent.com/pod-product-compliance
Lightning Source LLC
Chambersburg PA
CBHW061436300426
44114CB00014B/1704